Clinical Pocket Guide

Health & Physical Assessment in Nursing

2ND EDITION

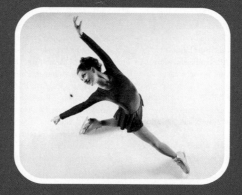

Colleen Barbarito, EdD, RN
Associate Professor
William Paterson University
Wayne, New Jersey

Donita D'Amico, MEd, RN
Associate Professor
William Paterson University
Wayne, New Jersey

D0090042

Pearson

Boston Columbus Indianapolis New York San Francisco Upper Saddle River
Amsterdam Cape Town Dubai London Madrid Milan Munich Paris Montreal Toronto
Delhi Mexico City São Paulo Sydney Hong Kong Seoul Singapore Taipei Tokyo

Library of Congress Cataloging-in-Publication Data

Barbarito, Colleen.

   Clinical Pocket Guide for Health & Physical Assessment in Nursing / Colleen Barbarito,
Donita D'Amico.

   p. ; cm.

   Other title: Health and physical assessment

   Rev. ed. of: Clinical handbook for health & physical assessment in nursing. c2007.

   Includes bibliographical references and index.

   ISBN-13: 978-0-13-511470-4 (alk. paper)

   ISBN-10: 0-13-511470-5 (alk. paper)

   1. Nursing assessment—Handbooks, manuals, etc.   2. Physical diagnosis—Handbooks,
manuals, etc.   I. Barbarito, Colleen.   II. D'Amico, Donita. Clinical handbook for health &
physical assessment in nursing.   III. Title.   IV. Title: Health and physical assessment.

   [DNLM: 1. Nursing Assessment—methods—Handbooks.   2. Physical Examination—
nursing—Handbooks.   WY 49]

   RT48.D36 2012

   616.07'5--dc22

                                2010029930

Publisher: Julie Levin Alexander
Publisher's Assistant: Regina Bruno
Executive Acquisitions Editor: Pamela Fuller
Development Editor: Jill Rembetski, Marion
Waldman, iD8 Publishing Services, Inc.
Editorial Assistant: Lisa Pierce/Cynthia Gates
Managing Production Editor: Patrick Walsh
Production Liaison: Cathy O'Connell
Production Editor: Roxanne Klaas, S4Carlisle
Publishing Services
Manufacturing Manager: Ilene Sanford
Art Director: Christopher Weigand

Cover Designer: Robert Siani
Interior Designer: Nesbitt Graphics
Art Editor: Patricia Gutierrez
Director of Marketing: David Gesell
Marketing Manager: Phoenix Harvery
Marketing Specialist: Michael Sirinides
Composition: S4Carlisle Publishing Services
Printer/Binder: RR Donnelley/
Crawfordsville
Cover Printer: RR Donnelley/
Crawfordsville
Cover Image: Shutterstock

Notice: Care has been taken to confirm the accuracy of information presented in this book. The
authors, editors, and the publisher, however, cannot accept any responsibility for errors or
omissions or for consequences from application of the information in this book and make no
warranty, express or implied, with respect to its contents.

   The authors and publisher have exerted every effort to ensure that drug selections and dosages set
forth in this text are in accord with current recommendations and practice at time of publication.
However, in view of ongoing research, changes in government regulations, and the constant flow of
information relating to drug therapy and drug reactions, the reader is urged to check the package inserts
of all drugs for any change in indications of dosage and for added warnings and precautions. This is
particularly important when the recommended agent is a new and/or infrequently employed drug.

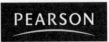

10 9 8 7 6 5 4 3 2 1
ISBN-10:   0-13-511470-5
www.pearsonhighered.com ISBN-13: 978-0-13-511470-4

Contents

Preface   v

CHAPTER 1
Health Assessment   1

CHAPTER 2
Techniques and Equipment   9

CHAPTER 3
General Survey   19

CHAPTER 4
The Health History   26

CHAPTER 5
Skin, Hair, and Nails   36

CHAPTER 6
Head, Neck, and Related Lymphatics   64

CHAPTER 7
Eye   78

CHAPTER 8
Ears, Nose, Mouth, and Throat   95

CHAPTER 9
Respiratory System   113

CHAPTER 10
Breasts and Axillae   130

CHAPTER 11
Cardiovascular System 141

CHAPTER 12
Peripheral Vascular System 153

CHAPTER 13
Abdomen 168

CHAPTER 14
Urinary System 184

CHAPTER 15
Male Reproductive System 196

CHAPTER 16
Female Reproductive System 211

CHAPTER 17
Musculoskeletal System 232

CHAPTER 18
Neurologic System 261

CHAPTER 19
Putting It All Together 294

CHAPTER 20
The Complete Health Assessment 300

CHAPTER 21
The Hospitalized Client 311

Photo Credits 318
Index 319

Preface

Clinical Pocket Guide for Health & Physical Assessment in Nursing is a resource that can be used by both novice students and professional nurses. For students who don't take a separate health assessment course who want to supplement their medical-surgical nursing text, the Clinical Pocket Guide is designed to be used as a health assessment primer; it guides the user through the steps of collecting health assessment data.

The focus of this text is comprehensive health assessment, which includes the collection of subjective and objective data. Subjective data encompasses both the client's health history and the focused interview. The nurse collects Objective data during the physical assessment.

To help readers use this guide effectively, the following features were developed for the body system chapters, chapters 5 through 18:

- The **Anatomy and Physiology Review** includes pertinent diagrams and illustrations.

- **Special Considerations** sections highlight differences in infants and children, pregnant women, and older adults.

- **Cultural Considerations** boxes alert the reader to variations related to cultural differences nurses encounter while performing the assessment.

- **Gathering the Data** guides the reader through the interviewing process, with specific questions.

- The **Physical Assessment** process includes Techniques, Normal Findings, Abnormal Findings, and Special Considerations.

- The sections on **Common Abnormal Findings** describe and illustrate common conditions.

The first two chapters of this guide introduce the concepts of assessment. Chapter 1 defines health and health assessment. In addition, it describes the steps of the nursing process, critical thinking, and documentation, using a variety of methods. Chapter 2 describes the techniques of inspection, palpation, percussion, and auscultation. It describes the role of the nurse and the identification of client cues, emphasizing a safe and clean environment.

Chapters 3 and 4 introduce the assessment process. Chapter 3, General Survey, describes the initiation of data collection. It includes components of the general survey, age-related considerations, measurement of the five vital signs, and a functional assessment. Chapter 4, The Health History, describes the health history and the component parts.

Chapter 19, "Putting It All Together," applies all the concepts of the preceding chapters. Chapter 20, "The Complete Health Assessment," describes the recommended procedure and pattern for completing a head-to-toe assessment. Chapter 21, "The Hospitalized Client," walks the reader through the recommended assessment procedure for the hospitalized client.

A sincere and deep expression of thanks is extended to our chapter contributors. Their time, effort, and expertise so willingly given for developing and writing chapters helped foster the project's success.

VickiLynn Coyle, RN, MS
Assistant Professor
William Paterson University
Wayne, New Jersey

Dawn Lee Garzon, PhD, APRN, BC, CPNP
Clinical Associate Professor
University of Missouri – St. Louis
Ladue, Missouri

Sheila Tucker, MA, RD, LDN
Dietician and Part-time Faculty Member
Boston College
Chestnut Hills, Massachusetts

About the Authors

Colleen Barbarito, EdD, RN

Colleen Barbarito received a nursing diploma from Orange Memorial Hospital School of Nursing, graduated with a baccalaureate degree from William Paterson College, and earned a master's degree from Seton Hall University, all in New Jersey. She received her Doctor of Education from Teachers College, Columbia University. Prior to a position in education, Dr. Barbarito's clinical experiences included medical-surgical, critical care, and emergency nursing. Dr. Barbarito has been a faculty member at William Paterson University since 1984, where she has taught physical assessment and a variety of clinical laboratory courses for undergraduate nursing students and curriculum development at the graduate level.

Dr. Barbarito coauthored three books with Donita D'Amico—*Modules for Medication Administration, Comprehensive Health Assessment: A Student Workbook,* and *Health & Physical Assessment in Nursing,* 1st edition. She published articles on anaphylaxis in *American Journal of Nursing* and *Coping with Allergies and Asthma.* Her research includes physical assessment and collaboration on revising a physical assessment project with results published as a brief in *Nurse Educator.*

Donita D'Amico, MEd, RN

Donita D'Amico earned her baccalaureate degree in nursing from William Paterson College. She earned a master's degree in Nursing Education at Teachers College, Columbia University, with a specialization in Adult Health. Ms. D'Amico has been a faculty member at William Paterson University for more than 25 years. Her teaching responsibilities include physical assessment, medical-surgical nursing, nursing theory, and fundamentals in the classroom, skills laboratory, and clinical settings.

Ms. D'Amico co-authored several textbooks, including *Health & Physical Assessment in Nursing,* 1st edition and its companion clinical handbook by Sims, D'Amico, Stiesmeyer, and Webster; as well as *Comprehensive Health Assessment: A Student Workbook* and *Modules for Medication Administration* with Dr. Colleen Barbarito.

1
Health Assessment

This chapter provides an overview of the aspects of nursing practice and nursing skills required for comprehensive health assessment. These include holistic assessment, nursing process, critical thinking, communication, and documentation. The skills and approaches required to meet the needs of diverse clients seeking advice and care in the changing healthcare system are illustrated throughout this text.

HEALTH

Traditionally, **health** has been thought of as the absence of disease. The terms *health* and *wellness* have been used interchangeably to describe the state when one is not sick. Today, these terms have clear distinctions in regard to definition and description of actions.

DEFINITIONS OF HEALTH

The World Health Organization (WHO) presented a definition of health that remains active and relevant today. Health is defined as a state of complete physical, mental, and social well-being (WHO, 1947). Further, the World Health Organization describes health from a holistic approach in which the individual is viewed as a total person interacting with others. The individual functions within his or her physical, psychologic, and social fields. These fields interact with each other and the external environment. The individual has the capability of maximizing the potential and fostering the most positive aspects of health.

The following definitions of health reflect the work of nursing theorists:

- A process and a state of being and becoming whole and integrated in a way that reflects person and environment mutuality (Roy & Andrews, 1999).

- The state of a person as characterized by soundness or wholeness of developed human structures and mental and bodily functioning that requires therapeutic self-care (Orem, 1971).

- A culturally defined, valued, and practiced state of well-being reflective of the ability to perform role activities (Leininger, 2007).

- A state of well-being and use of every power the person possesses to the fullest extent (Nightingale, 1860/1969).

Health is highly individualized and the definition one develops for oneself will be influenced by many factors. These factors will include but not be limited to age, gender, race, family, culture, religion, socioeconomic conditions, environment, previous experiences, and self-expectations.

Nurses must recognize that each client will have a personal definition for health, illness, and wellness. The behaviors one uses to maintain these changing states will be most individualized. Nurses must be aware of their own personal definition of health and at the same time accept and respect the client's definition of health, for this will influence practice. When health is defined in terms of physical change, the practice focus is on improvement of physical function. When health is considered to be reflective of physical, cultural, environmental, psychologic, and social factors, the focus of nursing practice is more holistic and wide ranging.

HEALTH ASSESSMENT

Health assessment may be defined as a systematic method of collecting data about a client for the purpose of determining the client's current and ongoing health status, predicting risks to health, and identifying health-promoting activities. The data include physical, social, cultural, environmental, and emotional factors that impact the overall well-being of the client. The health status will include wellness behaviors, illness signs and symptoms, client strengths and weaknesses, and risk factors. The scope of focus must be more than problems presented by the client. The nurse will use a variety of sources to gather the objective and subjective data. Knowledge of the natural and social sciences is a strong foundation for the nurse. Effective communication techniques and use of critical thinking skills are essential in helping the nurse to gather detailed, complete, relevant, objective, subjective, and measurable data needed to formulate a plan of care to meet the needs of the client. Health assessment includes the interview, physical assessment, documentation, and interpretation of findings. All planning for care is directed by interpretation of findings from objective and subjective data collected throughout the assessment process.

THE INTERVIEW
The **interview,** in which subjective data are gathered, includes the health history and focused interview. The data collected will come from primary and secondary sources. The primary source from which data are collected is the client, and the client is considered to be the direct source. An indirect or secondary source would include family members, caregivers, other members of the health team, and medical records.

Subjective data are items of information that the client experiences and communicates to the nurse. Perceptions of pain, nausea, dizziness, itching sensations, or feeling nervous are examples of subjective data. Only the client can describe these feelings. Subjective data are usually referred to as covert (hidden) data or as a symptom, when it is perceived by the client and cannot be observed by others. Family members or caregivers could report subjective data based on perceptions the client has shared with them. This information is most helpful when the client is very ill or unable to communicate and is required when the client is an infant or child. However, to ensure accuracy, the nurse must validate subjective data obtained from other sources. The accuracy of subjective data depends on the nurse's ability to clarify the information gathered with follow-up questions and to obtain supporting data from other pertinent sources.

THE HEALTH HISTORY
The purpose of the **health history** is to obtain information about the client's health in his or her own words and based on the client's own perceptions. Biographic data, perceptions about health, past and present history of illness and injury, family history, a review of systems, and health patterns and practices are the types of information included in the health history. The health history provides cues regarding the client's health and guides further data collection. The health history is the most important aspect of the assessment process.

THE FOCUSED INTERVIEW
The **focused interview** enables the nurse to clarify points, to obtain missing information, and to follow up on verbal and nonverbal cues identified in the health history. The nurse does not use a prepared set of questions for the focused interview. The nurse applies knowledge and critical thinking when asking specific and detailed questions or requesting descriptions of symptoms, feelings, or events. Therefore, the focused interview provides the means and opportunity to

expand the subjective database regarding specific strengths, weaknesses, problems, or concerns expressed by the client or required by the nurse to begin to make reliable judgments about information and observations as part of planning care. In-depth information about the focused interview in health assessment is included in each chapter of this text.

PHYSICAL ASSESSMENT

Physical assessment is hands-on examination of the client. Components of physical assessment are the survey and examination of systems. Objective data gathered during physical assessment, when combined with all other reliable sources of information, provide a sound database from which care planning may proceed. **Objective data** are observed or measured by the professional nurse. This is also known as overt data or a sign since they are detected by the nurse. These data can be seen, felt, heard, or measured by the professional nurse. For example, skin color can be seen, a pulse can be felt, a cough can be heard, and a blood pressure can be measured. These objective data are needed to validate subjective data and to complete the database.

INTERPRETATION OF FINDINGS

Interpretation of findings can be defined as making determinations about all of the data collected in the health assessment process. One must determine if the findings fall within normal and expected ranges in relation to the client's age, gender, and race and then the significance of the findings in relation to the client's health status and immediate and long-range, health-related needs. Interpretation of findings is influenced by a number of factors. These factors include the ability to obtain, recall, and apply knowledge; to communicate effectively; and to use a holistic approach. In a holistic approach, the nurse recognizes that developmental, psychological, emotional, family, cultural, and environmental factors will affect immediate and long-term actual and potential health goals, problems, and plans.

NURSING PROCESS

Nursing practice is concerned with health promotion, wellness, illness prevention, health restoration, and care for the dying. The nursing process in which the nurse uses comprehensive assessment to identify a client's health status and actual or potential needs guides the practice of nursing. The nursing process then directs the nurse in the development of plans and the use of nursing interventions to meet those identified needs. The **nursing process** is a systematic, rational, dynamic, and cyclic process used by the nurse for planning and providing care for the client. The steps of the nursing process are assessment, diagnosis, planning, implementation, and evaluation. The nursing process can be used in any setting, with clients of all ages, and in all levels of health and illness (Figure 1.1).

1. **Assessment,** the first step, is the collection, organization, and validation of subjective and objective data. The data collected form the database used by the nurse. As the data change, the nurse must update the database. The database will describe the physical, emotional, and spiritual health status of the client. Strengths and weaknesses are identified as are responses to any treatment modalities.

   Assessment begins at the moment the nurse meets the client and begins to gather information. Each piece of information collected about a client is a cue, because it hints at the total health status of the client. The baseline data act as a marker during future assessment. These data become a guide

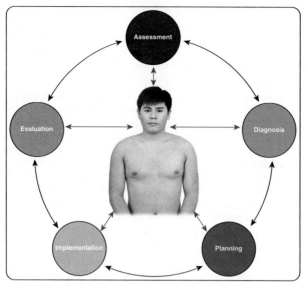

Figure 1.1 • Nursing process.

for the nurse as to what questions to ask and what additional information is needed.

2. **Diagnosis** is the second step of the nursing process. The nurse uses critical thinking and applies knowledge from the sciences and other disciplines to analyze and synthesize the data. Client strengths, risks, and weaknesses are clearly identified. Data are compared to normative values and standards. Normative values and standards include but are not limited to charts for growth and development, laboratory values (hemoglobin, hematocrit, total cholesterol, blood glucose, etc.), the degree of flexion in the joints, the rate and characteristics of pulses, blood pressure, heart sounds, skin texture, core body temperature, language development, role performance, and interdependent functions.

   Similar data are clustered or grouped together. The professional nurse makes a judgment after analysis and synthesis of collected data. This then becomes the nursing diagnosis, which is the basis for planning and implementing nursing care.

3. **Planning,** the third step, involves setting priorities, stating client goals or outcomes, and selecting nursing interventions, strategies, or orders to deal with the health status of the client. When possible, these activities need to include input from the client. Consultation or additional input may be needed from other healthcare professionals and family members. The developed nursing care plan acts as a guide for client care. This will help to enhance client strengths and help to negate, change, or prevent a weakness or problem for the client.

4. **Implementation** is the fourth step of the nursing process. Now the care plan is put into action. Putting the nursing interventions into action, the professional nurse determines the client's need for assistance or the ability to function independently to achieve the stated goals. The professional

nurse continues with the ongoing assessment of the client to update the database as behaviors change. The documentation of the implemented actions will include the client's response to nursing care. These actions will help meet the stated goals or outcomes, promote wellness, or convert illness to an improved state of health.

5. **Evaluation** is the final step of the nursing process. The professional nurse compares the present client status to achievement of the stated goals or outcomes. At this time the nurse will need to modify the nursing care plan. This modification can be to continue, change, or terminate the nursing care plan based on goal achievement.

CRITICAL THINKING

Critical thinking is a cognitive skill employed in all nursing activities that enhances the application of the nursing process. Alfaro-LeFevre (2003) defined and explained the critical thinking process. This work provided the foundation for the following discussion. **Critical thinking** is a process of purposeful and creative thinking about resolutions of problems or the development of ways to manage situations. It demands that nurses avoid bias and prejudice in their approach while using all of the knowledge and resources at their disposal to assist clients in achieving health goals or maintaining well-being.

When critically thinking about the client's health status, problems, or situations, one applies essential elements and skills. The five essential elements of critical thinking are collection of information, analysis of the situation, generation of alternatives, selection of alternatives, and evaluation. Figure 1.2 depicts the elements of critical thinking. Each element has working skills to help the nurse be complete, thorough, and competent with the cognitive processes of critical thinking. Critical thinking skills are linked with each of the essential elements.

1. **Collection of information,** the first of the elements in critical thinking, involves the five skills of identifying assumptions, organizing data collection, determining the reliability of the data, identifying relevant versus irrelevant data, and identifying inconsistencies in the data. In use of this first skill, the nurse must be able to identify assumptions that can misguide or misdirect the assessment and intervention processes. For example, when interviewing a client, one must not assume that lack of eye contact indicates lack of attention, dishonesty, or apathy when it occurs in Asian, Native American, and other individuals.

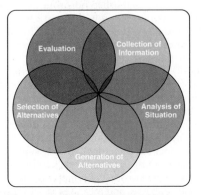

Figure 1.2 • Elements of critical thinking.

The second skill of collection of information is organizing data collection. Collection of subjective and objective data must be carried out in an organized manner. In health assessment the nurse first determines the client's current health status, level of distress, and ability to participate in the assessment process. The aim of data gathering in a client in acute distress is rapid identification of the problem and significant predisposing and contributory factors in order to select and initiate interventions to alleviate the distress. In nonacute situations, assessment follows an accepted and organized framework of survey, interview, and physical assessment.

The third skill of collection of information is determining the reliability of the data. One must recall that client information is valuable if it is reliable and accurate. The client is generally the best source of information, especially historic. However, physical and psychologic factors may interfere with that capability. Information is then sought from a family member or caregiver who can provide reliable information. Other reliable sources of information include charts, medical records, and notes from other health professionals. One must also be certain that objective data are accurate. Measuring devices must be standardized, calibrated, and applied correctly.

A wealth of information is obtained when carrying out a comprehensive health assessment. One then applies the fourth critical thinking skill, which is to determine the relevance of the information in relation to the client's current, evolving, or potential condition or situation. Consider the relevance of nonimmunization or contraction of German measles in a male client seeking care for a fracture versus a 26-year-old sexually active female having an annual examination.

Identifying inconsistencies is the last of the skills associated with the element of collection of information. The nurse must be able to recognize discrepancies in the information. Further, one must determine if the inconsistency is a result of an oversight, misunderstanding, linguistic factor, or cultural factor. Indication of confusion, memory impairment, and subtle or overt communication indicating discomfort with a topic or area of questioning must also be considered.

2. **Analysis of the situation** includes the following five skills: distinguish data as normal or abnormal, cluster related data, identify patterns in the data, identify missing information, and draw valid conclusions. The first of the skills is distinguishing normal from abnormal data. The nurse uses knowledge of human behavior as well as anatomy and physiology to compare findings with established norms in these areas. The nurse will use standards for laboratory results, diagnostic testing, charts, scales, and measures related to development and aging. The data must be analyzed in relation to expected ranges for age, gender, genetic background, and culture of the client.

When critically thinking, the nurse will then cluster related information by sorting and categorizing information into groupings that may include but are not limited to cues, symptoms, body systems, or health practices.

Once the clustering has been completed, the nurse must apply the third skill of identifying patterns in the information. Use of this skill enables the nurse to get an idea about what is happening with the client and to determine if more information is required. At this point the nurse would identify missing information, the fourth skill. Missing information would include but is not limited to onset of symptoms, medication history, family history of similar problems, and measures the client has taken to alleviate the problems. Additional information would include laboratory studies of hematologic, metabolic, or hormonal function.

The nurse has acquired information necessary to apply the last skill of drawing valid conclusions. This skill requires using all of one's knowledge and reasoning skills to draw logical conclusions about a problem or situation. The critical thinking process continues as the nurse works with the client to develop a treatment plan for his or her problem.

3. **Generation of alternatives** incorporates the skills of articulating options and establishing priorities. Articulation of options is simply stating possible paths to follow or actions to take to resolve a problem. Once the options have been enumerated, the nurse and client work together to establish priorities. This process must reflect the acuity of the problem and the client's ability to interpret the information required to weigh the advantages and disadvantages of each of the options in relation to health, lifestyle, cultural, and socioeconomic factors.

4. **Selection of alternatives** is the next element of critical thinking, and linked with it are the skills of developing outcomes and developing plans. Outcomes are statements of what the client will do or be able to do in a specific time period. The plan includes all of the actions required by the client independently or in coordination with healthcare professionals and others to achieve the stated outcomes. A plan is developed to guide the client toward meeting expectations in the stated outcomes.

5. **Evaluation** is the last element in critical thinking. This element includes the skills of determining if the expected outcomes have been achieved and reviewing the application of each of the critical thinking skills to be sure that omissions and misinterpretations did not occur. In addition, the nurse must evaluate thinking and judgment in the situation. One must be sure that decisions and actions were based on knowledge and the use of reliable resources and information. Furthermore, one must be sure that acts are based on moral and ethical principles and that the effects of values and biases have been considered.

DOCUMENTATION

Documentation of data from health assessment creates a client record or becomes an addition to an existing health record. The **client record** is a legal document used to plan care, to communicate information between and among healthcare providers, and to monitor quality of care.

Documentation is used to communicate information between and among the health professionals involved in the care of the client. In order for that communication to be effective documentation must be accurate, confidential, appropriate, complete, and detailed. When documenting, the nurse must use standard and accepted abbreviations, symbols, and terminology and must reflect professional and organizational standards.

Accuracy means that documentation is limited to facts or factual accounts of observations rather than opinions or interpretations of observations. When recording subjective data, it is important to use quotation marks and quote a client exactly rather than interpret the statement. In health assessment, accuracy also requires the use of accurate measurement and location of symptoms and physical findings.

Confidentiality means that information sharing is limited to those directly involved in client care. Information is considered appropriate for inclusion in a health record only if it has direct bearing on the client's health. Complete documentation means that all information required to develop a plan of care for the client has been included. Methods for documentation include narrative notes, problem-oriented charting, scales, flow sheets or check sheets, charting by exception, focus documentation, and computer documentation.

Narrative Notes. When implementing narrative notes, the nurse utilizes words, phrases, sentences, and paragraphs to record information. The information may be recorded in chronologic order from initial contact through conclusion of the assessment, or in categories according to the type of data collected. The narrative record includes words, sentences, phrases, or lists to indicate judgments made about the data, plans to address concerns, and actions taken to meet the health needs of the client.

Problem-Oriented Charting. Problem-oriented records include the SOAP and APIE methods. The letters SOAP refer to recording **S**ubjective data, **O**bjective data, **A**ssessment, and **P**lanning. Subjective data are those reported by the client or reliable informant. Objective data are derived from the physical examination, client records, and reports. Assessment refers to conclusions drawn from the data. Planning indicates the actions to be taken to resolve problems or address client needs. The letters APIE refer to **A**ssessment, **P**roblem, **I**ntervention, and **E**valuation. When using this method, documentation of assessment includes combining the subjective and objective data. The nurse will draw conclusions from the data, identify and record the problem or problems, and plan to address these problems. Interventions are documented as they are carried out. Evaluation refers to documentation of the response to the plan.

Flow Sheets. Documentation of health assessment data can be accomplished through the use of scales, check sheets, or flowcharts. These forms are usually formatted for a specific purpose or need. They may use columns or categories for recording data and may include lists of expected findings with associated qualifiers for ranges of normal or abnormal findings. Charts and check sheets often provide space for narrative descriptions or comments.

Focus Documentation. Focus documentation is a method that does not limit documentation to problems, but can include client strengths. This type of documentation is intended to address a specific purpose or focus, that is, a symptom, strength, or need. A comprehensive health assessment may result in one or more foci for documentation. The format for focus documentation is a column to address subjective and objective data, nursing action, and client response.

Charting by Exception. Charting by exception is a system in which documentation is limited to exceptions from pre-established norms or significant findings. Flow sheets with appropriate information and parameters are completed. This type of documentation eliminates much of the repetition involved in narrative and other forms of documentation.

Computer Documentation. Computer-generated documentation may include all of the previously mentioned methods for recording data. The amount and types of information to be documented vary according to the computer program and the policies and standards of the agency in which computer documentation is utilized.

2
Techniques and Equipment

Concepts to be considered when assessing the overall health status of the client include but are not limited to health, wellness, growth and development, culture, and psychosocial considerations. Much of the data gathered in relation to these concepts are subjective and are obtained through client interviews during the health history and focused interview sessions. Objective data must be gathered as part of the **database.** This is accomplished through the physical assessment of the client.

BASIC TECHNIQUES OF PHYSICAL ASSESSMENT

When performing physical assessment, the nurse will utilize four basic techniques to obtain objective and measurable data. These techniques are inspection, palpation, percussion, and auscultation and are performed in an organized manner. This pattern of organization varies when assessing the abdomen. The sequence for abdominal assessment is inspection, auscultation, percussion, and palpation. Percussion and palpation could alter the natural sounds of the abdomen; therefore, it is important to auscultate and listen to the unaltered sounds.

INSPECTION
Inspection is the skill of observing the client in a deliberate, systematic manner. It begins the moment the nurse meets the client and continues until the end of the client-nurse interaction. Inspection begins with a survey of the client's appearance and a comparison of the right and left sides of the client's body, which should be nearly symmetric. As the nurse assesses each body system or region, he or she inspects for color, size, shape, contour, symmetry, movement, or drainage. When inspecting a large body region, the nurse should proceed from general overview to specific detail. One should remember to look at the client, listen for natural sounds, and use the sense of smell to detect odors. Use of each of the senses enhances the findings.

Although the nurse will perform most of the inspection without the help of instruments, some special tools for visualizing certain body organs or regions are important. For example, the ophthalmoscope is used to inspect the inner aspect of the eye.

PALPATION
Palpation is the skill of assessing the client through the sense of touch to determine specific characteristics of the body. These characteristics include size, shape, location, mobility of a part, position, vibrations, temperature, texture, moisture, tenderness, and edema. The nurse must learn how much pressure to use during palpation with the examination hand. Too much pressure may produce pain for the client. Too little pressure may not permit the nurse to perceive the data accurately. This is a skill that requires practice and is developed over time.

The hand has several sensitive areas; therefore, it is important to use the part of the hand most responsive to body structures and functions. The nurse will use the fingertips, finger pads, base of the fingers, palmar surface of the fingers, and the dorsal and ulnar surfaces of the hand (Figure 2.1).

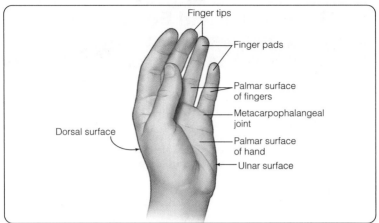

Figure 2.1 • Sensitive areas of the hand.

The finger pads are used for discrimination of underlying structures and functions such as pulses, superficial lymph nodes, or crepitus. Vibratory tremors felt through the chest wall are known as **fremitus.** Fremitus can be vocal, when the client speaks, or tussive, during coughing. Vibrations are best perceived by the examiner when using the base of the fingers (metacarpophalangeal joints). The palmar aspect of the fingers is used to determine position, consistency, texture, size of structures, pain, and tenderness. The dorsal surface of the fingers is most sensitive to temperature. The ulnar surface of the hand, including the finger, is most sensitive to vibrations such as fremitus. Remember, the dominant hand is always more sensitive than the nondominant hand. The fingertips are used in percussion and are discussed later in this chapter.

Light Palpation. During palpation, the nurse should use light, moderate, or deep pressure depending on the depth of the structure being assessed and the thickness of the layers of tissue overlying the structure. One must always begin with light palpation. This is the safest, least uncomfortable method and allows the client to become accustomed to the nurse's touch. Light palpation is used to assess surface characteristics, such as skin texture, pulse, or a tender, inflamed area near the surface of the skin. For light palpation, the finger pads of the dominant hand are placed upon the surface of the area to be examined. The hand is moved slowly and the finger pads, at a depth of 1 cm (0.39 in.), form circles on the skin during assessment, as demonstrated in Figure 2.2.

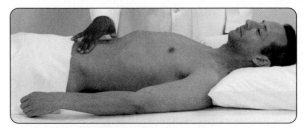

Figure 2.2 • Light palpation.

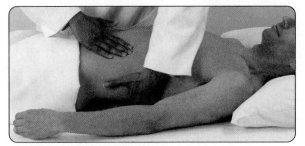

Figure 2.3 • Moderate palpation.

Moderate Palpation. Moderate palpation is used to assess most of the other structures of the body. For moderate palpation, the nurse uses moderate pressure, places the palmar surface of the fingers of the dominant hand over the structure to be assessed, and presses downward approximately 1 to 2 cm (0.39 to 0.78 in.), rotating the fingers in a circular motion. Now the nurse can determine the depth, size, shape, consistency, and mobility of organs as well as any pain, tenderness, or pulsations that might be present (Figure 2.3).

Deep Palpation. Deep palpation is used to palpate an organ that lies deep within a body cavity such as the kidney or spleen, or when overlying musculature is thick, tense, or rigid such as in obesity or with abdominal guarding. The nurse should use more than moderate pressure by placing the palmar surface of the fingers of the dominant hand on the skin surface. The extended fingers of the nondominant hand are placed over the fingers of the dominant hand, pressing and guiding the fingers downward. This technique provides extra support and pressure and allows the nurse to palpate at a deeper level, from 2 to 4 cm (0.75 to 1.5 in.). All palpation must be used with caution; however, greatest caution must be used with deep palpation. Deep palpation can cause pain and disrupt underlying pathology (Figure 2.4).

The nurse should proceed slowly, using smooth, deliberate movements, and avoid abrupt changes. Most clients will be more relaxed if the nurse talks to them during the examination, explaining each movement in advance. For example, during an abdominal assessment, the nurse might say, "I'm going to place my hand on your abdomen next. Tell me if you feel any discomfort and I will stop right away. How does it feel when I press down in this area?" It is a good

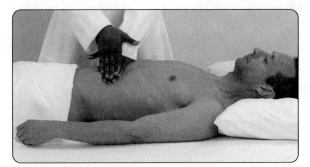

Figure 2.4 • Deep palpation.

idea to touch each area before palpating it. This touch informs the client that the examination of the area is about to begin and may prevent a startled reaction. Known painful areas of the body are usually the last area to be palpated.

PERCUSSION

Percussion is the third technique used by the nurse to obtain data when performing physical assessment. **Percussion** comes from the Latin word *percutire,* meaning "to strike through." Therefore, the nurse strikes through a body part with an object, fingers, or reflex hammer, ultimately producing a measurable sound. The striking or tapping of the body produces sound waves. As these waves travel toward underlying structures, they are heard as characteristic tones. The procedure is similar to a musician striking a drum, creating a vibration heard as a musical tone. Percussion is used to determine the size and shape of organs and masses, and whether underlying tissue is solid or filled with fluid or air.

Three methods of percussion can be used: direct percussion, blunt percussion, and indirect percussion. The part of the body to be percussed indicates the method to be used.

Direct Percussion. *Direct percussion* is the technique of tapping the body with the fingertips of the dominant hand. It is used to examine the thorax of an infant and to assess the sinuses of an adult, as illustrated in Figure 2.5.

Blunt Percussion. *Blunt percussion* involves placing the palm of the nondominant hand flat against the body surface and striking the nondominant hand with the dominant hand. A closed fist of the dominant hand is used to deliver the blow. This method is used for assessing pain and tenderness in the gallbladder, liver, and kidneys, as shown in Figure 2.6.

Indirect Percussion. *Indirect percussion* is the technique most commonly used because it produces sounds that are clearer and more easily interpreted. A hammer or tapping finger used to strike an object is called a **plexor,** derived from the Greek word *plexis.* **Pleximeter,** from the Greek word *metron,* meaning

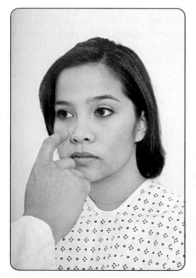

Figure 2.5 • Direct percussion.

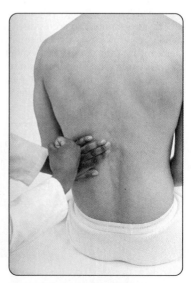

Figure 2.6 • Blunt percussion.

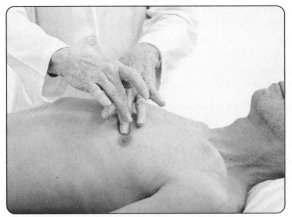

Figure 2.7 • Indirect percussion.

"measure," refers to the device that accepts the tap or blow from a hammer (Figure 2.7).

To perform indirect percussion, the hyperextended middle finger of the nondominant hand is placed firmly over the area being examined. This finger is the pleximeter. It is important to keep the other fingers and the palm of this hand raised in order to avoid contact with the body surface. Pressure from the other fingers and palm on the adjacent surface muffles tones being produced. Using only wrist action of the dominant hand to generate motion, the nurse delivers two sharp blows with the plexor. The plexor is the fingertip of a flexed middle finger of the dominant hand. The plexor makes contact with the distal phalanx of the pleximeter and is immediately removed. When the plexor maintains contact with the distal phalanx, the sound waves are muffled. Enough force should be used to generate vibrations and ultimately a sound without causing injury to the client or self. Some helpful percussion hints are:

- Ensure that motion is from the wrist, not the forearm or plexor finger.
- Release the plexor finger immediately after the delivery of two sharp strikes.
- Ensure that only the pleximeter makes contact with the body.
- Use the tip of the plexor finger, **NOT** the finger pad, to deliver the blow.
- Use two strikes and then reposition the pleximeter. Delivery of more than two rapid consecutive strikes creates the "woodpecker syndrome" and sounds are muffled.

Sounds. The amount of air in the underlying structure being percussed is responsible for the tone being produced. The more dense the tissue is, the softer and shorter the tone. The less dense the tissue is, the louder and longer the tone. The five percussion sounds are classified as follows:

1. **Tympany** is a loud, high-pitched, drumlike tone of medium duration characteristic of an organ that is filled with air. It is heard commonly over the gastric bubble in the stomach or over air-filled intestines.
2. **Resonance** is a loud, low-pitched, hollow tone of long duration. It is the normal finding over the lungs.

3. **Hyperresonance** is an abnormally loud, low tone of longer duration than resonance. It is heard when air is trapped in the lungs.

4. **Dullness** is a high-pitched tone that is soft and of short duration. It is usually heard over solid body organs such as the liver.

5. **Flatness** is a high-pitched tone, very soft, and of very short duration. It occurs over solid tissue such as muscle or bone.

Percussion sounds have characteristic features the professional nurse learns to interpret. These features include intensity, pitch, duration, and quality.

Intensity or *amplitude* of a sound refers to the softness or loudness of the sound. The louder the sound is, the greater the intensity or amplitude of the sound. This is influenced by the amount of air in the structure and the ability of the structure to vibrate.

Pitch or *frequency* of the sound refers to the number of vibrations of sound per second. Slow vibrations produce a low-pitched sound while a high-pitched sound comes from more rapid vibrations.

Duration refers to the length of time of the produced sound. This time frame ranges from very short to very long with variation in between.

Quality refers to the recognizable overtones produced by the vibration. This will be described as clear, hollow, muffled, or dull.

AUSCULTATION

Auscultation is the skill of listening to the sounds produced by the body. When auscultating, one uses both the unassisted sense of hearing and special instruments such as a stethoscope. Body sounds that can be heard with the ears alone include speech, coughing, respirations, and percussion tones. Many body sounds are extremely soft, and a stethoscope is needed to hear them. Stethoscopes work not by amplifying sounds but by blocking out other noises in the environment.

Auscultating body sounds requires a quiet environment in which the nurse can listen not just for the presence or absence of sounds, but also for the characteristics of each sound. External distractions such as radios, televisions, and loud equipment should be eliminated whenever possible. The nurse should avoid rubbing against client's clothes or drapes, or touching the stethoscope tubing since these actions produce sounds that will obscure the sounds of the body. It is important to keep the client warm, because shivering is uncomfortable and also obscures body sounds.

Sounds are described in terms of intensity, pitch, duration, and quality. For example, the nurse might note that a client's respirations are loud, high-pitched, long, and raspy. Many times the nurse will hear more than one sound at a time. It is important to focus on each sound and identify the characteristics of each sound. Closing the eyes and concentrating on each sound might help the nurse focus on the sound.

EQUIPMENT

Throughout physical assessment the nurse will use various instruments and pieces of equipment. These will help in visualizing, hearing, and measuring data. It is the responsibility of the nurse to know how to operate and when to use all equipment for client safety. Before beginning the physical assessment, the nurse should gather all the equipment together, organize it, and place it within easy reach. Table 2.1 gives a complete list of the equipment needed for a typical physical assessment. Some of the more complex items on the list are discussed in greater detail below or in later chapters.

Table 2.1	**Equipment Used during the Physical Assessment**

EQUIPMENT	
Cotton balls or wisps	Ruler, marked in centimeters
Cotton-tipped applicators	Skin-marking pen
Culture media	Slides
Dental mirror	Specimen containers
Doppler ultrasonic stethoscope	Sphygmomanometer
Flashlight	Sterile safety pin
Gauze squares	Stethoscope
Gloves	Tape measure, flexible, marked in centimeters
Goggles	Test tubes
Lubricant	Thermometer
Nasal speculum	Tongue blade
Ophthalmoscope	Tuning fork
Otoscope	Vaginal speculum
Penlight	Vision chart
Reflex hammer	Watch with second hand

STETHOSCOPE

The stethoscope is used to auscultate body sounds such as blood pressure, heart sounds, respirations, and bowel sounds. The stethoscope has three parts: the binaurals (earpieces), the flexible tubing, and the end piece. The end piece contains the diaphragm and the bell.

The flat end piece, called the diaphragm, screens out low-pitched sounds and, therefore, is best for transmitting high-pitched sounds such as lung sounds and normal heart sounds. The nurse should place the diaphragm evenly and firmly over the client's exposed skin. The deep, hollow end piece, called the bell, detects low-frequency sounds such as heart murmurs. It is placed lightly against the client's skin so that it forms a seal but does not flatten to a diaphragm. Either end piece may be held against the client's skin between the index and middle fingers of the examiner. Friction on the diaphragm or bell from coarse body hair may cause a crackling sound easily confused with abnormal breath sounds. This problem can be avoided by wetting the hair before auscultating the area. Stethoscopes usually include an assortment of interchangeable diaphragms and bells in different sizes for different purposes; for example, smaller diaphragm pieces are used for examining children.

DOPPLER ULTRASONIC STETHOSCOPE

A Doppler ultrasonic stethoscope uses ultrasonic waves to detect sounds that are difficult to hear with a regular stethoscope, such as fetal heart sounds and peripheral pulses.

OPHTHALMOSCOPE

An ophthalmoscope is used to inspect internal eye structures. Its main components are the handle, which holds the battery, and the head, which houses the aperture selector, viewing aperture, lens selector disk, lens indicator, lenses of varying powers of magnification, and mirrors.

The light source shines light through the viewing aperture, which is adjusted to select one of five apertures.

1. The large aperture is used most often. It emits a large, full spot for viewing dilated pupils.

2. The small aperture is used for undilated pupils.

3. The red-free filter shines a green beam used to examine the optic disc for pallor or hemorrhaging, which appears black with this filter.

4. The grid allows the examiner to assess the size, location, and pattern of any lesions.

5. The slit allows for examination of the anterior eye and aids in assessing the elevation or depression of lesions.

The lens selector dial must be rotated to bring the inner eye structures into focus. While looking through the viewing aperture, one rotates the lens selection dial to adjust the convergence or divergence of the light. At the zero setting, the lens neither converges nor diverges the light. The lens dial is moved clockwise to access the numbers in black, which range from +1 to +40. These lenses improve visualization in a client who is farsighted. The lens dial is moved counterclockwise to access the red numbers, which range from –1 to –20. These lenses improve visualization if the client is nearsighted.

OTOSCOPE

The otoscope is used to inspect internal ear structures. The main components of the otoscope are the handle, which is similar to that of the ophthalmoscope, the light, the lens, and specula of various sizes. The specula are used to narrow the beam of light. The nurse should select the largest one that will fit into the client's ear canal. If a nasal speculum is not available, the otoscope can be used to inspect the nose. In this case, the nurse should use the shortest, broadest speculum and insert it gently into the client's naris.

PROFESSIONAL RESPONSIBILITIES

Throughout all aspects of the assessment process, the nurse provides a safe and comfortable environment for the client. The nurse must identify cues presented by the client and apply critical thinking to determine the relevance of these data. The safe external environment created by the nurse includes comfort, warmth, privacy, and the use of Standard Precautions.

CUES

In addition to developing the skills of inspection, palpation, percussion, and auscultation, the nurse must be able to recognize the relative significance of the many visual, palpable, or auditory cues that may be present during an assessment. **Cues** are bits of information that hint at the possibility of a health problem. In other words, the nurse needs to know what to look for. To become skilled at cue recognition, nurses should cultivate their senses until they readily perceive even slight cues. For example, some things that are noticed during an initial survey or inspection of the client may hint at an underlying health problem. Swelling (edema) of the legs provides a cue to assess for heart problems. Bruising (ecchymosis) of the skin is a cue to ask the client about recent falls, trauma, injury, anticoagulant medication, or a bleeding problem. Grimacing, guarding (protective posture), or wincing when a client moves or a body part is moved during assessment are cues to examine for underlying joint and muscle problems or masses. Cues that suggest hearing loss include not following directions, looking at the examiner's lips during conversation, or speaking in a loud voice. Asymmetry of facial expression is a cue to assess function of the cranial nerves. Odors are cues to suggest a problem with hygiene or drainage from an orifice or wound. Cue recognition develops with practice, but beginners can acquire the skill by observing an experienced nurse, by practicing on partners, by studying the visual aids in this text, and by using the many videos, animations, skills, and clinical simulations available on the Companion Web site of the accompanying textbook.

PROVIDING A SAFE AND COMFORTABLE ENVIRONMENT

The physical assessment may be performed in a variety of settings, including a clinic, a hospital room, a school nurse's office, a corporate health services office, or a client's home. No matter where the location, the nurse is responsible for preparing a setting that is conducive to the client's comfort and privacy. The examination room should be warm, private, and free from distractions and interruptions. Overhead lighting must ensure good visibility and be free of distortion. A portable lamp to highlight body surfaces and contours may be needed.

The client should be positioned on a sturdy examination table with a firm surface that is covered with a clean sheet or paper cover. Though not as efficient, a firm bed will suffice if an examination table is not available. The table must be placed to allow the nurse easy access to both sides of the client's body. The table's height should allow the nurse to perform the examination without stooping. The nurse should also have a stool to sit on during certain parts of the examination and a small table or stand to hold the examination equipment.

The examination should be individualized according to the client's personal values and beliefs. Some clients, for example, may request that a family member be present during the examination. Some may ask for a nurse of the same sex. Some female clients may object to breast and vaginal examinations, regardless of the gender of the examiner, and some male clients may refuse penile, scrotal, and rectal examinations. A thorough assessment of the client's culture, religious beliefs, and environment, as described in chapters that follow, may help the nurse to anticipate these needs. Although explaining the reason for a certain procedure may help the client understand its benefit, a nurse must never attempt to influence or coerce the client to agree to any procedure. In all cases, the nurse must document which procedures took place and any that were refused.

TECHNIQUES AND EQUIPMENT IN ASSESSMENT OF THE OBESE CLIENT

Since the prevalence of obesity in the United States is rising, nurses must be prepared to address the special needs of the obese client during a comprehensive assessment. Equipment used for assessment must be appropriate for accurate data collection and to ensure client safety.

To ensure both comfort and safety chairs in the waiting and examination areas must be wide and sturdy. Examination tables should be wide and sturdy, with hand bars or footstools to help the client move onto the table. Examination tables should be bolted to the floor to avoid tipping.

Because of the weight of the chest wall and fat in the intercostal muscles, obese clients are unable to lie flat and deep breathing may be inhibited. The examination table must be adjustable to accommodate this problem.

Extra large examination gowns should be available. Scales with a capacity of greater than 350 pounds are required. Blood pressure cuffs must have a bladder width of 40% to 50% of the circumference of the arm and a length of 80% of the circumference of the arm. A large adult sized cuff, a thigh cuff, or special cuffs designed for the obese client must be considered for accurate measurement of the blood pressure. Comprehensive assessment of the obese client requires adjustments in the use and selection of equipment and techniques.

STANDARD PRECAUTIONS

Throughout the physical assessment, the professional nurse is required to apply the principles of asepsis. The Centers for Disease Control and Prevention (CDC) and the Occupational Safety and Health Administration (OSHA) have provided guidelines to protect the client and healthcare workers. Hand washing, use of gloves, use of protective barriers, disposal of sharps, handling of specimens, and proper disposal of body wastes are included in the guidelines. Each healthcare agency has created agency policies based on these guidelines. A nurse working at an agency is responsible for knowing the policies and following the guidelines.

3
General Survey

The **general survey** begins during the interview phase of a comprehensive health assessment. While collecting subjective data, the nurse observes the client while developing initial impressions about the individual's health and formulating strategies for the physical assessment. The observation includes what is seen, heard, or smelled during the initial phase of assessment. Clues that are uncovered during the general survey will guide the nurse during later assessment of body regions and systems.

COMPONENTS OF THE GENERAL SURVEY

The general survey is composed of four major categories of observation: physical appearance, mental status, mobility, and behavior of the client.

1. PHYSICAL APPEARANCE
The client's physical appearance provides immediate and important cues to the level of individual wellness. Body shape and build may indicate the client's general level of wellness. The body should be symmetric and the proportions regular: The client's arm span should approximate the height, and the distance from the pubis to the crown of the head should roughly equal the distance from the pubis to the sole of the foot. The client's height and weight should be within normal ranges for age and body build. Extreme thinness or obesity may indicate an eating disorder. The nurse must consider the client's lifestyle, socioeconomic level, and environment.

2. MENTAL STATUS
The nurse assesses the client's mental status while the client is responding to questions and giving information for the health history. The nurse notes the client's affect and mood, level of anxiety, orientation, and speech. Findings in these areas may be evaluated further during the assessment of the client's psychosocial status and neurologic system. The nurse assesses clients for orientation to person, place, and time.

3. MOBILITY
The nurse observes the client's gait, posture, and range of motion (the complete movement possible for a joint). Normally, the client walks in a rhythmic, straight, upright position with arms swinging at each side of the body. The shoulders are level and straight. Difficulty with gait and posture, such as stumbling, shuffling, limping, or the inability to stand erect, calls for further evaluation. Range of motion should be fluid and appropriate to the age of the client.

4. BEHAVIOR OF THE CLIENT
An assessment of the client's behavior includes information about the following factors: dress and grooming, body odors, facial expression, mood and affect, ability to make eye contact, and level of anxiety. The way in which clients dress may provide clues to their sense of self-esteem and body image.

The nurse observes the client for cleanliness and personal hygiene. The client who is dirty or has a strong body odor or poor dental hygiene may be depressed, have poor self-concept, lack knowledge about personal hygiene practices, or have difficulty managing hygiene because of obesity. The nurse assesses the client's emotional state by noting what the client says, the client's body language, facial expression, and the appropriateness of the client's behavior in relation to the situation and circumstances. The nurse also assesses the client for apprehension, fear, and nervousness. Like affect and mood, the client's level of anxiety is revealed through speech, body language, and facial expression. To obtain a relative impression of the level of anxiety, clients may be asked to rate their feelings of anxiety on a scale of 0 to 10. The nurse uses the client's response as an indicator of the need for further assessment and as a baseline for future assessment of anxiety levels.

The nurse assesses the client's speech for quantity, volume, content, articulation, and rhythm. The client should speak easily and fluently to the nurse or to an interpreter. Disorganized speech patterns, silence, or constant talking may indicate normal nervousness or shyness, or may signal a speech defect, neurologic deficit, depression, or another disorder.

AGE-RELATED CONSIDERATIONS

It is important to consider the developmental stage of the child or adolescent when assessing for each of the previous factors. The nurse should note the child's interaction with the parents or caretakers. Their relationship should exhibit mutual warmth and caring. Signs of child abuse include clinging to a parent or strong attachment to a parent because of fear of parental anger; absence of separation anxiety in a child who, because of developmental stage, would ordinarily demonstrate it; avoidance of eye contact between caretaker and child; a caretaker's demonstration of disgust with a child's behavior, illness, odor, or stool; flinching when people move toward the child; and regression to infantile behavior.

The dress, grooming, and personal hygiene of an older adult may be affected by limitations in mobility from arthritis, cardiovascular disease, and other disorders, or by a lack of funds. The gait of an older adult is often slower and the steps shorter. To maintain balance, older adults may hold their arms away from the body or use a cane. The posture of an older adult may look slightly stooped because of a generalized flexion, which also causes the older adult to appear shorter. A loss in height may also be due to thinning or compression of the intervertebral disks.

MEASURING HEIGHT AND WEIGHT

The nurse measures the client's height and weight to establish baseline data and to help determine health status.

HEIGHT

The nurse uses a measuring stick attached to a platform scale or to a wall to measure height. The client should look straight ahead while standing as straight as possible with heels together and shoulders back. When using a platform scale, the nurse raises the height attachment rod above the client's head, then extends and lowers the right-angled arm until it rests on the crown of the head. The measurement is read from the height attachment rod. When using a measuring stick, the nurse should place an L-shaped level on the crown of the client's head at a right angle to the measuring stick.

WEIGHT

A standard platform scale is used to measure the weight of older children and adults. If using a digital scale, the nurse simply reads the weight from the lighted display panel. Otherwise, the scale is calibrated by moving both weights to 0 and turning the knob until the balance beam is level. The nurse moves the large and small weights to the right and takes the reading when the balance beam returns to level. Special bed and chair scales are available for clients who cannot stand. Obese clients require scales that have a capacity of greater than

350 pounds (159 kg). Average height and weight for adult men and women are available in charts prepared by governmental agencies and insurers.

AGE-RELATED CONSIDERATIONS

To measure an infant's length, the nurse places the child in a supine position on an examining table that is equipped with a ruler, headboard, and adjustable footboard. The nurse positions the head against the headboard, extends the infant's leg nearest the ruler, and adjusts the footboard until it touches the infant's foot. The space between the headboard and footboard represents the length of the infant.

Infants are weighed on a modified platform scale with curved sides to prevent injury. The scale measures weight in grams and ounces. The nurse places the unclothed baby on the scale on a paper drape and watches the baby to prevent a fall. Measurements are taken to the nearest 10 g (0.5 oz).

MEASURING VITAL SIGNS

Vital signs include body **temperature, pulse, respiratory rate, blood pressure,** and **pain.** Measurement of oxygen saturation may be included when taking vital signs.

MEASURING BODY TEMPERATURE

The nurse should measure the client's core temperature, or the **temperature** of the deep tissues of the body (e.g., the thorax and abdominal cavity). This temperature remains relatively constant at about 37°C, or 98.6°F. The routes for measuring core temperature are oral, rectal, axillary, and tympanic.

MEASURING THE PULSE RATE

The left ventricle of the heart contracts with every beat, forcing blood from the heart into the systemic arteries. The force of the blood against the walls of the arteries generates a wave of pressure that is felt at various points in the body as a **pulse.**

Location of Pulse Points. The apical pulse is felt at the apex of the heart. Figure 3.1 illustrates the location of the apical pulse for a child under 4 years, a child 4 to 6 years, and an adult. The peripheral pulse is the pulse as felt in the body's periphery, for example, in the neck, wrist, or foot. Figure 3.2 shows eight sites where the peripheral pulse is most easily palpated.

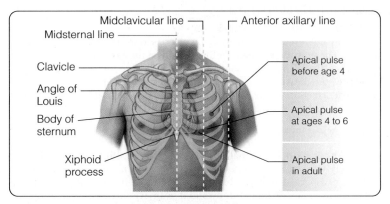

Figure 3.1 • Location of the apical pulse in a child under age 4, a child age 4 to 6, and an adult.

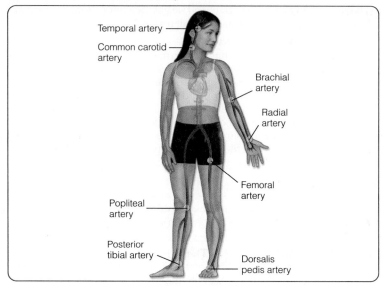

Figure 3.2 • Body sites where the peripheral pulse is most easily palpated.

MEASURING RESPIRATORY RATE

Counting the number of respirations per minute assesses **respiratory rate.** The nurse observes the full respiratory cycle (one inspiration and one expiration) for rate and pattern of breathing. The client's respiratory rate is assessed by counting the number of breaths for 30 seconds and then multiplying by 2. If the nurse detects irregularities or difficulty breathing, the respirations are counted for one full minute.

Oxygen Saturation. **Oxygen saturation** of the hemoglobin is measured using a pulse oximeter. The pulse oximeter uses a sensor and a photodetector to determine the light sent and absorbed by the hemoglobin. The reported percentage represents the light absorbed by oxygenated and deoxygenated hemoglobin. A value of 95% to 100% is considered normal, while a value of 70% is considered to be life threatening.

MEASURING BLOOD PRESSURE

Blood ebbs and flows within the systemic arteries in waves, causing two types of pressure. The **systolic pressure** is the pressure of the blood at the height of the wave, when the left ventricle contracts. This is the first number recorded in a blood pressure measurement. The **diastolic pressure** is the pressure between the ventricular contractions, when the heart is at rest. This is the second number recorded in a blood pressure measurement.

PAIN—THE FIFTH VITAL SIGN

Assessment of **pain** is essential in comprehensive health assessment. Pain is an entirely subjective and personal experience. When pain is present, it impacts every aspect of an individual's health and well-being. Pain can be acute and chronic, severe or mild, but overall it is an experience unique to the individual. The perception of pain and the ways in which the individual responds to pain vary according to age, gender, culture, and developmental level. When conducting a pain assessment, the nurse must consider all factors influencing the individual's experience with pain.

PAIN ASSESSMENT

The nurse typically initiates pain assessment because many individuals do not discuss their pain until asked about it. Pain assessment consists of two phases. The first phase is a pain history, and the second phase is observation of behaviors and responses to pain.

Pain History. A pain history includes collection of data about the location, intensity, quality, pattern, precipitating factors, actions aimed at relief of pain, impact on activities of daily living (ADLs), coping strategies, and emotional responses. A suggested method for assessment of physical complaints, including pain, is the acronym OLDCART & ICE. Figure 3.3 describes the meanings of the letters in the OLDCART & ICE acronyms. The following discusses the factors related to each of the aspects of the pain assessment.

Onset. The nurse asks the client to discuss and describe when the pain began.

Location. The nurse should ask the client to point to the specific location of pain. Charts in which body outlines are depicted are a useful method for children and adults to accurately identify the site of pain. When recording the location, the body outline charts may be used. The nurse is also expected to record locations, using appropriate terminology in relation to the proximity or distance from known landmarks (e.g., pain in substernal area 3 cm (1.18 in) below the xiphoid process).

Duration. The client is asked to describe the length of time the pain lasts. Included would be a determination of the pain as constant or intermittent. If the pain is intermittent, the nurse must assess the length of time without pain or between episodes of pain.

Characteristics. The characteristics of the pain are assessed by asking the client to apply an adjective to the pain. For example, pain may be experienced as burning, stabbing, piercing, or throbbing. Children may have difficulty describing pain; therefore, it is important to use familiar terminology, such as "boo-boo," "feel funny," or "hurt." The nurse must use quotation marks to record the description of the pain in the exact words spoken by the client.

OLDCART & ICE Acronym
O = Onset
L = Location
D = Duration
C = Characteristics
A = Aggravating Factors
R = Relieving Factors
T = Treatment
&
I = Impact on ADLs
C = Coping Strategies
E = Emotional Response

Figure 3.3 • OLDCART & ICE.

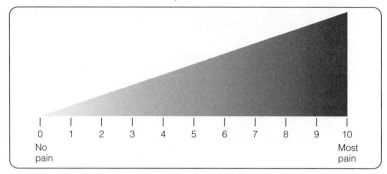

Figure 3.4 • Pain rating intensity scale.

The intensity of pain is most accurately assessed through the use of **pain rating scales** (Figure 3.4). Most scales use a numerical rating of 0 to 5 or 0 to 10, with 0 indicating the absence of pain. Descriptors accompany the number ratings in many scales. The descriptors assist the client to "quantify" the intensity of the pain. For children and adults who cannot read or are unable to numerically rate their pain, faces rating scales are available. Numbers accompany each facial expression so that pain intensity can be identified. Pain scales are available for non–English-speaking clients and for diverse populations at **http://painconsortium.nih.gov/pain_scales/index.html** and **http://pain-topics.org/clinical_concepts/assess.php**.

Aggravating Factors. A variety of factors can precipitate pain. These aggravating factors include activity, exercise, turning, breathing, swallowing, urinating, and temperature, or other climactic changes. Fear, anxiety, and stress can also aggravate pain.

Relieving Factors. Assessment of pain includes gathering data about the measures taken by the client to relieve or alleviate the pain. The nurse will inquire about the use of medications; home and folk remedies; and alternative or complementary therapies, such as acupuncture, massage, and imagery. The nurse must also gather data about the effectiveness of the measures.

Treatment. This assessment includes gathering data about pharmacologic and nonpharmacologic treatments for pain.

Impact on Activities of Daily Living. Assessment of the impact of pain on ADLs enables the nurse to understand the severity of the pain and the impact of the pain on the client's quality of life. ADLs include work, school, household and family management, mobility and transportation, leisure activities, and marital and family relationships. The nurse may ask the client to rate the impact of the pain on each of the ADLs.

Coping Strategies. There are a variety of ways in which individuals cope with pain. Various coping strategies include but are not limited to prayer, yoga, tai chi, chi quong, support groups, distraction, relaxation techniques, or withdrawal. The strategies are often unique to the individual or reflect cultural values and beliefs. The nurse attempts to identify coping strategies employed by the client and to determine if they are effective in pain management.

Emotional Responses. An assessment of the client's emotional response to pain is important. Pain, especially chronic or debilitating pain, can result in depression, anxiety, and physical and emotional exhaustion. The emotional response to pain is often related to the type, intensity, and duration of pain.

Observation. The observation phase of the pain assessment includes the direct observation of the client's behavior and physiologic responses.

Behavior. A variety of behaviors indicate the presence of pain. Many of these behaviors are nonverbal or consist of vocalizations. Behaviors indicative of pain include facial grimacing, moaning, crying or screaming, guarding or immobilization of a body part, tossing and turning, and rhythmic movements.

Physiologic Responses. The site of the pain and the duration of the pain influence physiologic responses to pain. The sympathetic nervous system is stimulated in the early stage of acute pain. The response is demonstrated in elevation of blood pressure, pulse and respiratory rates, pallor, and diaphoresis. Parasympathetic stimulation often accompanies visceral pain. This results in lowered blood pressure and pulse rate, and warm dry skin.

FUNCTIONAL ASSESSMENT DURING THE GENERAL SURVEY

The **functional assessment** is an observation to gather data while the client is performing common or routine activities. During the general survey of a healthy client, the nurse will observe the client while performing the following common activities: walking into the examination room, taking a seat for the interview, and moving the arms and hands to arrange clothing or to shake hands as an introduction. The nurse will also observe the facial expression while these acts occur. From this brief encounter, the nurse applies knowledge to begin to gather and interpret data about the client's mobility and strength, and the symmetry of the face and parts of the body.

4
The Health History

The health assessment interview provides an opportunity to gather detailed information about events and experiences that have contributed to a client's current state of health. The **health history** is a comprehensive record of the client's past and current health. The health history is gathered during the initial health assessment interview, which usually occurs at the client's first visit to a healthcare facility and is updated with each additional visit.

COMMUNICATION SKILLS

Communication is the exchange of information between individuals. Effective communication skills play an important role in developing a nurse-client relationship, conducting the health assessment interview, and collecting data for the health history. Communication is also important in educating, guiding, facilitating, directing, and counseling the client. The nurse cannot develop trust, establish rapport, or carry out nursing interventions for clients without knowledge of communication techniques.

Interactional skills are actions that are used to obtain and disseminate information, develop relationships, and promote understanding of self and others. Nurses use a variety of interactional skills during the communication process to gather assessment data from the client, family, significant others, and healthcare personnel. The interactional skills that are helpful during an interview are summarized in Table 4.1. The nurse uses these interactional techniques to help the client communicate information thoroughly and also to confirm that the nurse has understood the client's communication correctly.

BARRIERS TO EFFECTIVE CLIENT INTERACTION

In some situations the nurse may unknowingly hinder the flow of information by using nontherapeutic interactions (interactions that are harmful rather than helpful). Nontherapeutic interactions interfere with the communication process by making the client uncomfortable, anxious, or insecure. Some interactions that can be most harmful if used during the health assessment interview are false reassurance, interrupting or changing the subject, passing judgment, cross-examination, use of technical terms, and insensitivity.

False reassurance occurs when the nurse assures the client of a positive outcome with no basis for believing in it. False reassurance deprives clients of the right to communicate their feelings.

Interrupting the client or changing the subject shows insensitivity to the client's thoughts and feelings. In most cases this happens when the nurse is ill at ease with the client's comments and is unable to deal with their content.

Judgmental statements convey a strong message that the client must live up to the nurse's value system to be accepted. These statements imply nonacceptance and discourage further interaction.

Table 4.1 Interactional Skills

SKILL/DEFINITION	TECHNIQUE	EXAMPLES
Attending Giving the client undivided attention.	• Use direct eye contact if appropriate for culture. Look at the client during the conversation. • Lean toward the client slightly. • Select quiet area with no distractions for interview. • Convey unhurried manner; avoid fidgeting and looking at watch.	Nurse arranges with peers for no interruptions during interview. Nurse sits facing client, remains alert, and focuses on what client is saying.
Paraphrasing Restating the client's basic message to test whether it was understood.	• Listen for the client's basic message. • Restate the client's message in your own words. • Ask the client if your words are an accurate restatement of the message.	*Client:* "I toss and turn all night. Sometimes I can't get to sleep at all. I don't know why this is happening. I've always been a deep sleeper." *Nurse:* "It sounds like you're not getting enough sleep. Is that right?"
Direct Leading Directing the client to obtain specific information or to begin an interaction.	• Decide what area you want to explore. • Tell the client what you want to discuss. • Encourage the client to follow your lead.	"Let's discuss the pain in your back." "When did your symptoms begin?"
Focusing Helping the client zero in on a subject or get in touch with feelings.	• Use focusing when the client strays from the topic or uses tangential speech. • Listen for themes, issues, or feelings in the client's rambling conversation. • Ask the client to give more information about a specific theme, issue, or feeling. • Encourage the client to emphasize feelings when giving this information.	"Describe how you feel when you can't sleep." "Did you say you were angry and frustrated before you went to bed? Go over that again."

(continued)

Table 4.1 Interactional Skills (continued)

SKILL/DEFINITION	TECHNIQUE	EXAMPLES
Questioning Gathering specific information on a topic through the process of inquiry.	• Use open-ended questions whenever possible. Avoid using questions that can be answered with "yes," "no," "maybe," or "sometimes." • Ask the client to express feelings about what is being discussed. • Ask questions that help the client gain insight.	"What did you mean when you said your back was breaking?" "How did you feel after you talked to your boss?"
Reflecting Letting the client know that the nurse empathizes with the thoughts, feelings, or experiences expressed.	• Take in the client's feelings from verbal and nonverbal body language. • Determine which combination of "cues" you should reflect back to the client. • Reflect the "cues" back to the client. • Observe the client's response to the reflected feelings, experience, or content.	*Feelings:* "It sounds like you're feeling lonely." "It must really be frustrating not to be able to get enough sleep." *Experience:* "You're yawning. You must be tired." "You act as if you're in pain." *Content:* "You think you're going to die." "You believe the medication is helping."
Summarizing Tying together the various messages that the client has communicated throughout the interview.	• Listen to verbal and nonverbal content during the interview. • Summarize feelings, issues, and themes in broad statements. • Repeat them to the client, or ask the client to repeat them to you.	"Let's review the health problems you've identified today."

Cross-examination refers to asking question after question during an assessment interview and may cause the client to feel threatened; the client may seek refuge by revealing less information. Because all interviews include many questions, the nurse should be careful not to make clients feel that they are being cross-examined with an endless barrage of questions. It is helpful to pause between questions.

Technical terms, such as *anterior* and *posterior,* are useful for nursing and medical personnel but are more confusing to the client than the terms *front* and *back.* Whenever possible, the nurse should use lay rather than technical terms and avoid jargon, slang, or clichés. It is best to avoid the use of initials and acronyms unless they are commonly accepted as everyday language. For instance, most clients will understand the term *AIDS* but not *prn* (as necessary).

Sensitive issues refer to topics that are considered sensitive and personal. The client may feel uncomfortable providing information about such concerns as abuse, homelessness, emotional and psychologic problems, use of drugs and alcohol, self-image, sexuality, or religion. Discomfort with these issues may cause the client to lapse into silence. It is important to be sensitive to the client's need for silence. The client may need to reflect on what was said or to come to grips with emotions the question has evoked before proceeding. The nurse also watches for nonverbal signs, such as tear-filled eyes or wringing of hands, which indicate the client's need to pause for a moment.

THE INFLUENCE OF CULTURE ON NURSE-CLIENT INTERACTIONS

Differences in culture and the ways in which they are demonstrated have a significant impact on the interactions that occur in the nurse-client relationship. The professional nurse must be prepared to recognize and adapt the interactional processes to cultural differences. Further, nurses must not allow their own cultural values and practices to bias the impressions of the client, nor to impair the interaction.

DIVERSITY

Communication depends on a combination of factors such as culture, ethnicity, religion, nationality, education, health status, and level of intelligence. When two people differ in any of these ways, each must be more open to the other person's way of thinking and foster mutual understanding. The nurse is careful not to bring cultural stereotypes to the communication process.

THE HEALTH HISTORY INTERVIEW

The health history interview is the exchange of information between the nurse and the client. This information, along with the data from the physical assessment, is used to develop nursing diagnoses and design the nursing care plan. Unlike other types of interviews nurses conduct, the health history interview is a formal, planned interaction to inquire about the client's health patterns, ADLs, past health history, current health issues, self-care activities, wellness concerns, and other aspects of the client's health status. In most situations, nurses use a special health history tool to collect assessment data. The health history is a critical component of the comprehensive health interview.

THE PRIMARY SOURCE

The primary and best source of information for the health assessment interview is the client. The client is the only one who can describe personal symptoms,

Box 4.1	Guidelines for Interviewing Clients Who Do Not Speak English

- Be open to ways you can communicate effectively. Imagine yourself entering a care setting where few people speak your language. Your sensitivity to this fear and unease will be your greatest strength in providing quality care for your client.
- Determine what language your client speaks. Your first assumption may not be correct. For example, South American immigrants may speak one of a variety of Native American dialects, Portuguese, or Spanish.
- Make sure the client can read and write, as well as speak, in the native language. Be alert for any confusion.
- Learn key foreign phrases that will help you communicate with the client.
- Find friends, relatives, neighbors, or other nurses who can help you translate. Try to obtain a phone number for this person. You may need immediate help with a question or emergency.
- Find out if your healthcare facility has access to translators. It is best to have an official translator when you give instructions or obtain consent.
- Look at your *client* while telling the translator what to say. This helps your client feel connected to you and conveys meaning through body language and facial expression.
- Use clear simple language. For example, do not tell the translator to ask for a clean-catch specimen; instead explain what you mean step by step.
- Pause frequently for the translator.
- Ask the translator to provide the proper context for any colloquial expressions your client may use.

If You Cannot Find a Translator

- Develop cards with phrases or illustrations to aid communication. Have several translators review the cards before using them.
- Use written handouts for client teaching. These can be developed or purchased. Look for handouts with plenty of diagrams.

experiences, and factors leading to the current health concern. In some situations, the client may be unable or unwilling to provide information.

SECONDARY SOURCES

A **secondary source** is a person or record that provides additional information about the client. The nurse uses secondary sources when the client is unable or unwilling to communicate. For example, the parent or caregiver is the source of information for a child who cannot communicate. Secondary sources are used to augment and validate previously obtained data. The most commonly used secondary sources are significant others to whom the client has expressed thoughts and feelings about lifestyle or health status, and medical and other records containing descriptions of the client's subjective experience. Whenever possible, the nurse should obtain the client's permission before requesting information from another person. Client privacy is protected under the Health Insurance Portability and Accountability Act (HIPAA). HIPAA regulations expressly permit the use of professional judgment and experience in solicitation of information from secondary sources under emergency circumstances or when the client is incapacitated. The interviewing nurse should not overlook the attending physician and other healthcare personnel who have cared for the client as excellent secondary sources of information.

PHASES OF THE HEALTH ASSESSMENT INTERVIEW

The health assessment interview is divided into three phases: preinteraction, the initial or formal interview, and the focused interview. The first two phases provide information the nurse uses along with information from the physical assessment to develop the total client database, formulate nursing diagnoses, and initiate the nursing care plan. The third phase, the focused interview, occurs throughout all stages of the nursing process. Its purpose is to gather, clarify, and update additional client data as they become available.

Phase I: Preinteraction. The **preinteraction** phase is the period before first meeting with the client. During this time, the nurse collects data from the medical record, previous health risk appraisals, health screenings, therapists, dietitians, and other healthcare professionals who have cared for, taught, or counseled the client, and family members or friends. The nurse reviews the client's name, age, sex, nationality, medical and social history, and current health concern.

Phase II: The Initial Interview. The **initial interview** is a planned meeting in which the nurse interviewer gathers information from the client. In most cases, the nurse uses a health history form to collect the data to avoid overlooking any area of information. The nurse gathers information about every facet of the client's health status and state of wellness at this time. These data will be used to develop hypothetical nursing diagnoses. The nurse should inform the client what to expect.

Phase III: The Focused Interview. The nurse uses the **focused interview** throughout the physical assessment, during treatment, and while caring for the client. The purpose of the focused interview is to clarify previously obtained assessment data, gather missing information about a specific health concern, update and identify new diagnostic cues as they occur, guide the direction of a physical assessment as it is being conducted, and identify or validate probable nursing diagnoses. When obtaining subjective data about client symptoms, many nurses find it helpful to use an acronym to guide the interview. One acronym is OLDCART & ICE. When using the acronym, the nurse will elicit information about the onset, location, duration, characteristics, aggravating factors, relieving factors, and treatment of symptoms, as well as the impact of symptoms on ADLs, the coping strategies used to deal with symptoms, and emotional responses to the symptoms. See chapter 3, Figure 3.3 on page 23.

THE HEALTH HISTORY

The goal of the interview process is to obtain a health history containing information about the client's health status. The nursing health history focuses on the client's physical status, patterns of daily living, wellness practices, and self-care activities as well as psychosocial, cultural, environmental, and other factors that influence health status (Table 4.2). The information in a nursing health history is used along with the subsequent data from the physical assessment to develop a set of nursing diagnoses that reflect the client's health concerns.

COMPONENTS OF THE HEALTH HISTORY

Most healthcare settings have developed nursing and medical health history forms for collecting and organizing the data and ensuring that the interviewer does not omit any information. The information gathered for each of the components of the health history serves a purpose in health assessment and in

Table 4.2	Health History Format

I. Biographic Data	**IV. Family History**
Name	Immediate Family
Address	Extended Family
Age	Genogram
Date of Birth	**V. Psychosocial History**
Birthplace	Occupational History
Gender	Education
Marital Status	Financial Background
Race	Roles and Relationships
Ethnic Identity/Culture	Family
Religion and Spirituality	Social Structure /
Occupation	Emotional Concerns
Health Insurance	Self-Concept
Source of Information / Reliability	**VI. Review of Body Systems**
II. Present Health or Illness	Skin, Hair, and Nails
Reason for Seeking Care	Head, Neck, and Lymphatics
Health Beliefs and Practices	Eyes
Health Patterns	Ears, Nose, Mouth, and Throat
Medications, Prescription and Over	Respiratory
the Counter	Breasts and Axillae
III. Past History	Cardiovascular
Medical	Peripheral Vascular
Surgical	Abdomen
Hospitalization	Urinary
Outpatient Care	Male Reproductive
Childhood Illnesses	Female Reproductive
Immunizations	Musculoskeletal
Mental and Emotional Health	Neurologic
Allergies	
Substance Use	

application of the nursing process for each client. Responses to the questions asked in the health history provide specific information about the individual. The nurse will use professional judgment in determining the significance of the responses, the need for follow-up questioning, and the relevance of information to meeting the health needs of the client.

Biographic Data. The biographic data include the client's name and address, age and date of birth, birthplace, gender, marital status, race, religion, occupation, information about health insurance, and the reliability of the source of information. When possible, the client completes a form that elicits these data. Otherwise, the interviewing nurse documents it. Gathering biographic data is an important initial step in understanding the client. The biographic data provide a data set from which the nurse can begin to make judgments. The biographic data will be used to relate and compare individual characteristics to established expectations and norms for physical and emotional health. Furthermore, the biographic data provide information about social and environmental characteristics that impact physical and emotional health.

Present Health-Illness. The history of present health or illness includes information about all of the client's current health-related issues, concerns, and problems. The history includes determination of the reason for seeking care, as well as identification of health beliefs and practices, health patterns, health goals, and information about medication and therapies.

- *Reason for Seeking Care.* The client usually gives the reason for seeking care when the nurse asks, "Why are you seeking help today?" or "What is bothering you?" The reason for seeking care, sometimes written as the chief complaint, is an important part of the health history picture.

- *Health Beliefs and Practices.* A person's beliefs about health and illness are influenced by heritage, exposure to information, and experiences. Culture and heritage influence an individual's perceptions about internal and external factors that contribute to health and cause illness and the practices the individual follows to prevent and treat health problems.

- *Health Patterns.* A **health pattern** is a set of related traits, habits, or acts that affect a client's health. The description of the client's health patterns plays a key role in the client's total health history because it is the "lifestyle thread" that, woven throughout the fabric of the health history, gives it depth, detail, and definition.

    Health patterns also refer to the types and frequency of health care in which a client participates. The nurse will ask questions related to the frequency of healthcare visits, preventive and screening measures used by the client including laboratory and other diagnostic testing, and the results if known.

- *Medications.* Information about the use of medications is obtained during this part of the health history. The information should include the use of prescription and over-the-counter (OTC) medications. The nurse should determine the name, dose, purpose, duration, frequency, and desired or undesired effects of each of the medications. The medication history includes the use of home remedies, folk remedies, herbs, teas, vitamins, dietary supplements, or other substances.

Past History. The past history includes information about childhood diseases; immunizations; allergies; blood transfusions; major illnesses; injuries; hospitalizations; labor and deliveries; surgical procedures; mental, emotional, or psychiatric health problems; and the use of alcohol, tobacco, and other substances. Many health history forms include a checklist of the most commonly occurring illnesses or surgical procedures to help the client recall information.

Information about the client's emotional, mental, or psychiatric health should include the description of the problem. Information about allergies and the use of illicit drugs, caffeine, alcohol, and tobacco is included in the health history. Information about allergies should include determination of the allergy as food, drug, or environmentally occurring as well as the symptoms, treatment, and personal adaptation. When gathering information about the use of alcohol, tobacco, caffeine, and illicit drugs, the nurse will want to know the type, amount, duration, and frequency of use of each substance.

Family History. The family history is a review of the client's family to determine if any genetic or familial patterns of health or illness might shed light on the client's current health status. The nurse should encourage the client to recall as many generations as possible to develop a complete picture. The nurse documents information collected from the client and the family in a family genogram. A **genogram** is a pictorial representation of family relationships

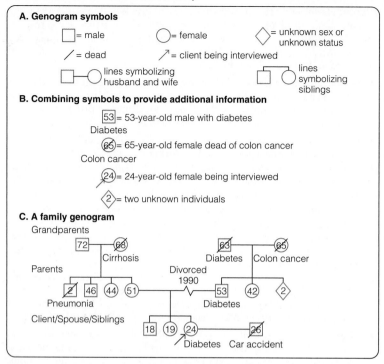

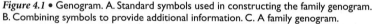

Figure 4.1 • Genogram. A. Standard symbols used in constructing the family genogram. B. Combining symbols to provide additional information. C. A family genogram.

and medical history. The family genogram, also known as a pedigree or family tree, is the most effective method of recording the large amount of data gathered from a family's health history (Figure 4.1).

Psychosocial History. The psychosocial history includes information about the client's occupational history, educational level, financial background, roles and relationships, ethnicity and culture, family, spirituality, and self-concept. Determining the client's level of education establishes expectations related to the ability to comprehend verbal and written language. The client's financial situation, that is, the ability to obtain health insurance or pay for health services, has an impact on health, health practices, and health-seeking behaviors. The nurse will also gather information about the client's roles and relationships, family, ethnicity and culture, spirituality, and self-concept.

Ethnic Identity and Culture. Information about ethnicity and culture is gathered because it enables the nurse to determine physical and social characteristics that influence healthcare decisions. Ethnicity or culture influences a number of health-related factors for the client. These factors include health beliefs, health practices, verbal and nonverbal methods of communication, roles and relationships in the family and society, perceptions of healthcare professionals, diet, dress and rituals, and rites associated with birth, marriage, child rearing, and death. Spirituality refers to the individual's sense of self in relation to others and a higher being, and what one believes gives meaning to life.

Box 4.2	Review of Body Systems

- Skin, Hair, and Nails
- Head, Neck, and Related Lymphatics
- Eyes
- Ears, Nose, Mouth, and Throat
- Respiratory System
- Breasts and Axillae
- Cardiovascular System
- Peripheral Vascular System
- Abdomen
- Urinary System
- Reproductive System
- Musculoskeletal System
- Neurologic System

Review of Body Systems. The focus of this portion of the health history is to uncover current and past information about each body system and its organs. The nurse asks the client about system function and any abnormal signs or symptoms, paying special attention to gathering information about the functional patterns of each system. Some health history formats use a cephalocaudal or head-to-toe approach for collecting data. In this approach, one considers regions of the body rather than systems. Other formats use an approach related to a nursing theory. Regardless of the method, each area of the body must be reviewed until all systems are covered in each region.

DOCUMENTATION

The data collected during the interview are recorded in the nurse's health history. The type of recording is often influenced by the agency or facility in which the interview is carried out. Forms for documentation are varied and include checklists, fill-in forms, and narrative records. The nurse's health history becomes part of the client record and is a legal document. Principles of documentation must be applied.

The subjective data are recorded using quotes. The nurse uses communication skills to elicit as much detail as possible about each area and topic within the health history. The nurse should ask the client to explain his or her meaning of words such as "good," "average," "okay," "normal," and "adequate." The nurse must be sure to record what the client intended by use of such terms. When recording data, the information must be presented in a clear and concise manner. For example, the nurse would use dates and write them in descending order from present to past when providing details about events.

5
Skin, Hair, and Nails

The integumentary system consists of the skin and the accessory structures, the sweat and oil glands, the hair, and the nails.

ANATOMY AND PHYSIOLOGY REVIEW

The skin is composed of the epidermal, dermal, and subcutaneous layers. The cutaneous glands, which are located in the dermal layer, release secretions to lubricate the skin and to assist in temperature regulation. The outermost portion of skin comprises the epidermis, a layer of epithelial tissue. The **dermis** is a layer of connective tissue that lies just below the epidermis. **Subcutaneous tissue** (or **hypodermis**) is a loose connective tissue that stores approximately half of the body's fat cells.

Cutaneous glands are formed in the stratum basale and push deep into the dermis. They release their secretions through ducts onto the skin surface. There are two types of sweat (or sudoriferous) glands: eccrine and apocrine. **Eccrine glands** are more numerous and more widely distributed. They produce a clear fluid called perspiration. **Apocrine glands** are found primarily in the axillary and anogenital regions. They are dormant until the onset of puberty. Apocrine glands produce a secretion made up of water, salts, fatty acids, and proteins, which is released into hair follicles. **Oil glands, or sebaceous glands,** are distributed over most of the body except the palms of the hands and soles of the feet. They produce *sebum,* an oily secretion composed of fat and keratin that is usually released into hair follicles. The layers of the skin and the accessory structures are depicted in Figure 5.1.

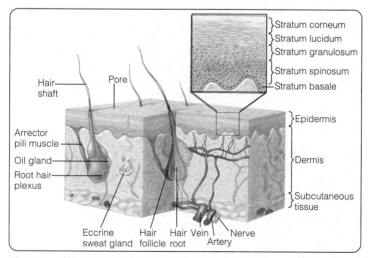

Figure 5.1 • Skin structure. Three-dimensional view of the skin, subcutaneous tissue, glands, and hairs.

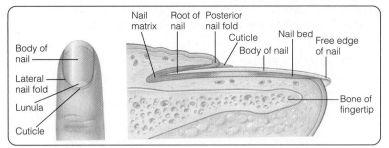

Figure 5.2 • Structure of a nail.

HAIR

A **hair** is a thin, flexible, elongated fiber composed of dead, keratinized cells that grow out in a columnar fashion (see Figure 5.1). Each hair shaft arises from a follicle. Nerve endings in the follicle are sensitive to the slightest movement of the hair. Each hair follicle also has an arrector pili muscle that causes the hair to contract and stand upright when a person is under stress or exposed to cold.

NAILS

Nails are thin plates of keratinized epidermal cells that shield the distal ends of the fingers and toes (Figure 5.2). Nail growth occurs at the nail matrix, as new cells arise from the basal layer of the epidermis. As the nail cells grow out from the matrix, they form a transparent layer, called the body of the nail, which extends over the nail bed. The nail body appears pink because of the blood supply in the underlying dermis. A moon-shaped crescent called a **lunula** appears on the nail body over the thickened nail matrix. A fold of epidermal skin called a **cuticle** protects the root and sides of each nail.

SPECIAL CONSIDERATIONS

Throughout the assessment process, the nurse gathers subjective and objective data reflecting the client's state of health. Factors to be considered when collecting the data include but are not limited to age, developmental level, race, ethnicity, work history, living conditions, social economics, and emotional well-being.

INFANTS AND CHILDREN

At birth, the newborn's skin typically is covered with **vernix caseosa,** a white, cheeselike mixture of sebum and epidermal cells. Infants may have areas of tiny white facial papules, called **milia,** due to sebum that collects in the openings of hair follicles. **Mongolian spots** are gray, blue, or purple spots in the sacral and buttocks areas of newborns. The subcutaneous fat layer is poorly developed in infants and the eccrine sweat glands do not secrete until the first few months of life. The fine, downy hair of the newborn, called **lanugo,** is replaced within a few months by vellus hair. Throughout childhood, the epidermis thickens, pigmentation increases, and more subcutaneous fat is deposited, especially in females during puberty. During adolescence, both the sweat glands and the oil glands increase their production. This predisposes the development of acne. Pubic and axillary hair appears during adolescence, and males may develop facial and chest hair.

THE PREGNANT FEMALE

Pigmentation of the skin commonly increases during pregnancy, especially in the areolae, nipples, vulva, and perianal area. Approximately 70% of pregnant women develop hyperpigmented patches on the face referred to as **chloasma,** melasma gravidum, or "the mask of pregnancy." Some pregnant clients may also have a dark line called a **linea nigra** running from the umbilicus to the pubic area, increased pigmentation of the areolae and nipples, and darkened moles and scars. These are all normal findings.

Many pregnant females develop striae gravidarum (stretch marks) across the abdomen. These usually fade after pregnancy but do not disappear entirely.

THE OLDER ADULT

As the skin ages, the epidermis thins and stretches out, and collagen and elastin fibers decrease, causing decreased skin elasticity and increased skin wrinkling. The skin becomes slack and may sag, especially beneath the chin and eyes, in the breasts of females, and in the scrotum of males. Decreased production of sebum leads to dryness of both the skin and the hair.

Older clients may develop senile *lentigines* (liver spots), which look like hyperpigmented freckles. Cherry angiomas are small, bright red spots common in older adults. They increase in number with age. Cutaneous tags may appear on the neck and upper chest, and cutaneous horns may occur on any part of the face. The hair becomes increasingly gray as melanin production decreases. Hair thins as the number of active hair follicles decreases. Facial hair may become more coarse.

The nails may show little change, or they may show the effects of decreased circulation in the body extremities, appearing thicker, harder, yellowed, oddly shaped, or opaque. They may be brittle and peeling and may be prone to splitting and breaking.

PSYCHOSOCIAL CONSIDERATIONS

Stress may exacerbate certain skin conditions such as rashes or acne. Stress may also be a factor in compulsive behaviors such as hair twisting or plucking (trichotillomania) and nail biting, signaled by nails that have no visible free edge or that have short, jagged edges. A lack of cleanliness of the skin, hair, or nails also may result from emotional distress, poor self-esteem, or a disturbed body image.

Changes in skin color may be difficult to evaluate in clients with dark skin. It is helpful to inspect areas of the body with less pigmentation, such as the lips, oral mucosa, sclerae, palms of the hands, and conjunctivae of the inner eyelids. (See Table 5.1 for evaluating color variations in light and dark skin.)

CULTURAL CONSIDERATIONS

Assessment and findings are influenced by culture. See the cultural considerations box for specific examples.

The focused interview for the integumentary system concerns data related to the structures and functions of that system. Subjective data related to the condition of the skin, hair, and nails are gathered during the focused interview.

Table 5.1 Color Variations in Light and Dark Skin

COLOR VARIATION/ LOCALIZATION	POSSIBLE CAUSES	APPEARANCE IN LIGHT SKIN	APPEARANCE IN DARK SKIN
Pallor *Loss of color in skin due to the absence of oxygenated hemoglobin.* Widespread, but most apparent in face, mouth, conjunctivae, and nails.	May be caused by sympathetic nervous stimulation resulting in peripheral vasoconstriction due to smoking, a cold environment, or stress. May also be caused by decreased tissue perfusion due to cardiopulmonary disease, shock and hypotension, lack of oxygen, or prolonged elevation of a body part. May also be caused by anemia.	White skin loses its rosy tones. Skin with natural yellow tones appears more yellow; may be mistaken for mild jaundice.	Black skin loses its red undertones and appears ash-gray. Brown skin becomes yellow-tinged. Skin looks dull.
Absence of Color *Congenital or acquired loss of melanin pigment.* Congenital loss is typically generalized, and acquired loss is typically patchy.	Generalized depigmentation may be caused by albinism. Localized depigmentation may be due to vitiligo or tinea versicolor, a common fungal infection.	Albinism appears as white skin, white or pale blond hair, and pink irises. Vitiligo appears as patchy milk-white areas, especially around the mouth. Tinea versicolor appears as patchy areas paler than the surrounding skin.	Albinism appears as white skin, white or pale blond hair, and pink irises. Vitiligo is very noticeable as patchy milk-white areas. Tinea versicolor appears as patchy areas paler than the surrounding skin.
Cyanosis *Mottled blue color in skin due to inadequate tissue perfusion with oxygenated blood.* Most apparent in the nails, lips, oral mucosa, and tongue.	Systemic or central cyanosis is due to cardiac disease, pulmonary disease, heart malformations, and low hemoglobin levels. Localized or peripheral cyanosis is due to vasoconstriction, exposure to cold, and emotional stress.	The skin, lips, and mucous membranes look blue-tinged. The conjunctivae and nail beds are blue.	The skin may appear a shade darker. Cyanosis may be undetectable except for the lips, tongue, and oral mucous membranes, nail beds, and conjunctivae, which appear pale or blue-tinged.

(continued)

Table 5.1 Color Variations in Light and Dark Skin *(continued)*

COLOR VARIATION/ LOCALIZATION	POSSIBLE CAUSES	APPEARANCE IN LIGHT SKIN	APPEARANCE IN DARK SKIN
Reddish Blue Tone *Ruddy tone due to an increased hemoglobin and stasis of blood in capillaries.* Most apparent in the face, mouth, hands, feet, and conjunctivae.	Polycythemia vera, an overproduction of red blood cells, granulocytes, and platelets.	Reddish purple hue.	Difficult to detect. The normal skin color may appear darker in some clients. Check lips for redness.
Erythema *Redness of the skin due to increased visibility of normal oxyhemoglobin.* Generalized, or on face and upper chest, or localized to area of inflammation or exposure.	Hyperemia, a dilatation and congestion of blood in superficial arteries. Due to fever, warm environment, local inflammation, allergy, emotions (blushing or embarrassment), exposure to extreme cold, consumption of alcohol, dependent position of body extremity.	Readily identifiable over entire body or in localized areas. Local inflammation and redness are accompanied by higher temperature at the site.	Generalized redness may be difficult to detect. Localized areas of inflammation appear purple or darker than surrounding skin. May be accompanied by higher temperature, hardness, swelling.
Jaundice *Yellow undertone due to increased bilirubin in the blood.* Generalized, but most apparent in the conjunctivae and mucous membranes.	Increased bilirubin may be due to liver disease, biliary obstruction, or hemolytic disease following infections, severe burns, or resulting from sickle cell anemia or pernicious anemia.	Generalized. Also visible in sclerae, oral mucosa, hard palate, fingernails, palms of hands, and soles of the feet.	Visible in the sclerae, oral mucosa, junction of hard and soft palate, palms of the hands, and soles of the feet.

Carotenemia *Yellow-orange tinge caused by increased levels of carotene in the blood and skin.* Most apparent in face, palms of the hands, and soles of the feet.	Excess carotene due to ingestion of foods high in carotene such as carrots, egg yolks, sweet potatoes, milk, and fats. Also may be seen in clients with anorexia nervosa or endocrine disorders such as diabetes mellitus, myxedema, and hypopituitarism.	Yellow-orange tinge most visible in palms of the hands and soles of the feet. No yellowing of sclerae or mucous membranes.	Yellow-orange seen in forehead, palms, soles. No yellowing of sclerae or mucous membranes.
Uremia *Pale yellow tone due to retention of urinary chromogens in the blood.* Generalized, if perceptible.	Chronic renal disease, in which blood levels of nitrogenous wastes increase. Increased melanin may also contribute, and anemia is usually present as well.	Generalized pallor and yellow tinge, but does not affect conjunctivae or mucous membranes. Skin may show bruising.	Very difficult to discern because the yellow tinge is very pale and does not affect conjunctivae or mucous membranes. Rely on laboratory and other data.
Brown *An increase in the production and deposition of melanin.* Generalized or localized.	May be due to Addison's disease or a pituitary tumor. Localized increase in facial pigmentation may be caused by hormonal changes during pregnancy or the use of birth control pills. More commonly due to exposure to ultraviolet radiation from the sun or from tanning booths.	With endocrine disorders, general bronzed skin. Hyperpigmentation in nipples, palmar creases, genitals, and pressure points. Sun exposure causes red tinge in pale skin, and olive-toned skin tans with little or no reddening.	With endocrine disorders, general deepening of skin tone. Hyperpigmentation in nipples, genitals, and pressure points. Sun exposure leads to tanning in various degrees from brown to black.

Cultural Considerations

- Skin color variations exist in all cultures. Assessment for oxygenation, jaundice, and petechiae in dark-skinned clients requires examination of nail bed refill, sclera, and mucous membranes, respectively.
- Caucasians are at greater risk for skin cancers than are darker-skinned clients.
- African Americans have an increased incidence of chronic inflammatory skin diseases.
- Sparse body hair is common in Asian Americans, especially those of Vietnamese descent.
- Asian males have less facial hair than males of other cultures.
- African Americans have a tendency to develop keloid formations.
- Chinese, Native American, and African American newborns have increased incidence of Mongolian spots on the sacral area.
- Pseudofolliculitis (razor bumps) is more frequent in African American males.
- Melasma (mask of pregnancy) occurs more frequently in dark-skinned African American women.
- Dark-skinned individuals may have pigmented streaks in the nails.
- Linguistic and cultural factors must be considered to avoid miscommunication and misinterpretation of information about diagnosis when caring for many immigrant populations.
- Indian females may have nose piercing.
- Arabic and Indian females use henna as a skin adornment.
- Sikhs are prohibited from removing or cutting hair on any part of the body.
- Religions or cultural practices of covering the head and hair are common in Muslims and Orthodox Jews.
- Touching the head is prohibited in the Vietnamese culture.
- Tattoos and body piercing can be part of cultural or religious practices.
- Tattoos and body piercing are increasing among adolescents in the American cultures.
- Females may require the presence of another female during physical assessment of the skin, especially when the examiner is not of the same sex.
- One must be sensitive to cultural issues about disrobing for the assessment of the skin.

Gathering the Data

FOCUSED INTERVIEW QUESTIONS

Skin

1. Describe your skin today. How does it compare to 2 months ago? How does it compare to 2 years ago? What changes have you noticed such as dryness, oiliness, the development of lesions?

2. Do you or any member of your family have a history of allergies, rashes, or other skin problems?

3. Have you noticed a change in the size, color, shape, or appearance of any moles or birthmarks? Have you noticed any other lesions, lumps, bumps, tender spots, or painful areas on your body?

4. Do you use a lotion with sun protection factor (SPF) when spending time in the sun? Do you remember having a sunburn that left blisters?

5. Do you now have or have you ever had a tattoo(s)?

6. Do you now have or have you ever had piercing of any part of your body?

QUESTIONS REGARDING INFANTS AND CHILDREN

1. Does the child have a rash? If so, what seems to cause it? Have you introduced any new foods into your child's diet? How do you clean the child's diaper area? How do you wash the child's diapers?

QUESTIONS FOR THE PREGNANT FEMALE

1. What changes have you noticed in your skin since you became pregnant?

QUESTIONS FOR THE OLDER ADULT

1. What changes have you noticed in your skin in the past few years?

Hair

1. Describe your hair now. How does it compare to 2 months ago? How does it compare to 2 years ago? Have you ever had problems with your hair?

QUESTIONS REGARDING INFANTS AND CHILDREN

1. Has the child shared hair combs, brushes, or pillows with other children?

Nails

1. Describe your nails now. How do they compare to 2 months ago? How do they compare to 2 years ago? Have you ever had problems with your nails?

2. Have you noticed any pain, swelling, or drainage around your cuticles?
3. Do you wear nail enamel? Do you wear artificial fingernails, tips, or wraps?

QUESTIONS REGARDING INFANTS AND CHILDREN

1. Does the child have any habits such as pulling or twisting the hair, rubbing the head, or biting the nails?

QUESTIONS FOR THE PREGNANT FEMALE

1. Have your nails changed? If so, what are the changes?

Physical Assessment

EQUIPMENT

examination gown and drape
magnifying glass
examination light
penlight

examination gloves clean and nonsterile
centimeter ruler
Wood's lamp (filtered ultraviolet light)
for special procedures

HELPFUL HINTS

* A warm, private environment will reduce client anxiety.
* Provide special instructions and explain the purpose for removal of clothing, jewelry, hairpieces, nail enamel.
* Maintain the client's dignity by using draping techniques.
* Monitor one's verbal responses to skin conditions that already threaten the client's self-image.
* Be sensitive to cultural issues. In some cultures touching or examination by members of the opposite sex is prohibited.
* Covering the head, hair, face, or skin may be part of religious or cultural beliefs. Provide careful explanations regarding the need to expose these areas for assessment.
* Direct sunlight is best for assessment of the skin; if it is not available, lighting must be strong and direct. Tangential lighting may be helpful in assessment of dark-skinned clients.
* Use Standard Precautions throughout the assessment.

Physical assessment of the skin, hair, and nails follows an organized pattern. It begins with a survey and inspection of the skin, followed by palpation of the skin. Inspection and palpation of the hair and nails are then carried out. When lesions are present, measurements are used to identify the size of the lesions and the location in relation to accepted landmarks.

TECHNIQUES AND NORMAL FINDINGS	ABNORMAL FINDINGS SPECIAL CONSIDERATIONS

INSPECTION OF THE SKIN

1. **Observe for cleanliness and use the sense of smell to determine body odor.**
   * Body odor is produced when bacterial waste products mix with perspiration on the skin surface. During heavy physical activity, body odor increases. Amounts of urea and ammonia are excreted in perspiration.

▶ Urea and ammonia salts are found on the skin of clients with kidney disorders.

TECHNIQUES AND NORMAL FINDINGS	ABNORMAL FINDINGS SPECIAL CONSIDERATIONS

2. **Observe the client's skin tone.**
   - Evaluate any widespread color changes such as cyanosis, pallor, erythema, or jaundice. For example, always assess cyanotic clients for vital signs and level of consciousness.

     Use Table 5.1 to evaluate color variations in light and dark skin.
   - The amount of melanin and carotene pigments, the oxygen content of the blood, and the level of exposure to the sun influence skin color. Dark skin contains large amounts of melanin, while fair skin has small amounts. The skin of most Asians contains a large amount of carotene, which causes a yellow cast.

   ► Cyanosis or pallor indicates abnormally low plasma oxygen, placing the client at risk for altered tissue perfusion. Pallor is seen in anemia.

3. **Inspect the skin for even pigmentation over the body.**
   - In most cases, increased or decreased pigmentation is caused by differences in the distribution of melanin throughout the body. These are normal variations. For example, the margins of the lips, areolae, nipples, and external genitalia are more darkly pigmented. Freckles and certain *nevi* (congenital marks) occur in people of all skin colors in varying degrees.

   ► For unknown reasons, some people develop patchy depigmented areas over the face, neck, hands, feet, and body folds. This condition is called **vitiligo.** Skin is otherwise normal. Vitiligo occurs in all races in all parts of the world but seems to affect dark-skinned people more severely. Clients with vitiligo may suffer a severe disturbance in body image.

4. **Inspect the skin for superficial arteries and veins.**
   - A fine network of veins or a few dilated blood vessels visible just beneath the surface of the skin are normal findings in areas of the body where skin is thin (e.g., the abdomen and eyelids).

PALPATION OF THE SKIN

1. **Determine the client's skin temperature.**
   - Use the dorsal surface of your hand, which is most sensitive to temperature. Palpate the forehead or face first. Continue to palpate inferiorly, including the hands and feet, comparing the temperature on the right and left side of the body (Figure 5.3).

   ► The temperature of the skin is higher than normal in the presence of a systemic infection or metabolic disorder such as hyperthyroidism, after vigorous activity, and when the external environment is warm.

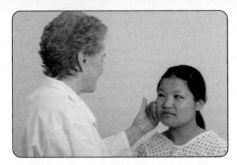

Figure 5.3 • Palpating skin temperature.

- Local skin temperature is controlled by the amount and rate of blood circulating through a body region. Normal temperatures range from mildly cool to slightly warm.
- The skin on both sides of the body is warm when tissue is perfused. Sometimes the hands and feet are cooler than the rest of the body, but the temperature is normally similar on both sides.

2. **Assess the amount of moisture on the skin surface.**
   - Inspect and palpate the face, skin folds, axillae, palms, and soles of the feet, where perspiration is most easily detected.

   ▶ **Diaphoresis** (profuse sweating) occurs during exertion, fever, pain, and emotional stress and in the presence of some metabolic disorders such as hyperthyroidism. It may also indicate an impending medical crisis such as a myocardial infarction.

   - A fine sheen of perspiration or oil is not an abnormal finding, nor is moderately dry skin, especially in cold or dry climates.

   ▶ Severely dry skin typically is dark, weathered, and fissured. Generalized dryness may occur in an individual who is dehydrated or has a systemic disorder such as hypothyroidism.

   ▶ Dry, parched lips and mucous membranes of the mouth are clear indicators of systemic dehydration. Dry skin over the lower legs may be due to vascular insufficiency.

| **TECHNIQUES AND NORMAL FINDINGS** | **ABNORMAL FINDINGS**
SPECIAL CONSIDERATIONS |

3. **Palpate the skin for texture.**
   - Use the palmar surface of fingers and finger pads when palpating for texture. Normal skin feels smooth, firm, and even.

▶ The skin may become excessively smooth and velvety in clients with hyperthyroidism, whereas clients with hypothyroidism may have rough, scaly skin.

4. **Palpate the skin to determine its thickness.**
   - The outer layer of the skin is thin and firm over most parts of the body except the palms, soles of the feet, elbows, and knees, where it is thicker. Normally, the skin over the eyelids and lips is thinner.

▶ Very thin, shiny skin may signal impaired circulation.

5. **Palpate the skin for elasticity.**
   - Elasticity is a combination of turgor (resiliency, or the skin's ability to return to its normal position and shape) and mobility (the skin's ability to be lifted).
   - Using the forefinger and thumb, grasp a fold of skin beneath the clavicle or on the medial aspect of the wrist (Figure 5.4).

▶ When skin turgor is decreased, the skinfold "tents" (holds its pinched formation) and slowly returns to the former position (see Figure 5.4). Decreased turgor occurs when the client is dehydrated or has lost large amounts of weight.

▶ Increased skin turgor may be caused by scleroderma, literally "hard skin," a condition in which the underlying connective tissue becomes scarred and immobile.

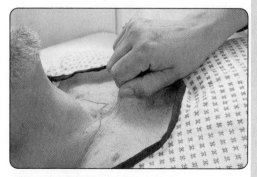

Figure 5.4 • Palpating for skin elasticity.

   - Notice the reaction of the skin both as you grasp and as you release. Healthy skin is mobile and returns rapidly to its previous shape and position.
   - Finally palpate the feet, ankles, and sacrum. Edema is present if your palpation leaves a dent in the skin.
   - Grade any edema on a four-point scale: 1 indicates mild edema, and 4 indicates deep edema (Figure 5.5).

▶ **Edema** is a decrease in skin mobility caused by an accumulation of fluid in the intercellular spaces. Edema makes the skin look puffy, pitted, and tight. It may be most noticeable in the skin of the hands, feet, ankles, and sacral area.

TECHNIQUES AND NORMAL FINDINGS

ABNORMAL FINDINGS
SPECIAL CONSIDERATIONS

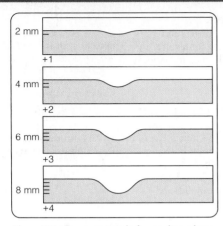

Figure 5.5 • Four-point scale for grading edema.

- Note that because the fluid of edema lies above the pigmented and vascular layers of the skin, skin tone in the client with edema is obscured.

6. **Inspect and palpate the skin for lesions.**
   - Lesions of the skin are changes in normal skin structure. **Primary lesions** develop on previously unaltered skin. Lesions that change over time or because of scratching, abrasion, or infection are called **secondary lesions.**
   - Carefully inspect the client's body, including skin folds and crevices, using a good source of light. In the obese client this requires lifting the breasts, and careful examination of skin under folds in the abdomen, back, and perineal areas.
   - When lesions are observed, palpate lesions between the thumb and index finger. Measure all lesion dimensions (including height, if possible) with a small, clear, flexible ruler.
   - Document lesion size in centimeters. If necessary, use a magnifying glass or a penlight for closer inspection.

▶ The periumbilical and flank areas of the body should be observed for the presence of **ecchymosis** (bruising). Ecchymoses in the periumbilical area may signal bleeding somewhere in the abdomen (Cullen's sign). Ecchymoses in the flank area are associated with pancreatitis or bleeding in the peritoneum (Grey Turner's sign).

| TECHNIQUES AND NORMAL FINDINGS | ABNORMAL FINDINGS SPECIAL CONSIDERATIONS |

- Shine a Wood's lamp on the skin to distinguish fluorescing lesions.
  - Assess any drainage for color, odor, consistency, amount, and location. If indicated, obtain a specimen of the drainage for culture and sensitivity.
- Some fungal infections including tinea capitis do not fluoresce.
- Healthy skin is typically smooth and free of lesions; however, some lesions, such as freckles, insect bites, healed scars, and certain birthmarks, are expected findings.
- Use the ABCDE method to evaluate lesions

ABCDE Criteria for Melanoma Assessment

A = Asymmetry
B = Border irregularity
C = Color variegation
D = Diameter greater than 6 mm
E = Evolving changes*

*Evolving changes includes changes in size, shape, symptoms (itching, tenderness), surface (bleeding), and shades of color.

7. **Palpate the skin for sensitivity.**
   - Palpate the skin in various regions of the body and ask the client to describe the sensations.
   - Give special attention to any pain or discomfort that the client reports, especially when palpating skin lesions.
   - Ask the client to describe the sensation as closely as possible, and document the findings.
   - The client should not report any discomfort from your touch.

▶ Physical abuse should be suspected if the client has any of the following: bruises or welts that appear in a pattern suggesting the use of a belt or stick; burns with sharply demarcated edges suggesting injury from cigarettes, irons, or immersion of a hand in boiling water; additional injuries such as fractures or dislocations; or multiple injuries in various stages of healing. A nurse must be especially sensitive if the client is fearful of family members, is reluctant to return home, and has a history of previous injuries. When any of these diagnostic cues is evident, it is important to obtain medical assistance and follow the state's legal requirements to notify the police or local protective agency.

▶ The injection of drugs into the veins of the arms or other parts of the body results in a series of small scars called *track marks* along the course of the blood vessel. A nurse who sees track marks and suspects substance abuse should refer the client to a mental health or substance abuse professional.

ALERT! *Localized hot, red, swollen painful areas indicate the presence of inflammation and possible infection. These areas should not be palpated, because the slightest disturbance may spread the infection deeper into skin layers.*

TECHNIQUES AND NORMAL FINDINGS	ABNORMAL FINDINGS SPECIAL CONSIDERATIONS

INSPECTION OF THE SCALP AND HAIR

1. **Observe for cleanliness.**
   - Ask the client to remove any hairpins, hair ties, barrettes, wigs, or hairpieces and to undo braids. If the client is unwilling to do this, examine any strands of hair that are loose or undone.
   - Part and divide the hair at 1-in. intervals and observe.
   - A small amount of **dandruff** (dead, scaly flakes of epidermal cells) may be present.

   ▶ Excessive dandruff occurs with psoriasis or seborrheic dermatitis. Dandruff should be distinguished from head lice.

2. **Observe the client's hair color.**
   - Like skin color, hair color varies according to the level of melanin production. Graying is influenced by genetics and may begin as early as the late teens in some clients.

   ▶ Graying of the hair in patches may indicate a nutritional deficiency, commonly of protein or copper.

3. **Assess the texture of the hair.**
   - Roll a few strands of hair between your thumb and forefinger.
   - Hold a few strands of hair taut with one hand while you slide the thumb and forefinger of your other hand along the length of the strand.
   - Hair may be thick or fine and may appear straight, wavy, or curly.

   ▶ Hypothyroidism and other metabolic disorders, as well as nutritional deficiencies, may cause the hair to be dull, dry, brittle, and coarse.

4. **Observe the amount and distribution of the hair throughout the scalp.**
   - The amount of hair varies with age, gender, and overall health. Healthy hair is evenly distributed throughout the scalp.
   - In most men and women, atrophy of the hair follicles causes hair growth to decline by the age of 50. Male pattern baldness, a genetically determined progressive loss of hair beginning at the anterior hairline, has no clinical significance. It is the most frequent reason for hair loss in men.

   ▶ When hair loss occurs in women, it is thought to be caused by an imbalance in adrenal hormones.

   ▶ Widespread hair loss may also be caused by illness, infections, metabolic disorders, nutritional deficiencies, and chemotherapy. Patchy hair loss (**alopecia areata**) may be due to infection.

- Remember to assess the amount, texture, and distribution of body hair. Some practitioners prefer to perform this assessment with the regions of the body.

5. **Inspect the scalp for lesions.**
   - Dim the room light and shine a Wood's lamp on the client's scalp as you part the hair.
   - The healthy scalp is free from lesions and areas of fluorescent glow.

▶ Gray, scaly patches with broken hair may indicate the presence of a fungal infection such as ringworm.
▶ Infestation by **pediculosis capitis** (head lice) is signaled by tiny, white, oval eggs (nits) that adhere to the hair shaft.

ASSESSMENT OF THE NAILS

1. **Assess for hygiene.**
   - Confirm that the nails are clean and well groomed.

▶ Dirty fingernails may indicate a self-care deficit but could also be related to a person's occupation.

2. **Inspect the nails for an even, pink undertone.**
   - Small, white markings in the nail are normal findings and indicate minor trauma.

▶ The nails appear pale and colorless in clients with peripheral arteriosclerosis or anemia. The nails appear yellow in clients with jaundice, and dark red in clients with *polycythemia*. Fungal infections may cause the nails to discolor. Horizontal white bands may occur in chronic hepatic or renal disease. A darkly pigmented band in a single nail may be a sign of a melanoma in the nail matrix and should be referred to a physician for further evaluation.

3. **Assess capillary refill.**
   - Depress the nail edge briefly to blanch, and then release. Color returns to healthy nails instantly upon release.

▶ The nail beds appear blue, and color return is sluggish in clients with cardiovascular or respiratory disorders.

4. **Inspect and palpate the nails for shape and contour.**
   - Perform the Schamroth technique to assess clubbing.

     Ask the client to bring the dorsal aspect of corresponding fingers together, creating a mirror image.
   - Look at the distal phalanx and observe the diamond-shaped opening created by nails. When clubbing is present, the diamond is not formed and the distance increases at the fingertip (Figure 5.6).

▶ *Clubbing of the fingernails* occurs when there is hypoxia or impaired peripheral tissue perfusion over a long period of time. It may also occur with cirrhosis, colitis, thyroid disease, or long-term tobacco smoking. The ends of the fingers become enlarged, soft, and spongy, and the angle between the skin and the nail base is greater than 160 degrees (Figure 5.7).

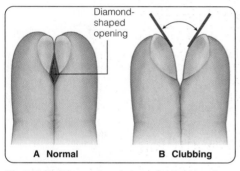

Diamond-shaped opening

A Normal   **B Clubbing**

Figure 5.6 • Schamroth technique. A. Healthy nail. B. Clubbing.

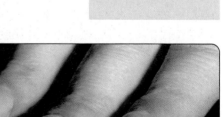

Figure 5.7 • Clubbing of fingernails.

| TECHNIQUES AND NORMAL FINDINGS | ABNORMAL FINDINGS SPECIAL CONSIDERATIONS |

- The nails normally form a slight convex curve or lie flat on the nail bed. When viewed laterally, the angle between the skin and the nail base should be approximately 160 degrees (Figure 5.8).

▶ *Spoon nails* form a concave curve and are thought to be associated with iron deficiency.

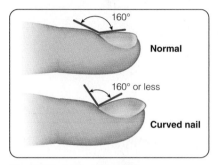

Figure 5.8 • Angle of fingernail.

5. **Palpate the nails to determine their thickness, regularity, and attachment to the nail bed.**
   - Healthy nails are smooth, strong, and regular and are firmly attached to the nail bed, with only a slight degree of mobility.

▶ Nails may be thickened in clients with circulatory disorders. **Onycholysis,** separation of the nail plate from the nail bed, occurs with trauma, infection, or skin lesions.

6. **Inspect and palpate the cuticles.**
   - The cuticles are smooth and flat in healthy nails.

▶ *Hangnails* are jagged tears in the lateral skin folds around the nail. An untreated hangnail may become inflamed and lead to a **paronychia,** an infection of the cuticle.

Abnormal Findings

PRIMARY LESIONS

Macule, Patch

A macule, patch is a flat, nonpalpable change in skin color. Macules are smaller than 1 cm, with a circumscribed border (Figure 5.9), and patches are larger than 1 cm and may have an irregular border.

Examples: Macules: freckles, measles, and petechiae. Patches: Mongolian spots, port-wine stains, vitiligo, and chloasma.

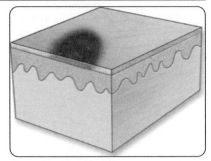

Figure 5.9 • Macule.

Papule, Plaque

A papule, plaque is an elevated, solid palpable mass with circumscribed border (Figure 5.10). Papules are smaller than 0.5 cm; plaques are groups of papules that form lesions larger than 0.5 cm.

Examples: Papules: elevated moles, warts, and lichen planus. Plaques: psoriasis, actinic keratosis, and also lichen planus.

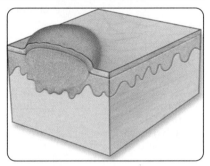

Figure 5.10 • Papule, plaque.

Nodule, Tumor

A nodule, tumor is an elevated, solid, hard or soft palpable mass extending deeper into the dermis than a papule (Figure 5.11). Nodules have circumscribed borders and are 0.5 to 2 cm; tumors may have irregular borders and are larger than 2 cm.

Examples: Nodules: small lipoma, squamous cell carcinoma, fibroma, and intradermal nevi. Tumors: large lipoma, carcinoma, and hemangioma.

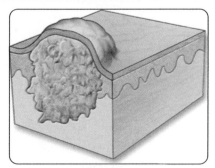

Figure 5.11 • Nodule, tumor.

Vesicle, Bulla

A vesicle, bulla is an elevated, fluid-filled, round or oval-shaped, palpable mass with thin, translucent walls and circumscribed borders (Figure 5.12). Vesicles are smaller than 0.5 cm; bullae are larger than 0.5 cm.

Examples: Vesicles: herpes simplex/zoster, early chickenpox, poison ivy, and small burn blisters. Bullae: contact dermatitis, friction blisters, and large burn blisters.

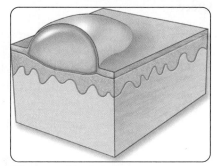

Figure 5.12 • Vesicle, bulla.

SECONDARY LESIONS

Lichenification

Lichenification is a rough, thickened, hardenesd area of epidermis resulting from chronic irritation such as scratching or rubbing (Figure 5.13).

Examples: Chronic dermatitis.

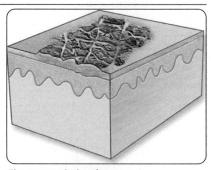

Figure 5.13 • Lichenification.

Scales

Scales are shedding flakes of greasy, keratinized skin tissue. Color may be white, gray, or silver. Texture may vary from fine to thick (Figure 5.14).

Examples: Dry skin, dandruff, psoriasis, and eczema.

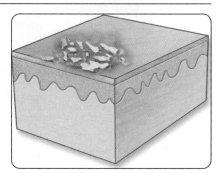

Figure 5.14 • Scales.

Ulcer

An ulcer is a deep, irregularly shaped area of skin loss extending into the dermis or subcutaneous tissue (Figure 5.15). It may bleed or leave a scar.

Examples: Decubitus ulcers (pressure sores), stasis ulcers, chancres.

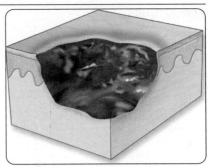

Figure 5.15 • Ulcer.

Keloid

A keloid is an elevated, irregular, darkened area of excess scar tissue caused by excessive collagen formation during healing (Figure 5.16). It extends beyond the site of the original injury. There is higher incidence in people of African descent.

Examples: Keloid from ear-piercing or surgery.

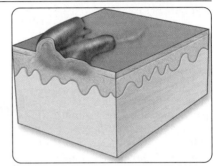

Figure 5.16 • Keloid.

CONFIGURATIONS AND SHAPES OF LESIONS

Annular

Annular lesions are lesions with a circular shape (Figure 5.17).

Examples: Tinea corporis, pityriasis rosea.

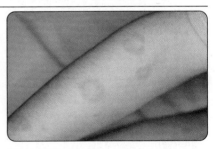

Figure 5.17 • Annular lesions.

Confluent

Confluent lesions are lesions that run together (Figure 5.18).

Examples: Urticaria.

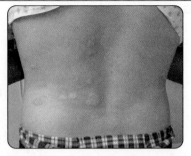

Figure 5.18 • Confluent lesions.

Discrete

Discrete lesions are lesions that are separate and discrete (Figure 5.19).

Examples: Malluscum.

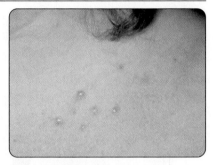

Figure 5.19 • Discrete lesions.

Grouped

Grouped lesions are lesions that appear in clusters (Figure 5.20).

Examples: Contact dermatitis.

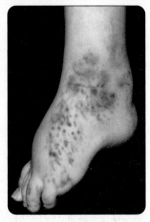

Figure 5.20 • Grouped lesions.

Gyrate

Gyrate lesions are lesions that are coiled or twisted (Figure 5.21).

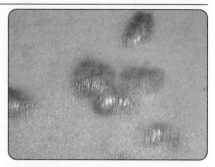

Figure 5.21 • Gyrate lesions.

Target

Target lesions are lesions with concentric circles of color (Figure 5.22).

Examples: Erythema multiforme.

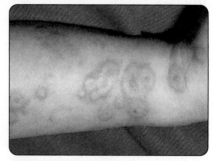

Figure 5.22 • Target lesions.

Linear

Linear lesions are lesions that appear as lines (Figure 5.23).

Examples: Scratches.

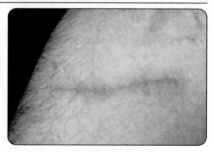

Figure 5.23 • Linear lesions.

Polycyclic

Polycyclic lesions are lesions that are circular but united (Figure 5.24).

Examples: Psoriasis.

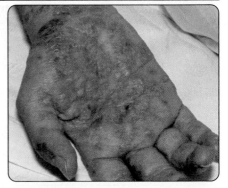

Figure 5.24 • Polycyclic lesions.

Zosteriform

Zosteriform lesions are arranged in a linear manner along a nerve route (Figure 5.25).

Examples: Herpes zoster.

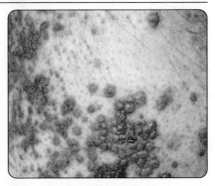

Figure 5.25 • Zosteriform lesions.

COMMON SKIN LESIONS

Tinea

Tinea, sometimes known as ringworm, is a fungal infection affecting the body (tinea corporis), the scalp (tinea capitis), or the feet (tinea pedis, also known as athlete's foot). Secondary bacterial infection may also be present. The appearance of the lesions varies, and they may present as papules, pustules, vesicles, or scales (Figure 5.26).

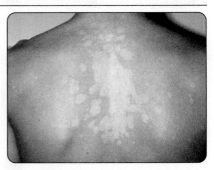

Figure 5.26 • Tinea corporis (also called ringworm).

Measles (Rubeola)

Measles is a highly contagious viral disease that causes a rash of red to purple macules or papules (Figure 5.27). The rash begins on the face, then progresses over the neck, trunk, arms, and legs. It does not blanch. It may be accompanied by tiny white spots that look like grains of salt (called Koplik's spots) on the oral mucosa. It occurs mostly in children.

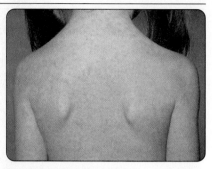

Figure 5.27 • Measles (rubeloa).

German Measles (Rubella)

German measles is a highly contagious disease caused by a virus. Typically it begins as a pink, papular rash that is similar to measles but paler (Figure 5.28). Like measles, it begins on the face, then spreads over the body. Unlike measles, it may be accompanied by swollen glands. It is not accompanied by Koplik's spots. It occurs mostly in children.

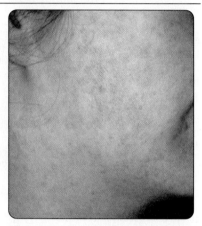

Figure 5.28 • German measles (rubella).

Chickenpox (Varicella)

Chickenpox is a mild infectious disease caused by the herpes zoster virus. It begins as groups of small, red, fluid-filled vesicles usually on the trunk (Figure 5.29) and progresses to the face, arms, and legs. Vesicles erupt over several days, forming pustules, then crusts. The condition may cause intense itching. It occurs mostly in children.

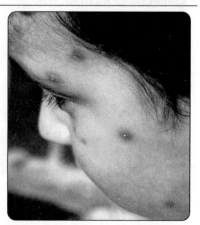

Figure 5.29 • Chickenpox (varicella).

Herpes Simplex

Herpes simplex is a viral infection that causes characteristic lesions on the lips and oral mucosa (Figure 5.30). Lesions progress from vesicles to pustules, and then crusts. Herpes simplex also occurs in the genitals.

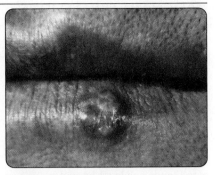

Figure 5.30 • Herpes simplex.

Herpes Zoster

Herpes zoster is an eruption of dormant herpes zoster virus, which typically has invaded the body during an attack of chickenpox. Clusters of small vesicles form on the skin along the route of sensory nerves. Vesicles progress to pustules and then crusts (Figure 5.31). It causes intense pain and itching. The condition is more common and more severe in older adults.

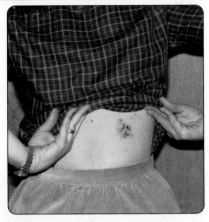

Figure 5.31 • Herpes zoster (shingles).

Impetigo

Impetigo is a bacterial skin infection that usually appears on the skin around the nose and mouth (Figure 5.32). It is contagious and common in children. It may begin as a barely perceptible patch of blisters that breaks, exposing red, weeping area beneath. A tan crust soon forms over this area, and the infection may spread out of the edges.

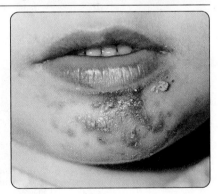

Figure 5.32 • Impetigo.

MALIGNANT SKIN LESIONS

Squamous Cell Carcinoma

Squamous cell carcinoma arises from the cells of the stratum spinosum. It begins as a reddened, scaly papule, then forms a shallow ulcer with a clearly delineated, elevated border (Figure 5.33). It commonly appears on the scalp, ears, backs of the hands, and lower lip, and is thought to be caused by exposure to the sun. It grows rapidly.

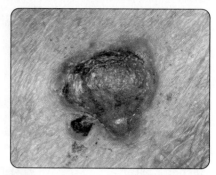

Figure 5.33 • Squamous cell carcinoma.

Kaposi's Sarcoma

Kaposi's sarcoma is a malignant tumor of the epidermis and internal epithelial tissues. Lesions are typically soft, blue to purple, and painless (Figure 5.34). Other characteristics are variable: they may be macular or papular and may resemble keloids or bruises. Kaposi's sarcoma is common in people who are HIV positive.

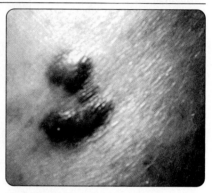

Figure 5.34 • Kaposi's sarcoma.

ABNORMALITIES OF THE HAIR

Tinea Capitis

Tinea capitis, commonly known as ringworm, is patchy hair loss on the head with pustules on the skin (Figure 5.35). This highly contagious fungal disease is transmitted from the soil, from animals, or from person to person.

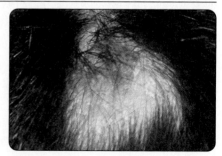

Figure 5.35 • Tinea capitis (scalp ringworm).

Folliculitis

Folliculitis, infections of hair follicles, appears as pustules with underlying erythema (Figure 5.36).

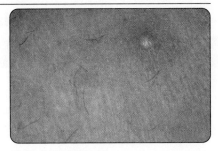

Figure 5.36 • Folliculitis.

ABNORMALITIES OF THE NAILS

Paronychia

Paronychia is an infection of the skin adjacent to the nail, usually caused by bacteria or fungi (Figure 5.37). The affected area becomes red, swollen, and painful, and pus may ooze from it.

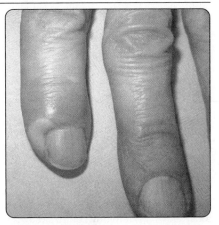

Figure 5.37 • Paronychia.

Clubbing

In clubbing, the nail appears more convex and wide (Figure 5.38). The nail angle is greater than 160 degrees. It occurs in chronic respiratory and cardiac conditions in which oxygenation is compromised.

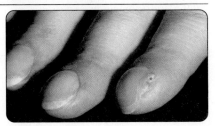

Figure 5.38 • Nail clubbing.

6

Head, Neck, and Related Lymphatics

The head and neck region is in many ways the most important region in the body. Several systems are integrated in the head and neck. For example, the musculoskeletal system permits movement of the neck and face, while the bones protect the brain, spinal cord, and eyes.

ANATOMY AND PHYSIOLOGY REVIEW

The structures of the head include the skull and facial bones. The vertebrae, hyoid bone, cartilage, muscles, thyroid gland, and major blood vessels are found within the neck. A large supply of lymph nodes is located in the head and neck region.

HEAD

The skull is a protective shell made up of the bones of the cranium (Figure 6.1) and face. The major bones of the cranium are the frontal, parietal, temporal, and occipital bones. These bones are connected to each other by means of **sutures,** or nonmovable joints.

The skin, muscles, and bones of the face provide landmarks for assessment, as do the bones of the skull. The eyebrows, appendages of the skin, are over the supraorbital margins of the skull. The lateral canthus of the eye forms a straight line with the pinna, and the nasolabial folds are equal (Figure 6.2).

NECK

The neck is formed by the seven cervical vertebrae, ligaments, and muscles, which support the cranium. The first cervical vertebra (C_1), commonly called the **atlas,** carries the skull. The second cervical vertebra (C_2), commonly called the **axis,** allows for movement of the head (see Figure 6.1). The greatest mobility is at the level of C_4, C_5, and C_6. The seventh cervical vertebra (vertebra prominens) has the largest spinous process.

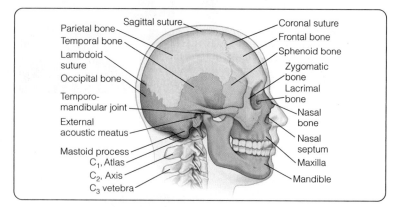

Figure 6.1 • Bones of the head and neck.

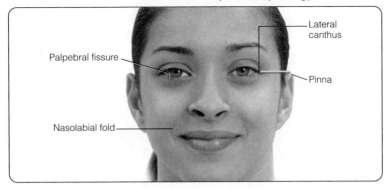

Figure 6.2 • Facial landmarks.

This vertebral process is visible and easily palpated, making it a definite landmark during client assessment.

The sternocleidomastoid and trapezius muscles are the primary muscles of the neck. The sternocleidomastoid muscles originate at the manubrium of the sternum and the medial portion of the clavicles. Each trapezius muscle originates on the occipital bone of the skull and spine of several vertebrae. These two muscle groups form the anterior and posterior triangles of the neck (Figure 6.3).

The hyoid bone is suspended in the neck (Figure 6.4) above the larynx. The base of the tongue rests on the curved body of this bone. This serves as a landmark for assessing structures of the neck, especially the trachea and thyroid gland.

The thyroid cartilage is the largest cartilage of the larynx. The cricoid cartilage, C-shaped ring, is the first cartilage ring anchored to the trachea. The trachea descends from the larynx to the bronchi of the respiratory system. The trachea has slight mobility and flexibility (see Figure 6.4).

The **thyroid gland,** the largest gland of the endocrine system, is butterfly shaped. The isthmus of the thyroid connects the right and left lobes of the thyroid gland. The thyroid gland lies over the trachea, and the sternocleidomastoid muscles cover the lateral aspects of the lobes (see Figure 6.4).

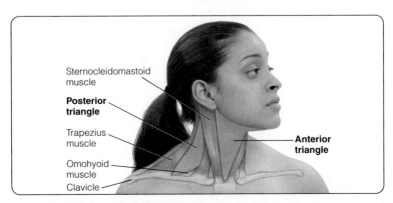

Figure 6.3 • Triangles of the neck.

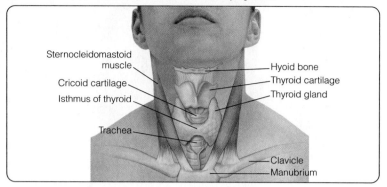

Figure 6.4 • Structures of the neck.

LYMPHATICS

A large supply of lymph nodes is located in the head and neck region of the body. The lymph nodes are clustered along lymphatic vessels that infiltrate tissue capillaries and pick up excess fluid called *lymph.*

SPECIAL CONSIDERATIONS

Throughout the assessment process, the nurse gathers subjective and objective data reflecting the client's state of health. Factors to be considered when collecting the data include but are not limited to age, developmental level, race, ethnicity, work history, living conditions, social economics, and emotional well-being.

INFANTS AND CHILDREN

An infant's head should be measured at each visit until 2 years of age. The newborn's head is about 34 cm (13 to 14 in.), and this is generally equal to the chest circumference. The shape of the head may indicate *molding.* Suture lines should be open as are the fontanels. The anterior fontanel is diamond shaped, and the posterior fontanel is triangular in shape. Slight pulsations in the fontanels are normal. The neck of the newborn is short with many skin folds and begins to lengthen over time. The thyroid is difficult to palpate on an infant, but it can be accomplished on a child using two or three fingers.

THE PREGNANT FEMALE

The pregnant female may develop blotchy pigmented spots (melasma) on her face, facial edema, and enlargement of the thyroid. All of these symptoms are considered normal and subside after childbirth. The pregnant female may also complain of headaches during the first trimester, which may be related to increased hormones; however, severe persistent headaches should be evaluated.

THE OLDER ADULT

The older adult loses subcutaneous fat in the face. The loss of teeth and improperly fitting dentures provide a change to facial expressions and symmetry. Rigidity of the cervical vertebrae is common, causing limited range of motion of the neck. The thyroid gland produces fewer hormones with age.

CULTURAL CONSIDERATIONS

Assessment and findings are influenced by culture. See the cultural considerations box for specific examples.

Cultural Considerations

- Covering of the hair or face is required in some cultures, such as Muslim and Sikh.
- Hypothyroidism occurs more frequently in Caucasians and Mexican Americans than in African Americans.
- Immigrants from countries in which millet is a staple food are more likely to have goiter.

- Facial malformations may occur in infants with fetal alcohol syndrome. Fetal alcohol syndrome (FAS) occurs more frequently in Native Americans, Alaska Natives, and African Americans than in other cultural groups.

PSYCHOSOCIAL CONSIDERATIONS

A client who is under a great deal of stress may be prone to headaches, neck pain, and mouth ulcers. Other indications of psychosocial disturbances include tics (involuntary muscle spasms), hair twisting or pulling, lip biting, and excessive blinking.

Gathering the Data

The focused interview for the head and neck concerns data related to the head, the face, and structures of the neck including the thyroid, trachea, and lymph nodes. Subjective data are gathered during the focused interview.

FOCUSED INTERVIEW QUESTIONS

1. Have you ever been diagnosed with an illness affecting your head, face, or neck?
2. Have you ever had any problem with your thyroid gland? Have you had thyroid surgery? Are you currently taking thyroid medication?
3. Describe any recent or past injury to your head.
4. Have you had any dizziness, loss of consciousness, seizures, or blurred vision? When did each symptom occur? How long did the symptom last? What did you do to relieve the symptom? Does the treatment help?
5. Do you have headaches? If so, please tell me about them.

QUESTIONS REGARDING INFANTS AND CHILDREN

1. Did you use alcohol or recreational drugs during your pregnancy?
2. Have you noticed any depression or bulging over the infant's "soft spots" (fontanels)?

QUESTIONS FOR THE PREGNANT FEMALE

1. Do you have frequent headaches?
2. Do you have a history of thyroid disease? If yes, what is the disease and treatment?

Physical Assessment

Physical assessment of the head and neck requires the use of inspection, palpation, and auscultation. Knowledge of normal parameters and expected findings is essential to interpreting data as the nurse performs the assessment.

EQUIPMENT

examination gown

clean, nonsterile examination gloves

glass of water

stethoscope

HELPFUL HINTS

* Explain what is expected of the client for each step of the assessment.
* Tell the client the purpose of each procedure and when and if discomfort will accompany any examination.
* Identify and remedy language or cultural barriers at the outset of the client interaction.
* Explain to the client the need to remove any items that would interfere with the assessment, including jewelry, hats, scarves, veils, hairpieces, and wigs.
* Use Standard Precautions.

TECHNIQUES AND NORMAL FINDINGS

ABNORMAL FINDINGS SPECIAL CONSIDERATIONS

THE HEAD

1. **Inspect the head and scalp.**
   * Note size, shape, symmetry, and integrity of the head and scalp. Identify the prominences—frontal, parietal, and occipital—that determine the shape and symmetry of the head.
   * Part the hair and look for scaliness of the scalp, lesions, or foreign bodies.
   * Check hair distribution and hygiene.

2. **Inspect the face.**
   * Note the facial expression and symmetry of structures. The eyes, ears, nose, and mouth should be symmetrically placed. The nasolabial folds should be equal. The palpebral fissures should be equal. The top of the ear should be equal to the canthi of the eyes (see Figure 6.2).

TECHNIQUES AND NORMAL FINDINGS	ABNORMAL FINDINGS SPECIAL CONSIDERATIONS

3. **Observe movements of the head, face, and eyes.**
   - All movements should be smooth and with purpose. Cranial nerves III, IV, and VI control movement of the eye. Cranial nerve V stimulates movement for mastication. Cranial nerve VII controls movement of the face.

   ▶ Jerky movements or tics may be the result of neurologic or psychologic disorders.

4. **Palpate the head and scalp.**
   - Note contour, size, and texture. Ask the client to report any tenderness as you palpate. Normally there is no tenderness with palpation.

   ▶ Note any tenderness, swelling, edema, or masses that require further evaluation.

5. **Confirm skin and tissue integrity.**
   - The skin should be intact.

   ▶ Note any alteration in skin or tissue integrity related to ulcerations, rashes, discolorations, or swellings.

6. **Palpate the temporal artery.**
   - Palpate between the eye and the top of the ear. The artery should feel smooth.

   ▶ Any thickening or tenderness could indicate inflammation of the artery.

7. **Auscultate the temporal artery.**
   - Use the bell of the stethoscope to auscultate for a bruit (a soft blowing sound). Bruits are not normally present.

   ▶ A bruit is indicative of stenosis (narrowing) of the vessel.

8. **Test the range of motion of the TMJ.**
   - Place your fingers in front of each ear and ask the client to open and close the mouth slowly. There should be no limitation of movement or tenderness. You should feel a slight indentation of the joint.

     Soft clicking noises on movement are sometimes heard and are considered normal.

   ▶ Any limitation of movement or tenderness on movement requires further evaluation.

   ▶ Crepitation, a crackling sound on movement, may indicate joint problems.

THE NECK

1. **Inspect the neck for skin color, integrity, shape, and symmetry.**
   - Observe for any swelling of the lymph nodes below the angle of the jaw and along the sternocleidomastoid muscle.
   - The head should be held erect with no tremors.

   ▶ Excessive rigidity of the neck may indicate arthritis. Inability to hold the neck erect may be due to muscle spasms. Swelling of the lymph nodes may indicate infection and requires further assessment.

TECHNIQUES AND NORMAL FINDINGS	ABNORMAL FINDINGS SPECIAL CONSIDERATIONS

In the obese client with a short neck, any assessments of structures in the neck can be difficult. Alternate methods may be required, for example, a Doppler stethoscope to assess pulses.

2. **Test range of motion of the neck.**
   - Ask the client to slowly move the chin to the chest, turn the head right and left, then touch the left ear to left shoulder and the right ear to right shoulder (without raising the shoulders). Then ask the client to extend the head back.

     There should be no pain and no limitation of movement.

▶ Any pain or limitation of movement could indicate arthritis, muscle spasm, or inflammation. Rapid movement and compression of cerebral vertebrae may cause dizziness.

3. **Observe the carotid arteries and jugular veins.**
   - The carotid artery runs just below the angle of the jaw, and its pulsations can frequently be seen.

▶ Any distention or prominence may indicate a vascular disorder.

4. **Palpate the trachea.**
   - Palpate the sternal notch. Move the finger pad of the palpating finger off the notch to the midline of the neck. Lightly palpate the area. You will feel the C rings (cricoid cartilage) of the trachea.

     Move the finger laterally, first to the right and then to the left. You have now identified the lateral borders of the trachea.

▶ Tracheal displacement is the result of masses in the neck or mediastinum, pneumothorax, or fibrosis.

   - The trachea should be midline, and the distance to the sternocleidomastoid muscles on each side should be equal. Place the thumb and index finger on each side of the trachea and slide them upward. As the trachea begins to widen, you have now identified the thyroid cartilage. Continue to slide your thumb and index finger high into the neck. Palpate the hyoid bone. The greater horns of the hyoid bone are most prominent. Confirm that the hyoid bone and tracheal cartilages move when the client swallows.

TECHNIQUES AND NORMAL FINDINGS	ABNORMAL FINDINGS SPECIAL CONSIDERATIONS

5. **Inspect the thyroid gland.**
   - The thyroid is not observable normally until the client swallows. Give the client a cup of water.
   - Distinguish the thyroid from other structures in the neck by asking the client to drink a sip of water.
   - The thyroid tissue is attached to the trachea, and, as the client swallows, it moves superiorly. You may want to adjust the lighting in the room if possible so that shadows are cast on the client's neck. This may help you to visualize the thyroid.

▶ If the client has any enlargement of the thyroid or masses near the thyroid, they appear as bulges when the client swallows.

6. **Palpate the thyroid gland from behind the client.**
   - Normally, the thyroid gland is nonpalpable, and so you need to be patient as you learn this technique.
   - Stand behind the client.
   - Ask the client to sit up straight, lower the chin, and turn the head slightly to the right.
   - This position causes the client's neck muscles to relax.
   - Using the fingers of your left hand, push the trachea to the right. Use light pressure during palpation, to avoid obliterating findings.
   - With the fingers of the right hand, palpate the area between the trachea and the sternocleidomastoid muscle. Slowly and gently retract the sternocleidomastoid muscle, then ask the client to drink a sip of water. Palpate as the thyroid gland moves up during swallowing (Figure 6.5). Normally, you will not feel the thyroid gland, although in some clients with long, thin necks, you may be able to feel the isthmus. Reverse the procedure for the left side.

▶ An enlarged thyroid gland may be due to a metabolic disorder such as hyperthyroidism. Palpable masses of 5 mm or larger are alterations in health. Their location, size, and shape should be documented, and the client should be evaluated further. In pregnancy, a slightly enlarged thyroid can be a normal finding. Most pathologic hyperthyroidism in pregnancy is caused by Graves' disease, an autoimmune disorder that causes increased production of thyroid hormones.

TECHNIQUES AND NORMAL FINDINGS	ABNORMAL FINDINGS SPECIAL CONSIDERATIONS

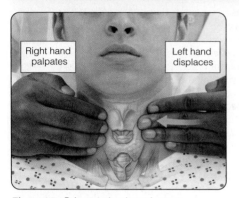

Figure 6.5 • Palpating the thyroid using a posterior approach.

7. **Palpate the thyroid gland from in front of the client.**
   - This is an alternative approach. Stand in front of the client. Ask the client to lower the head and turn slightly to the right. Using the thumb of your right hand, push the trachea to the right (Figure 6.6).

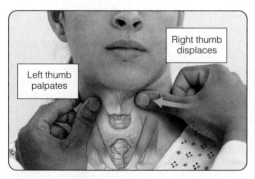

Figure 6.6 • Alternative technique for palpating the thyroid.

   - Place your left thumb and fingers over the sternocleidomastoid muscle and feel for any enlargement of the right lobe as the client swallows. Have water available to make swallowing easier. Reverse the procedure for the left side.

| TECHNIQUES AND NORMAL FINDINGS | ABNORMAL FINDINGS SPECIAL CONSIDERATIONS |

8. **Auscultate the thyroid.**
   - If the thyroid is enlarged, the area over the thyroid is auscultated to detect any bruits. In an enlarged thyroid, blood flows through the arteries at an accelerated rate, producing a soft, rushing sound. This sound can best be detected with the bell of the stethoscope.

▶ The presence of a bruit is abnormal and is an indication of increased blood flow.

9. **Palpate the lymph nodes of the head and neck.**
   - Palpate the lymph nodes by exerting gentle circular pressure with the finger pads of both hands. It is important to avoid strong pressure, which can push the nodes into the muscle and underlying structures, making them difficult to find. It is also important to establish a routine for examination; otherwise, it is possible to omit one or more of the groups of nodes. One suggested order of examination is depicted in Figure 6.7.

▶ Enlargement of lymph nodes is called lymphadenopathy and can be due to infection, allergies, or a tumor.

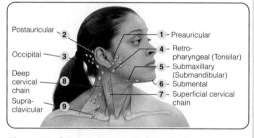

Figure 6.7 • Suggested sequence for palpating lymph nodes.

   - Ask the client to bend the head toward the side being examined to relax the muscles and make the nodes easier to palpate. If any lymph nodes are palpable, make a note of their location, size, shape, fixation or mobility, and tenderness.

Abnormal Findings

Abnormal findings in the head and neck include headaches, abnormalities in the size and contour of the skull, malformations or abnormalities of the face and neck, and thyroid disorders. Examples of common abnormalities of the head and neck are presented in the following pages.

HEADACHES

Classic Migraine

A classic migraine is usually preceded by an aura during which the client may feel depressed, restless, or irritable; see spots or flashes of light; feel nauseated; or experience numbing or tingling in the face or extremities. The pain of the migraine itself may be mild or debilitating, requiring the client to lie down in the darkness in silence. It is usually a pulsating pain that is localized to the side, front, or back of the head and may be accompanied by nausea, vertigo, tremors, and other symptoms. The acute phase of a classic migraine typically lasts from 4 to 6 hours.

Cluster Headache

A cluster headache is so named because numerous episodes occur over a period of days or even months and then are followed by a period of remission during which no headaches occur. Cluster headaches have no aura. Their onset is sudden and may be associated with alcohol consumption, stress, or emotional distress. They often begin suddenly at night with an excruciating pain on one side of the face spreading upward behind one eye. The nose and affected eye water, and nasal congestion is common. Cluster headaches may last for only a few minutes or up to a few hours.

Tension Headache

A tension headache, also known as a muscle contraction headache, is due to sustained contraction of the muscles in the head, neck, or upper back. The onset is gradual, not sudden, and the pain is usually steady, not throbbing. The pain may be unilateral or bilateral and typically ranges from the cervical region to the top of the head. Tension headaches may be associated with stress, overwork, dental problems, premenstrual syndrome, sinus inflammation, and other health problems.

ABNORMALITIES OF THE SKULL AND FACE

Bell's Palsy

Bell's palsy is a temporary disorder affecting cranial nerve VII and producing a unilateral facial paralysis (Figure 6.8). It may be caused by a virus. Its onset is sudden, and it usually resolves spontaneously in a few weeks without residual effects.

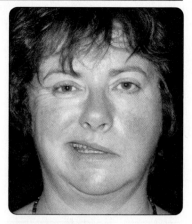

Figure 6.8 • Bell's palsy.

Down Syndrome

Down syndrome is a chromosomal defect causing varying degrees of mental retardation and characteristic facial features such as slanted eyes, a flat nasal bridge, a flat nose, a protruding tongue, and a short, broad neck (Figure 6.9).

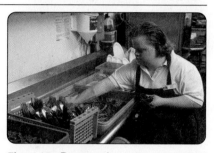

Figure 6.9 • Down syndrome.

Parkinson's Disease

A masklike expression occurs in Parkinson's disease (Figure 6.10). The disease is the result of a decrease in dopamine, a neurotransmitter.

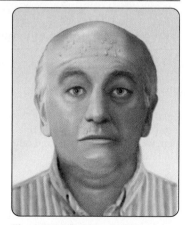

Figure 6.10 • Parkinson's disease.

Brain Attack

A brain attack, stroke, or cerebrovascular accident (CVA) can result in neurologic deficits that include facial paralysis (Figure 6.11).

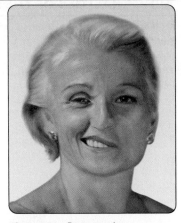

Figure 6.11 • Brain attack.

Torticollis

Torticollis is spasm of the sternocleidomastoid muscle on one side of the body, which often results from birth trauma (Figure 6.12). If left untreated, the muscle becomes fibrotic and permanently shortened.

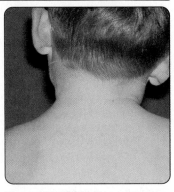

Figure 6.12 • Torticollis.

THYROID ABNORMALITIES

Hyperthyroidism

Hyperthyroidism is excessive production of thyroid hormones. Hyperthyroidism results in enlargement of the gland, exophthalmos (bulging eyes), fine hair, weight loss, diarrhea, and other alterations.

Goiter

A goiter is an enlargement of the thyroid gland.

Graves' Disease

Graves' disease is the most common type of hyperthyroidism. There is no known cause. Graves' disease may be an autoimmune response or related to hereditary factors.

Thyroid Adenoma

Thyroid adenoma refers to benign thyroid nodules that occur most frequently in older adults. There is no known cause for thyroid adenomas.

Thyroid Carcinoma

Thyroid carcinoma can occur following radiation of the thyroid, chronic goiter, or as a result of hereditary factors. Thyroid carcinomas are malignant tumors in hormone-producing cells or supporting cells. Excess thyroid hormone is produced in the tumors.

Hyperthyroidism and Medication

Excessive iodine in some medications may cause oversecretion of thyroid hormones.

Hypothyroidism

Hypothyroidism occurs when there is a decrease in production of thyroid hormones. The decrease in thyroid hormones results in lowered basal metabolism. The most common occurrence in hypothyroidism is loss of thyroid tissue as a result of iodine deficiency or an autoimmune response. It may be a result of decreased pituitary stimulation of the thyroid gland or lack of hypothalamic thyroid-releasing factor. Hypothyroidism occurs most frequently in females between the ages of 30 and 50.

Congenital Hypothyroidism

In congenital hypothyroidism, the thyroid is nonfunctioning at birth. If untreated it results in retardation of physical and mental growth.

Myxedema

This severe form of hypothyroidism causes nonpitting edema throughout the body and thickening of facial features. Complications of this disease affect major organ systems. Myxedema coma results in cardiovascular collapse, electrolyte disturbances, respiratory depression, and cerebral hypoxia.

Thyroiditis

Thyroiditis is an inflammation of the thyroid gland. This inflammation may cause release of stored hormones, resulting in temporary hyperthyroidism of weeks or months.

Postpartum Thyroiditis

Postpartum thyroiditis is a temporary condition occurring in 5% to 9% of females postpartum.

Hashimoto's Thyroiditis

Hashimoto's thyroiditis is an autoimmune disease that is thought to be hereditary and results in primary hypothyroidism.

7
Eye

The eyes, located in the orbital cavities of the skull, are the sensory organs responsible for vision. Vision is a major mechanism for experiencing the world.

ANATOMY AND PHYSIOLOGY REVIEW

EYE

The eye is a fluid-filled sphere having a diameter of approximately 2.5 cm (1 in.). The eye receives light waves and transmits these waves to the brain for interpretation as visual images. Most of the eye is set into and protected by the bony orbit of the skull (Figure 7.1).

The eye is composed of three layers: sclera, choroid, and retina. The **sclera,** the white fibrous part of the eye, is seen anteriorly. Its primary function is to support and protect the structures of the eye (Figure 7.2).

The **cornea** is the clear, transparent part of the sclera and forms the anterior one sixth of the eye. The **choroid,** the middle layer, is the vascular-pigmented layer of the eye. The **iris** is the circular, colored muscular aspect of this layer of the eye and is located in the anterior portion of the eye. The center of the iris is the pupil. The iris responds to light by making the pupil larger or smaller, thereby controlling the amount of light that enters the eye.

The third and innermost membrane, the **retina,** is the sensory portion of the eye. The retina, a direct extension of the optic nerve, helps to change light waves to neuroimpulses for interpretation as visual impulses by the brain.

The **optic disc,** on the nasal aspect of the retina, is round with clear margins. It is usually creamy yellow and is the point at which the optic nerve and retina meet. The center of this disc, the physiologic cup, is the point at which the vascular network enters the eye. The **macula** is responsible for central vision. The macula, with its yellow pitlike center called the *fovea centralis,* appears as a hyperpigmented spot on the temporal aspect of the retina.

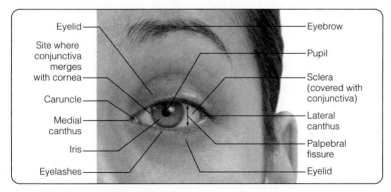

Figure 7.1 • Structures of the external eye.

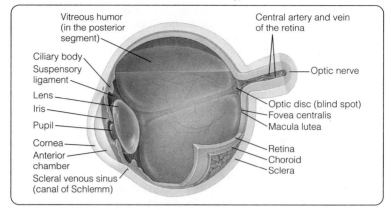

Figure 7.2 • Interior of the eye.

REFRACTION OF THE EYE

The **aqueous humor** is a clear, fluidlike substance found in the anterior segment of the eye that helps maintain ocular pressure. The aqueous humor is a refractory medium of the eye that is constantly being formed and is always flowing through the pupil and draining into the venous system. The **vitreous humor,** another refractory medium, is a clear gel located in the posterior segment of the eye. This gel helps maintain the intraocular pressure and the shape of the eye, and transmits light rays through the eye.

The **lens,** situated directly behind the pupil, is a biconvex (convex on both surfaces), transparent, and flexible structure. It separates the anterior and posterior segments of the eye. The ability of the lens to accommodate or change its shape permits light to focus properly on the retina and enhances fine focusing of images.

ACCESSORY STRUCTURES OF THE EYE

The eye has several external accessory structures. These include the eyebrows, eyelids or palpebrae, palpebral fissures, and medial and lateral canthus as depicted in Figure 7.1. The lacrimal apparatus consists of the lacrimal glands and ducts. Lacrimal secretions, tears, are secreted and spread over the conjunctiva when blinking. The tears enter the lacrimal puncta and drain via the many ducts into the posterior nasal passage. Each eye has six extrinsic or extraocular muscles to hold the eye in place within the bony orbit. With the coordination of these muscles, the individual experiences one-image sight. The muscles are innervated by cranial nerves III, IV, and VI.

SPECIAL CONSIDERATIONS

Vision and eye health are influenced by a number of factors including age, developmental level, race, ethnicity, occupation, socioeconomics, and emotional well-being.

INFANTS AND CHILDREN

At birth, the eyes of the neonate should be symmetric. The pupils are equal and respond to light. The iris is generally brown in dark-skinned neonates, and slate gray-blue in light-skinned neonates. By about the third month of age, the color of the eyes begins to change to a more permanent shade. The *red reflex* should be elicited from birth. Peripheral vision may be assessed by confrontation in children older than 3 years of age. It is important to assess extraocular muscle function as early as possible in young children because delay can lead to permanent visual damage. The corneal light reflex, Hirschberg's test, can be used to determine symmetry of muscle function.

THE PREGNANT FEMALE

The pregnant female may complain of dry eyes and may discontinue wearing contact lenses during her pregnancy. Changes in eyesight such as refraction changes requiring a new prescription for glasses or contact lenses, blurriness, or distorted vision can occur because of temporary changes in the shape of the eye during the last trimester of pregnancy and the first 6 weeks postpartum.

THE OLDER ADULT

By age 45, the lens of the eye loses elasticity, and the ciliary muscles become weaker, resulting in a decreased ability of the lens to change shape to accommodate for near vision. This condition is called **presbyopia.** The loss of fat from the orbit of the eye produces a drooping appearance. The lacrimal glands decrease tear production, and the client may complain of a burning sensation in the eyes. The cornea of the eye may appear cloudy, and the nurse may detect a deposit of white-yellow material around the cornea, called *arcus senilis.* This is a deposition of fat, but it is considered normal after age 45 to 50 and has no effect on vision. The pupillary light reflex is slower with age, and the pupils may be smaller in size.

PSYCHOSOCIAL CONSIDERATIONS

Decreased visual acuity and visual impairment can impact individuals across the age span. Visual impairment results in stress for individuals and families as they adapt to alterations in activities of daily living (ADLs) and as they navigate the healthcare and social service systems for diagnosis, treatment, and assistance.

CULTURAL CONSIDERATIONS

Assessment and findings are influenced by culture. See the cultural considerations box for specific examples.

Cultural Considerations

- Prevalence rates of age-related macular degeneration are higher in Caucasians than in other groups over 75 years of age.
- African American females have a higher incidence of age-related macular degeneration than males until the age of 75.
- Cataracts occur more frequently in Caucasian females than in other races.
- Glaucoma occurs more frequently in African Americans than in Hispanics and Caucasians.
- Hispanics have higher rates of visual impairments than other races.
- The prevalence of myopia is related to national origin and ethnicity. Myopia occurs more frequently in industrialized nations. Asians, Alaska Natives, and some Native American tribes have higher rates of myopia than other cultural groups.
- Individuals from underdeveloped nations have higher rates of blindness than those from other nations. The cause of blindness is associated with trachoma, vitamin A deficiency, river blindness, and other infectious diseases.
- Blindness can occur as a result of diabetic retinopathy. Rates of type 2 diabetes are higher in African Americans, Hispanic Americans, Asian Americans, Pacific Islanders, and Native Americans.

Gathering the Data

FOCUSED INTERVIEW QUESTIONS

1. Describe your vision today. Please describe any changes in your vision in the past few months.
2. What was the date of your last eye examination? What were the results of that examination?
3. Have you ever been diagnosed with a disease or visual disturbance of the eye?
4. Have you had an injury to the eye? Do you wear safety glasses?
5. Have you had eye surgery?
6. Are you taking any medications specifically for the eyes?
7. Have you had any eye pain? If yes, ask about location, onset, duration, frequency, treatment, severity.

QUESTIONS REGARDING INFANTS AND CHILDREN

1. Did the mother have any vaginal infections at the time of delivery?
2. Did the baby get eye ointment after birth?
3. Does the infant look directly at you? Does your infant follow objects with the eyes?
4. Has the child had a vision examination? When was the last eye examination?

QUESTIONS FOR THE PREGNANT FEMALE

1. Have you had any changes in your eyesight during your pregnancy?

QUESTIONS FOR THE OLDER ADULT

1. Are you routinely tested for glaucoma?

Physical Assessment

Physical assessment of the eyes follows an organized pattern. It begins with assessment of visual acuity and is followed by assessments of visual fields, muscle function, and external eye structures. The assessment of the eye concludes with the ophthalmoscopic examination.

EQUIPMENT

visual acuity charts (Snellen or E for distant vision, Rosenbaum for near vision)
opaque card or eye cover

penlight
cotton-tipped applicator
ophthalmoscope

HELPFUL HINTS

- Provide specific instructions about what is expected of the client. This would include telling the client clearly which eye to cover when conducting an assessment of visual acuity.
- The ability to read letters will determine the type of acuity chart to be used. Children and non-English-speaking clients can use the E chart or a chart with figures and images for visual acuity.
- An opaque card or eye cover is used for covering the eye in several assessments. The client must be instructed not to close or apply pressure to the covered eye.
- Several types of lighting are required. Visual acuity requires bright lighting, while the room is darkened to assess papillary responses and the internal eye.
- The room must provide 20 feet from the Snellen chart.
- The assessment may be conducted with the client seated or standing. The nurse stands or sits at eye level with the client.
- Use Standard Precautions.

TECHNIQUES AND NORMAL FINDINGS	ABNORMAL FINDINGS SPECIAL CONSIDERATIONS

TESTING VISUAL ACUITY

Testing Distance Vision

1. **Position the client.**
   - Position the client exactly 20 ft, or 6.1 meters (m), from the Snellen chart (Figure 7.3). The client may be standing or seated. the chart should be at the client's eye level.

2. **Ask the client to cover one eye with the opaque card or eye cover. Tell the client to read, left to right, from the top of the chart down to the smallest line of letters that the client can see.**

3. **Ask the client to cover the other eye and to read from the top of the chart down to the smallest line of letters that the client can see.**

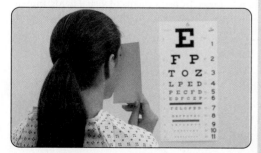

Figure 7.3 • Testing distant vision.

| TECHNIQUES AND NORMAL FINDINGS | ABNORMAL FINDINGS SPECIAL CONSIDERATIONS |

4. **Ask the client to read from the top of the chart down to the smallest line of letters that the client can see with both eyes uncovered.**

5. **If a client uses corrective lenses for distance vision, test first with eyeglasses or contact lenses. Then test without glasses or contact lenses.**

- The results are recorded as a fraction. The numerator indicates the distance from the chart (20 ft). The denominator indicates the distance at which a person with normal vision can read the last line.

- Normal vision is 20/20; therefore, at 20 ft the client can read the line numbered 20. If a client's vision is 20/30, the client reads at 20 ft what a person with normal vision reads at 30 ft. Observe while the client is reading the chart.

- If the client is unable to read more than one half of the letters on a line, record the number of the line above.

▶ Frowning, leaning forward, and squinting indicate visual or reading difficulties.

Inability to see objects at a distance is myopia. The smaller the fraction, the worse the vision. Vision of 20/200 is considered legal blindness.

Testing Near Vision

1. **Position the client.**
- The client is sitting with a Rosenbaum chart held at a distance of 12 to 14 in. (30.5 to 35.5 cm) from the eyes.

2. **Ask the client to cover one eye with the opaque card or eye cover.**

3. **Repeat the test with the other eye and then with both eyes uncovered. The results are recorded as a fraction. A normal result is 14/14 in each eye.**

4. **If a client uses corrective lenses for reading, test with the corrective lenses.**

▶ Inability to see objects at close range is called hyperopia. Presbyopia, the inability to accommodate for near vision, is common in persons over 45 years of age.

TESTING VISUAL FIELDS BY CONFRONTATION

1. **Position the client.**
- The client should be sitting 2 to 3 ft (0.6 to 0.9 m) from you and at eye level.

2. **Ask the client to cover one eye with a card while you cover your opposite eye with a card.**

TECHNIQUES AND NORMAL FINDINGS	ABNORMAL FINDINGS SPECIAL CONSIDERATIONS

3. Holding a penlight in one hand, extend your arm upward, and advance it in from the periphery to the midline point.

4. Be sure to keep the penlight equidistant between the client and yourself.

5. Ask the client to report when the object is first seen. Repeat the procedure upward, toward the nose, and downward. Then repeat the entire procedure with the other eye covered. This test assumes the examiner has normal peripheral vision.

▶ If the client is not able to see the object at the same time that the examiner does, there may be some peripheral vision loss. The client should be evaluated further.

TESTING THE SIX CARDINAL FIELDS OF GAZE

1. **Position the client.**
   - The client is sitting in a comfortable position. You are at eye level with the client.

2. **Instruct the client.**
   - Explain that you will be testing eye movements and the muscles of the eye. Explain that the client must keep the head still while following a pen or penlight that you will move in several directions in front of the client's eyes.

3. **Stand about 2 ft (0.6 m) in front of the client.**

4. **Letter "H" method.**
   - Starting at midline, move the penlight to the extreme left, then straight up, then straight down.
   - Drop your hand. Position the penlight against the midline.
   - Now move the penlight to the extreme right, then straight up, then straight down (Figure 7.4) then center before changing direction.

TECHNIQUES AND NORMAL FINDINGS	ABNORMAL FINDINGS SPECIAL CONSIDERATIONS

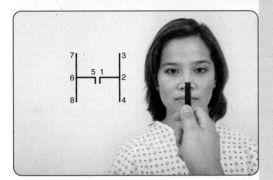

Figure 7.4 • Testing cardinal field of gaze.

5. **Assess the client's ability to follow your movements with the eyes. Nystagmus, rapid fluttering of the eyeball, occurs at completion of rapid lateral eye movement.**

▶ If nystagmus occurs during testing, there could be a weakness in the extraocular muscles or cranial nerve III.

ASSESSMENT OF CORNEAL LIGHT REFLEX

1. **Position the client.**
   • You will sit at eye level with the client.
2. **Instruct the client.**
   • Explain that you are examining the cornea of the eyes. Instruct the client to stare straight ahead while you hold a penlight 12 in. (30.5 cm) from both eyes.
3. **Shine the light into the eyes from a distance of 12 inches.**
   • The reflection of light should appear in the same spot on both pupils. This appears as a "twinkle" in the eye.

▶ If the reflection of light is not symmetric, there could be a weakness in the extraocular muscles.

PERFORM THE COVER TEST

1. **Position the client.**
   • You should be sitting at eye level with the client.

TECHNIQUES AND NORMAL FINDINGS	ABNORMAL FINDINGS SPECIAL CONSIDERATIONS

2. **Instruct the client.**
   - Explain that this test determines the balance mechanism (fusion reflex) that keeps the eyes parallel. Explain that the client will look at a fixed point while covering each eye. You will observe the eyes.

3. **Cover one eye with a card and observe the uncovered eye, which should remain focused on the designated point.**

▶ If there is a weakness in one of the eye muscles, the fusion reflex is blocked when one eye is covered and the weakness of the eye can be observed.

4. **Remove the card from the covered eye and observe the newly uncovered eye for movement. It should focus straight ahead.**

5. **Repeat the procedure with the other eye.**

INSPECTION OF THE PUPILS

1. **Position the client.**
   - In this and all subsequent tests, you will sit at eye level with the client.

2. **Instruct the client.**
   - Explain that you will be looking at the client's eyes to assess the size and shape of the pupils.

3. **Inspect the pupils.**
   - The pupils should be round, equal in size and shape, and in the center of the eye. This is controlled by cranial nerve III.

▶ Pupils that are not round and symmetric may indicate previous ocular surgery, increased intracranial pressure, or cranial nerve pathology.

EVALUATION OF PUPILLARY RESPONSE

1. **Instruct the client.**
   - Explain that you are testing the pupil's response to light. Tell the client that the room light must be dimmed. Explain that you will shine a light directly at each eye and that the client must stare straight ahead.

2. **Moving your penlight in from the client's side, shine light directly into one eye.**

TECHNIQUES AND NORMAL FINDINGS	ABNORMAL FINDINGS SPECIAL CONSIDERATIONS

3. **Observe the constriction in the illuminated pupil.**

- Also observe the simultaneous reaction (**consensual constriction**) of the other pupil. The direct reaction should be faster and greater than the consensual reaction.

▶ If the illuminated pupil fails to constrict, there is a defect in the direct pupillary response. If the unilluminated pupil fails to constrict, there is a defect in the consensual response, controlled by cranial nerve III (oculomotor).

TESTING FOR ACCOMMODATION OF PUPIL RESPONSE

1. **Instruct the client.**
   - Explain that you are testing muscles of the eye. Tell the client to shift the gaze from the far wall to an object held 4 to 5 in. (10 to 12 cm) from the client's nose.

2. **Ask the client to stare straight ahead at a distant point.**

3. **Hold a penlight about 4 to 5 in. (10 to 12 cm) from the client's nose; then ask the client to shift the gaze from the distant point to the penlight.**

   - The eyes should converge (turn inward) and the pupils should constrict as the eyes focus on the penlight. This pupillary change is **accommodation,** a change in size to adjust vision from far to near.
   - A normal response to pupillary testing is recorded as PERRLA (pupils equal, round, react to light, and accommodation).

▶ Lack of **convergence** (turning inward of the eye) and failure of the pupils to constrict indicates dysfunction of cranial nerves III, IV, and VI.

INSPECTION OF THE EXTERNAL EYE

1. **Stand directly in front of the client and focus on the external structures of the eye.** The eyebrows should be symmetric in shape and the eyelashes similar in quantity and distribution. The eyebrows and eyelashes should be free of flakes and drainage.

▶ Absence of the lateral third of the eyebrow is associated with hypothyroidism. Absent eyelashes may indicate pulling or plucking associated with obsessive-compulsive behavior.

TECHNIQUES AND NORMAL FINDINGS	ABNORMAL FINDINGS SPECIAL CONSIDERATIONS

2. **With the client's eyes open, confirm that the distances between the palpebral fissures are equal.** Confirm that the upper eyelid covers a small arc of the iris.

3. **Confirm that the eyelids symmetrically cover the eyeballs when closed.** The eyeball should be neither protruding nor sunken.

4. **Gently separate the eyelids and ask the client to look up, down, and to each side.** The conjunctiva should be moist and clear, with small blood vessels. The lens should be clear, and the sclera white. The irises should be round and both of the same color, although irises of different colors can be a normal finding.

5. **Inspect the cornea by shining a penlight from the side across the cornea.** The cornea should be clear with no irregularities. The pupils should be round and equal in size.

One eyelid drooping (**ptosis**) can be caused by a dysfunction of cranial nerve III (oculomotor). Eyes that protrude beyond the supra-orbital ridge can indicate a thyroid disorder; however, this trait may be normal for the client. Edema of the eyelids can be caused by allergies, heart disease, or kidney disease. Inability to move the eyelids can indicate dysfunction of the nervous system, including facial nerve paralysis.

PALPATION OF THE EYE

1. **Ask the client to close both eyes.**

2. **Using the first two or three fingers, gently palpate the lacrimal sacs, the eyelids, and the eyeballs.**

3. **Confirm that there is no swelling or tenderness and the eyeballs feel firm.**

▶ Swelling may be a symptom of infection, cardiovascular problems, or renal problems.

▶ Less than firm eyeballs can be an indication of dehydration.

EXAMINATION OF THE CONJUNCTIVA AND SCLERA UNDER THE EYELIDS

1. **Evert the lower eyelid by asking the client to look down, pressing the lower lid against the lower orbital rim, then asking the client to look up.**

   • The conjunctiva should be pink with no tenderness or irregularities. If you find any abnormality, examine the conjunctiva under the upper eyelid.

▶ Inflammation and edema of the conjunctiva indicate an infection or possible foreign body.

2. **Ask the client to close the eyes.**

3. **Evert the upper eyelid by placing a cotton-tipped applicator against the upper lid.**

4. **Grasp the eyelashes and pull the eyelid downward, forward, and up over the applicator. Inspect the conjunctiva.**

5. **Gently release and return the eyelid to the normal position when finished.**

INSPECTION OF THE FUNDUS WITH THE OPHTHALMOSCOPE

1. **Instruct the client.**
   - Explain that you will be using the ophthalmoscope to look into the inner deep part of the eye (**fundus**) and that the lights in the room will be dimmed. Explain that the client must stare ahead at a fixed point while you move in front with the ophthalmoscope. Tell the client to maintain a fixed gaze, as if looking through you. Explain that you will place your hand on the client's head so you both remain stable. (Refer to chapter 2 to review the parts of the ophthalmoscope.)

2. **To examine the right eye, hold the ophthalmoscope in your right hand with the index finger on the lens wheel.**

3. **Begin with the lens on the 0 diopter. With the light on, place the ophthalmoscope over your right eye.**

4. **Stand at a slight angle lateral to the client's line of vision.**

5. **Approach the client at about a 15-degree angle toward the client's nose.**

6. **Place your left hand on the client's shoulder or head.**

7. **Hold the ophthalmoscope against your head, directing the light into the client's pupil. Keep your other eye open.**

8. **Advance toward the client.**

TECHNIQUES AND NORMAL FINDINGS	ABNORMAL FINDINGS SPECIAL CONSIDERATIONS

9. As you look into the client's pupil, you will see the *red reflex*, which is the reflection of the light off the retina. Remember to examine the client's right eye with your right eye, and the client's left eye with your left eye. At this point you may need to adjust the lens wheel to bring the ocular structures into focus. Normally, you will see no shadows or dots interrupting the red reflex. If the light strays from the pupil, you will lose the red reflex. Adjust your angle until you see the red reflex again.

▶ Persistent absence of the red reflex may indicate a cataract, an opacity of the lens.

10. Keep advancing toward the client until the ophthalmoscope is almost touching the client's eyelashes.

11. Rotate the diopter wheel if necessary to bring the ocular fundus into focus.

12. If the client's vision is myopic, you will need to rotate the wheel into the minus numbers.

13. If the client's vision is hyperopic, rotate the wheel into the plus numbers.

14. Begin to look for the optic disc by following the path of the blood vessels. As they grow larger, they lead to the optic disc on the nasal side of the retina (Figure 7.5).

     The optic disc normally looks like a round or oval yellow-orange depression with a distinct margin. It is the site where the optic nerve and blood vessels exit the eye.

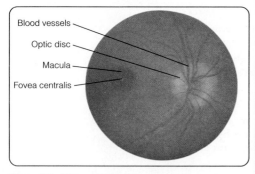

Figure 7.5 • The optic disc.

| TECHNIQUES AND NORMAL FINDINGS | ABNORMAL FINDINGS SPECIAL CONSIDERATIONS |

15. **Follow the vessels laterally to a darker circle. This is the macula, or area of central vision.**
    The fovea centralis, a small white spot located in the center of the macula, is the area of sharpest vision.

▶ Degeneration of the macula is common in older adults and results in impaired central vision. It may be due to hemorrhages, cysts, or other alterations.

16. **Systematically inspect these structures. A crescent shape around the margin of the optic disc is a normal finding. A *scleral crescent* is an absence of pigment in the choroid and is a dull white color. A pigment crescent, which is black, is an accumulation of pigment in the choroid.**

▶ Abnormalities of the retinal structures present as dark or opaque spots on the retina, an irregularly shaped optic disc, and lesions or hemorrhages on the fundus.

17. **Use the optic disc as a clock face for documenting the position of a finding, and the diameter of the disc (DD) for noting its distance from the optic disc.**

18. **Trace the path of a paired artery and vein from the optic disc to the periphery in the four quadrants of the eyeball.**

19. **Note the number of major vessels, color, width, and any crossing of the vessels.**

▶ An absence of major vessels in any of the four quadrants is an abnormal finding. Constricted arteries look smaller than two-thirds the diameter of accompanying veins. Crossing of the vessels more than 2 DD away from the optic disc requires further evaluation.

20. **Repeat the preceding procedure to examine the client's left eye, using your left hand and left eye.**

▶ Extremely tortuous vessels also require further evaluation.

Abnormal Findings

Abnormalities of the eye arise for a variety of reasons and can be associated with vision, eye movement, and the internal and external structures of the eye. The following sections address abnormal findings associated with the functions and structures of the eye.

Visual Acuity

Visual acuity is dependent upon the ability of the eye to refract light rays and focus them upon the retina. The shape of the eye is one determinant in the refractive and focusing processes of vision.

Emmetropia is the normal refractive condition of the eye in which light rays are brought into sharp focus on the retina.

Myopia (nearsightedness) is generally inherited and occurs when the eye is longer than normal. As a result, light rays focus in front of the retina.

Hyperopia (farsightedness) is also an inherited condition in which the eye is shorter than normal. In hyperopia the light rays focus behind the retina.

Astigmatism is often a familial condition in which the refraction of light is spread over a wide area rather than on a distinct point on the retina. In the normal eye, the cornea is round in shape, whereas in astigmatism the cornea curves more in one direction than another. As a result, light is refracted and focused on two focal points on or near the retina. Vision in astigmatism may be blurred or doubled.

Presbyopia is an age-related condition in which the lens of the eye loses the ability to accommodate. As a result, light is focused behind the retina, and focus on near objects becomes difficult.

ABNORMAL PUPILLARY RESPONSE

Adie's Pupil

Also known as tonic pupil, Adie's pupil is unilateral and sluggish pupillary response (Figure 7.6).

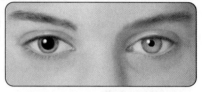

Figure 7.6 • Tonic pupil (Adie's pupil).

Cranial Nerve III Damage

Cranial nerve III damage results in a unilaterally dilated pupil (Figure 7.7). There is no reaction to light. Ptosis may be seen.

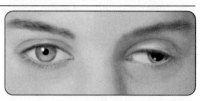

Figure 7.7 • Cranial nerve III damage.

Mydriasis

Mydriasis refers to fixed and dilated pupils (Figure 7.8). This condition may occur with sympathetic nerve stimulation, glaucoma, central nervous system damage, or deep anesthesia.

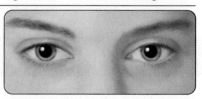

Figure 7.8 • Mydriasis.

Miosis

Miosis refers to fixed and constricted pupils (Figure 7.9). This condition may occur with the use of narcotics, with damage to the pons, or as a result of treatment for glaucoma.

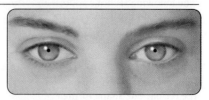

Figure 7.9 • Miosis.

ABNORMALITIES OF THE STRUCTURES OF THE EXTERNAL EYE

Acute Glaucoma

Acute glaucoma is a result of sudden increase in intraocular pressure resulting from blocked flow of fluid from the anterior chamber. The pupil is oval in shape and dilated (Figure 7.10). There is circumcorneal redness. The cornea appears cloudy and steamy. Pain is sudden in onset and is accompanied by decrease in vision and halos around lights. Acute glaucoma requires immediate intervention.

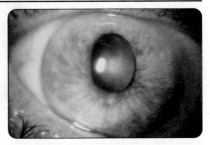

Figure 7.10 • Acute glaucoma.

Cataract

A cataract is an opacity in the lens (Figure 7.11). It usually occurs in aging.

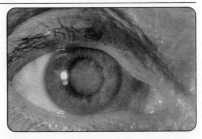

Figure 7.11 • Cataract.

Conjunctivitis

Conjunctivitis is an infection of the conjunctiva usually due to bacteria or virus but which may result from chemical exposure (Figure 7.12).

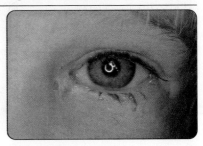

Figure 7.12 • Conjunctivitis.

ABNORMALITIES OF THE FUNDUS

Diabetic Retinopathy

Diabetic retinopathy refers to the changes that occur in the retina and vasculature of the retina including microaneurysms, hemorrhages, macular edema, and retinal exudates (Figure 7.13).

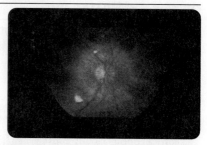

Figure 7.13 • Diabetic retinopathy.

Hypertensive Retinopathy

Hypertensive retinopathy refers to the changes in the retina and vasculature of the retina in response to elevations in blood pressure that accompany atherosclerosis, heart disease, and kidney disease (Figure 7.14). The changes include flame hemorrhages, nicking of vessels, and "cotton wool" spots that arise from infarction of the nerve fibers.

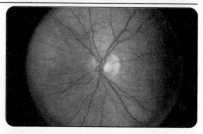

Figure 7.14 • Hypertensive retinopathy.

Macular Degeneration

Age-related macular degeneration (ARMD) is a degenerative condition of the macula, the central retina (Figure 7.15). Central vision is lost gradually while peripheral vision remains intact. The eyes are affected at different rates.

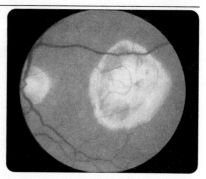

Figure 7.15 • Macular degeneration.

8

Ears, Nose, Mouth, and Throat

The structures of the ear, nose, mouth, and throat are responsible for the senses of hearing, smell, and taste. The interrelationships of the senses, and their structures, provide data for several body systems.

ANATOMY AND PHYSIOLOGY REVIEW

EAR

The ear is the sensory organ that functions in hearing and equilibrium. The external portion, or what most people think of as the ear, is called the **auricle** or **pinna.**

External Ear. The external large rim of the auricle is called the **helix.** The **tragus** is a stiff projection that protects the anterior meatus of the auditory canal. The **lobule** of the ear is a small flap of flesh at the inferior end of the auricle. The external auditory canal is about 1 in. in length, is S-shaped, and leads to the middle ear. It is lined with glands that secrete a yellow-brown wax called **cerumen.**

Middle Ear. The external ear and middle ear are separated by the **tympanic membrane,** or eardrum (Figure 8.1). This thin, translucent membrane is pearly gray in color and lies obliquely in the canal. Sound waves entering the auditory canal strike the membrane, causing it to vibrate. The vibrations are transferred to the **ossicles,** or bones of the middle ear: the malleus, the incus,

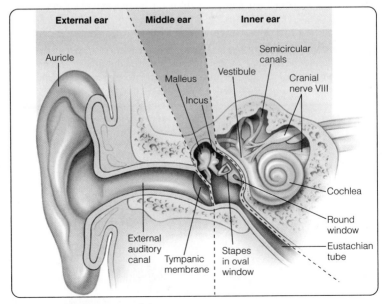

Figure 8.1 • The three parts of the ear.

and the stapes. The ossicles, in turn, transfer the vibration to the oval window of the inner ear. The **eustachian tube,** or auditory tube, connects the middle ear with the nasopharynx. These tubes help to equalize air pressure on both sides of the tympanic membrane. The middle ear functions to conduct sound vibrations from the external ear to the inner ear. It also protects the inner ear by reducing loud sound vibrations.

Inner Ear. The inner ear contains the bony labyrinth, which consists of a central cavity called the vestibule, three semicircular canals responsible for the sense of equilibrium, and the **cochlea,** a spiraling chamber that contains the receptors for hearing.

NOSE AND SINUSES

The nose is a triangular projection of bone and cartilage situated midline on the face. The nose consists of external and internal structures. Externally, the bridge of the nose is on the superior aspect of the nose, medial to each orbit of the eyes. Inferior to the bridge and free of attachment to the face is the tip of the nose. The nares, two oval external openings at the base of the nose, are surrounded by the columella and ala structures of cartilage. Each naris widens into the internal vestibule and nasal cavity. The nasal septum is a continuation of the columella dividing the nose into a right and left side.

The nasal mucosa with its rich blood supply helps filter inspired air and has a redder appearance than the oral mucosa. Three turbinates (superior, middle, and inferior) project from the medial wall into each side of the nasal cavity. These bony projections, covered with nasal mucosa, add surface area for cleaning, moistening, and warming air entering the respiratory tract. Each side of the posterior nasal cavity opens into the nasopharynx (Figure 8.2).

Mucous membranes line the **paranasal sinuses.** They are air-filled cavities that surround the nasal cavity and perform the same air processing functions of filtration, moistening, and warming. They are named for the bones of the skull in which they are contained: sphenoid, frontal, ethmoid, and maxillary.

MOUTH

The oral cavity, an oval-shaped cavity, is the beginning of the alimentary canal and digestive system (Figure 8.3). The oral cavity is divided into two parts by the teeth: the vestibule and the mouth. The vestibule, the anterior and smaller of the two regions, is composed of the lips, the buccal mucosa, the outer surface of the gums

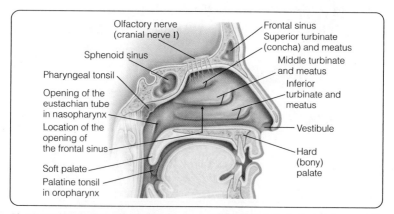

Figure 8.2 • Internal structure of the nose—lateral view.

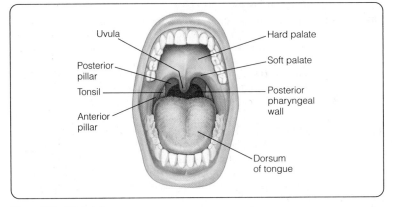

Figure 8.3 • Oral cavity.

and teeth, and the cheeks. At the posterior aspect of the teeth, the mouth is formed and includes the tongue, the hard and soft palate, the **uvula,** and the mandibular arch and maxillary arch. Thirty-two permanent teeth in the adult and 20 decidu-ous teeth in the child sit in the alveoli sockets of the mandible and maxilla.

The tongue, the organ for taste, sits on the floor of the mouth. Its base sits on the hyoid bone. The anterior portion of the tongue is attached to the floor of the mouth by the frenulum. The ventral surface (undersurface) of the tongue is smooth with visible vessels. The dorsal (top) surface of the tongue is rough and supports the papillae with speech and swallowing. Hard and soft palates form the roof of the mouth. The hard **palate,** formed by bones, is the anterior por-tion of the roof of the mouth. The uvula hangs from the free edge of the soft palate. Parotid, submandibular, and sublingual salivary glands are responsible for the production of saliva. The parotid glands are situated anterior to the ear within the cheek. Saliva enters the mouth via Stensen's duct located in the buccal mucosa opposite the second upper molar. The submandibular glands sit beneath the mandible at the angle of the jaw. Saliva from these glands enters the mouth via Wharton's duct. The orifice of these ducts is on either side of the frenulum on the floor of the mouth. The sublingual salivary glands, the small-est of the glands, are situated in the floor of the mouth and have many ducts that empty into the floor of the mouth.

THROAT

The throat, known as the pharynx, connects the nose, mouth, larynx, and esophagus and has three sections. The nasopharynx is behind the nose and above the soft palate. The adenoids and openings of the eustachian tubes are lo-cated in the nasopharynx. The oropharynx is behind the mouth and below the nasopharynx. It extends to the epiglottis and serves as a passageway for air and food. The tonsils are located behind the pillars (palatopharyngeal folds) on ei-ther side. The laryngopharynx is behind the larynx and is the passageway for the respiratory and digestive systems.

SPECIAL CONSIDERATIONS

The nurse must be aware that variations in findings from health assessment oc-cur in relation to age, developmental level, race, ethnicity, work history, living conditions, socioeconomics, and emotional well-being.

INFANTS AND CHILDREN

The infant's auditory canal is shorter than the adult's and has an upward curve. Children have a more horizontal auditory tube than adults, which leads to easier migration of organisms from infection in the throat to the middle ear. The nose of a child is too small to examine with a speculum. Both sets of teeth develop before birth. Eruption of permanent teeth begins at around age 6 and continues through adolescence. Salivation begins at 3 months of age. Drooling of saliva occurs for several months until swallowing saliva is learned.

THE PREGNANT FEMALE

Vessel changes of the middle ear may cause a feeling of fullness or earaches. Increased blood flow (hyperemia) to the sinuses can cause rhinitis (inflammation of the nasal cavity) and epistaxis (nosebleed). The sense of smell is heightened in pregnancy. Edema of the vocal cords may cause hoarseness or deepening of the voice.

THE OLDER ADULT

The older adult may have coarse hairs at the opening of the auditory meatus. The ears may appear more prominent, because cartilage formation continues throughout life. The tympanic membrane becomes paler in color and thicker in appearance with aging. Assessment of hearing may reveal a loss of high-frequency tones, which is consistent with aging. Over time, this loss often progresses to lower-frequency sounds as well. Gradual hearing loss with age is called **presbycusis.**

The lips and buccal mucosa of the mouth become thinner and less vascular. Gums are paler in color. The tongue develops more fissures, and motor function may become impaired, resulting in problems with swallowing. Senile tremors may cause slight protrusion of the tongue. Gums begin to recede, and some tooth loss may occur due to osteoporosis. If teeth are lost, the remaining teeth may drift. Lesions of the mouth may also develop from ill-fitting dentures.

PSYCHOSOCIAL CONSIDERATIONS

A client who is under a great deal of stress may be prone to mouth ulcers and lip biting. Tics (involuntary muscle spasms) and unconscious clenching of the jaw may indicate psychosocial disturbances.

CULTURAL CONSIDERATIONS

Assessment and findings are influenced by culture. See the cultural considerations box for specific examples.

Cultural Considerations

- Otitis media occurs more frequently and with greater severity in Hispanics and Native Americans than in other cultural groups.
- Cerumen appears dry and gray to brown in Asians and Native Americans.
- Cerumen appears moist and yellow-orange in African Americans and Caucasians.
- Cleft lip and palate occur with greatest frequency in Asians and least often in African Americans.
- Caucasians have the highest incidence of tooth decay.

Gathering the Data

FOCUSED INTERVIEW QUESTIONS

Ear

1. Describe your hearing. Have you noticed any change in your hearing? If so, tell me about: onset, character, and situations.
2. When was your last hearing test? Do you use a hearing aid?
3. Has any member of your family had ear problems or hearing loss?
4. Have you ever been diagnosed with a disease, infection affecting the ears, tinnitus, or vertigo?
5. Do you have any pain in your ears? If so, describe it.

QUESTIONS REGARDING INFANTS AND CHILDREN

1. Does the child have recurrent ear infections?
2. Does the child tug at his or her ears?
3. Does the child respond to loud noises?

QUESTIONS FOR THE PREGNANT FEMALE

1. Have you ever experienced a humming in your ears?
2. Have you experienced an earache or a feeling of fullness in your ears?

QUESTIONS FOR THE OLDER ADULT

1. Do you wear a hearing aid?
2. Do you have any difficulty operating the hearing aid?

Nose and Sinuses

1. Are you having any problems with your nose or sinuses? If so, describe them. Are you able to breathe through your nose?
2. Do you have or have you ever had nasal discharge, nosebleeds, surgery, or trauma to your nose?
3. Do you use recreational drugs?

QUESTIONS REGARDING INFANTS AND CHILDREN

1. Does the child put objects into his or her nose?

QUESTIONS FOR THE PREGNANT FEMALE

1. Have you had nosebleeds during your pregnancy? If so, how often?

Mouth and Throat

1. How would you describe the condition of your mouth, throat, and teeth? Have you noticed any changes in the last few months?
2. Do you have any problems swallowing?
3. Do your gums bleed frequently?
4. Have you noticed any hoarseness or loss of your voice?
5. Do you now or did you ever smoke a pipe, cigarettes, or cigars?

QUESTIONS REGARDING INFANTS AND CHILDREN

1. Does the child suck his or her thumb or a pacifier?

QUESTIONS FOR THE OLDER ADULT

1. Are you able to chew all types of food?
2. Do you experience dryness in your mouth?
3. Do you wear dentures?

Physical Assessment

Physical assessment of the ears, nose, mouth, and throat requires the use of inspection, palpation, percussion, and transillumination of sinuses. In addition, special assessment techniques include the use of the otoscope, tuning fork, and nasal speculum.

EQUIPMENT

examination gown
clean, nonsterile examination gloves
otoscope
tuning fork

nasal speculum
penlight
gauze pads
tongue blade

HELPFUL HINTS

* Provide specific instructions about what is expected of the client. The nurse would state whether the head must be turned or the mouth opened.
* Consider the age of the client. Response to directions varies across the life span.
* Pay attention to nonverbal cues throughout the assessment.
* Hearing difficulties may affect the data gathering process. Clarify problems and possible remedies before beginning the assessment. The client may use sign language, hearing aids, lip reading, or written communication.
* Explain the use of each piece of equipment throughout the assessment.
* Use Standard Precautions.

TECHNIQUES AND NORMAL FINDINGS	ABNORMAL FINDINGS SPECIAL CONSIDERATIONS

EAR

1. **Inspect the external ear for symmetry, proportion, color, and integrity.**
   * Confirm that the external auditory meatus is patent with no drainage. The color of the ear should match that of the surrounding area and the face, with no redness, nodules, swelling, or lesions.

▶ Any discharge, redness, or swelling may indicate an infection or allergy.

TECHNIQUES AND NORMAL FINDINGS	ABNORMAL FINDINGS SPECIAL CONSIDERATIONS

2. **Palpate the auricle and push on the tragus.**
   - Confirm that there are no hard nodules, lesions, or swelling. The tragus should be movable.
   - This technique should not cause pain.

▶ Pain could be the result of an infection of the external ear or temporomandibular joint dysfunction. Hard nodules (tophi) are uric acid crystal deposits, which are a sign of gout. Lesions with a history of long-term exposure to the sun may be cancerous.

3. **Palpate the mastoid process lying directly behind the ear.**
   - Confirm that there are no lesions, pain, or swelling.

4. **Inspect the auditory canal using the otoscope.**
   - For the best visualization, use the largest speculum that will fit into the auditory canal.
   - Ask the client to tilt the head away from you toward the opposite shoulder.
   - Hold the otoscope between the palm and first two fingers of the dominant hand. The handle may be positioned upward or downward (Figure 8.4).

▶ **Mastoiditis** is a complication of either a middle ear infection or a throat infection. Mastoiditis is very difficult to treat. It spreads easily to the brain since the mastoid area is separated from the brain by only a thin, bony plate.

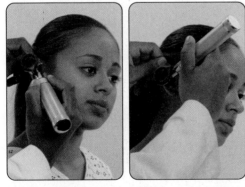

Figure 8.4 • Two techniques for holding and inserting an otoscope.

   - Use your other hand to straighten the canal.
   - In the adult client, pull the pinna up, back, and out to straighten the canal.
   - Be sure to maintain this position until the speculum is removed.
   - Instruct the client to tell you if any discomfort is experienced but not to move the head or suddenly pull away.

TECHNIQUES AND NORMAL FINDINGS	ABNORMAL FINDINGS SPECIAL CONSIDERATIONS

ALERT! *One must use care when inserting the speculum of the otoscope into the ear. The inner two thirds of the ear are very sensitive, and pressing the speculum against either side of the auditory canal will cause pain.*

- With the light on, use the upward or downward position of the handle to insert the speculum into the ear. The external canal should be open and without tenderness, inflammation, lesions, growths, discharge, or foreign substances.
- Note the amount of cerumen that is present, the texture, and the color.

▶ If the ear canal is occluded with cerumen, it must be removed.

5. **Examine the tympanic membrane using the otoscope.**
   - The membrane should be flat, gray, and translucent with no scars. A cone-shaped reflection of the otoscope light should be visible at the 5 o'clock position in the right ear and the 7 o'clock position in the left ear. The short process of the malleus should be seen as a shadow behind the tympanic membrane. The membrane should be intact.

   - If you cannot visualize the tympanic membrane, remove the otoscope, reposition the auricle, and reinsert the otoscope. Do not reposition the auricle with the otoscope in place.

▶ White patches on the tympanic membrane indicate scars from prior infections. If the membrane is yellow or reddish, it could indicate an infection of the middle ear. A bulging membrane may indicate increased pressure in the middle ear, whereas a retracted membrane may indicate a vacuum in the middle ear, due to a blocked eustachian tube.

6. **Perform the whisper test.**
   - This test evaluates hearing acuity of high-frequency sounds.
   - Ask the client to hold the heel of the hand over the left ear.
   - Cover your mouth so that the client cannot see your lips.
   - Standing at the client's side at a distance of 1 to 2 ft, whisper a simple phrase such as, "The weather is hot today." Ask the client to repeat the phrase. Then do the same procedure to test the right ear using a different phrase. The client should be able to repeat the phrases correctly.

▶ Inability to repeat the phrases may indicate a loss of the ability to hear high-frequency sounds.

TECHNIQUES AND NORMAL FINDINGS	ABNORMAL FINDINGS SPECIAL CONSIDERATIONS

7. **Perform the Rinne test.**
   - The Rinne test compares air and bone conduction. Hold the tuning fork by the handle and gently strike the fork on the palm of your hand to set it vibrating.
   - Place the base of the fork on the client's mastoid process. Ask the client to tell you when the sound is no longer heard.

   ▶ If the client hears the bone-conducted sound as long as or longer than the air-conducted sound, the client may have some degree of conductive hearing loss.

   - Note the number of seconds. Then immediately move the tines of the still-vibrating fork in front of the external auditory meatus. It should be 1 to 2 cm (about 1/2 in.) from the meatus.
   - Ask the client to tell you again when the sound is no longer heard. Again note the number of seconds. Normally, the sound is heard twice as long by air conduction than by bone conduction after bone conduction stops. For example, a normal finding is AC 30 seconds, BC 15 seconds.

8. **Perform the Weber test.**
   - The Weber test uses bone conduction to evaluate hearing in a person who hears better in one ear than in the other. Hold the tuning fork by the handle and strike the fork on the palm of the hand. Place the base of the vibrating fork against the client's skull. The midline of the anterior portion of the frontal bone is used. The midline of the forehead is an alternative choice (Figure 8.5).

   ▶ If the client hears the sound in one ear better than the other ear, the hearing loss may be due to either poor conduction or nerve damage. If the client has poor conduction in one ear, the sound is heard better in the impaired ear because the sound is being conducted directly through the bone to the ear, and the extraneous sounds in the environment are not being picked up. Conductive loss in one ear may be due to impacted cerumen, infection, or a perforated eardrum. If the client has a hearing loss due to nerve damage, the sound is referred to the better ear, in which the cochlea or auditory nerve is functioning better.

TECHNIQUES AND NORMAL FINDINGS	ABNORMAL FINDINGS SPECIAL CONSIDERATIONS

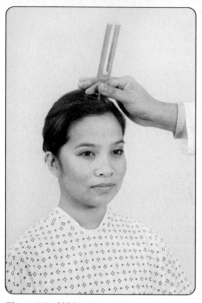

Figure 8.5 • Weber test.

- Ask the client if the sound is heard equally on both sides, or better in one ear than the other. The normal response is bilaterally equal sound, which is recorded as "no lateralization." If the sound is lateralized, ask the client to tell you which ear hears the sound better.

▶ The abnormal findings are recorded as "sound lateralizes to (right or left) ear."

9. **Perform the Romberg test.**
   - The Romberg test assesses equilibrium. Ask the client to stand with feet together and arms at sides, first with eyes opened and then with eyes closed.
   - Wait about 20 seconds. The person should be able to maintain this position, although some mild swaying may occur. Mild swaying is documented as a negative Romberg. It is important to stand nearby and prepare to support the client if there is a loss of balance.

▶ If the client is unable to maintain balance or needs to have the feet farther apart, there may be a problem with functioning of the vestibular apparatus.

TECHNIQUES AND NORMAL FINDINGS	ABNORMAL FINDINGS SPECIAL CONSIDERATIONS

NOSE AND SINUSES

1. **Inspect the nose for symmetry, shape, skin lesions, or signs of infection.**
   - Confirm that the nose is straight, the nares are equal in size, the skin is intact, and no drainage is present.

   ▶ If breathing is noisy or a discharge is present, the client may have an obstruction or an infection.

2. **Test for patency.**
   - Press your finger on the client's nostril to occlude one naris, and ask the client to breathe through the opposite side.
   - Repeat with the other nostril.
   - The client should be able to breathe through each naris.

   ▶ If the client cannot breathe through each naris, severe inflammation or an obstruction may be present.

   ▶ Ineffective breathing patterns or mouth breathing may be related to nasal swelling or trauma.

3. **Palpate the external nose for tenderness, swelling, and stability.**
   - Using two fingers, palpate the nose.
   - Note the smoothness and stability of the underlying soft tissue and cartilage.

4. **Inspect the nasal cavity using a nasal speculum.**
   - With your nondominant hand, stabilize the client's head. With the speculum in your dominant hand, insert the speculum with blades closed into the naris. Then separate the blades, dilating the naris. The speculum should be in the dominant hand for better control at the time of insertion to avoid hitting the sensitive septum.
   - With the client's head erect, inspect the inferior turbinates.
   - With the client's head tilted back, inspect the middle meatus and middle turbinates. Mucosa should be dark pink and smooth without swelling, discharge, bleeding, or foreign bodies. The septum should be midline, straight, and intact.
   - When finished with inspection, close the blades of the speculum and remove. Again, do not hit the sensitive septum.
   - Repeat on other side.

   ▶ If the mucosa is swollen and red, the client may have an upper respiratory infection. If mucosa is pale and boggy or swollen, the client may have chronic allergies. *A deviated septum* appears as an irregular lump in one nasal cavity. **Nasal polyps** are smooth, pale, benign growths found in many clients with chronic allergies.

TECHNIQUES AND NORMAL FINDINGS	ABNORMAL FINDINGS SPECIAL CONSIDERATIONS

5. **Palpate the sinuses.**
   - Begin by pressing your thumbs over the frontal sinuses below the superior orbital ridge. Palpate the maxillary sinuses below the zygomatic arches of the cheekbones (Figure 8.6).

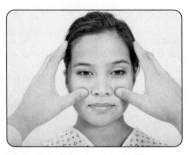

Figure 8.6 • Palpating the maxillary sinuses.

   - Observe the client for signs of discomfort. Ask the client to inform you of pain.

▶ Tenderness upon palpation may indicate chronic allergies or sinusitis.

6. **Percuss the sinuses.**
   - To determine if there is pain in the sinuses, directly percuss over the maxillary and frontal sinuses by lightly tapping with one finger (Figure 8.7).

▶ Pain may indicate sinus fullness, allergies, or infection.

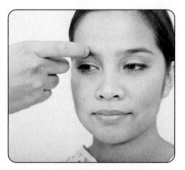

Figure 8.7 • Percussion of frontal sinuses.

TECHNIQUES AND NORMAL FINDINGS	ABNORMAL FINDINGS SPECIAL CONSIDERATIONS

7. Transilluminate the sinuses.
- If you suspect a sinus infection, the maxillary and frontal sinuses may be transilluminated.
- To transilluminate the frontal sinus, darken the room and hold a penlight under the superior orbit ridge against the frontal sinus area.
- Cover it with your hand. There should be a red glow over the frontal sinus area.

▶ If the sinus is filled with fluid, it will not transilluminate.

- To test the maxillary sinus, place a clean penlight in the client's mouth and shine the light on one side of the hard palate, then the other.
- There should be a red glow over the cheeks. Make sure the penlight is cleaned before using it again.
- An alternate technique is to place the penlight directly on the cheek and observe the glow of light on the hard palate.

MOUTH AND THROAT

Note: *Be sure to wear clean, nonsterile examination gloves for this part of the assessment.*

1. Inspect and palpate the lips.
- Confirm that the lips are symmetric, smooth, pink, moist, and without lesions. Makeup or lipstick should be removed.

2. Inspect the teeth.
- Observe the client's dental hygiene. Ask the client to clench the teeth and smile while you observe occlusion.
- Note dentures and caps at this time.
- The teeth should be white, with smooth edges, and free of debris. Adults should have 32 permanent teeth if wisdom teeth are intact.

▶ Lesions or blisters on the lips may be caused by the herpes simplex virus. These lesions are also known as **fever blisters** or **cold sores.** However, lesions must be evaluated for cancer, because cancer of the lip is the most common oral cancer. Pallor or cyanosis of the lips may indicate hypoxia.

▶ Loose, painful, broken, misaligned teeth, malocclusion, and inflamed gums need further evaluation.

TECHNIQUES AND NORMAL FINDINGS	ABNORMAL FINDINGS SPECIAL CONSIDERATIONS

3. **Inspect and palpate the buccal mucosa, gums, and tongue.**
   - Look into the client's mouth under a strong light.
   - Confirm that the tongue is pink and moist with papillae on the dorsal surface.
   - Ask the client to touch the roof of the mouth with the tip of the tongue. The ventral surface should be smooth and pink. Palpate the area under the tongue.
   - Check for lesions or nodules. Using a gauze pad, grasp the client's tongue and inspect for any lumps or nodules. The tissue should be smooth.
   - Use a tongue blade to hold the tongue aside while you inspect the mucous lining of the mouth and the gums.
   - Confirm that these areas are pink, moist, smooth, and free of lesions.
   - Confirm the integrity of both the soft and the hard palate.

▶ A smooth, coated, or hairy tongue is usually related to dehydration or disease. A small tongue may indicate undernutrition. Tremor of the tongue may indicate a dysfunction of the hypoglossal nerve (cranial nerve XII). Persistent lesions on the tongue must be evaluated further. Cancerous lesions occur most commonly on the sides or at the base of the tongue. The gums are diseased if there is bleeding, retraction, or overgrowth onto the teeth.

4. **Inspect the salivary glands.**
   - The salivary glands open into the mouth. Wharton's ducts (submandibular) open close to the lingual frenulum. Stensen's ducts (parotid) open opposite the second upper molars. Both ducts are visible, whereas the ducts of the sublingual glands are not visible.
   - Confirm that all salivary ducts are visible, with no pain, tenderness, swelling, or redness.
   - Touch the area close to the ducts with a sterile applicator, and confirm the flow of saliva.

▶ Pain or the lack of saliva can indicate infection or an obstruction.

5. **Inspect the throat.**
   - Use a tongue blade and penlight to inspect the throat.
   - Ask the client to open the mouth wide, tilt the head back, and say "aah." The uvula should rise in the midline.

TECHNIQUES AND NORMAL FINDINGS

**ABNORMAL FINDINGS
SPECIAL CONSIDERATIONS**

- Use the tongue blade to depress the middle of the arched tongue enough so that you can clearly visualize the throat, but not so much that the client gags. Ask the client to say "aah" again.
- Confirm the rising of the soft palate, which is a test for cranial nerve X.
- Confirm that the tonsils, uvula, and posterior pharynx are pink and are without inflammation, swelling, or lesions. Observe the tonsils behind the anterior tonsillar pillar. The color should be pink with slight vascularity present. Tonsils may be partially or totally absent.
- As you inspect the throat, note any mouth odors.
- Discard the tongue blade.

▶ Viral pharyngitis may accompany a cold. Tonsils may be bright red and swollen, and may have white spots on them.

Clients with diabetic acidosis have a sweet, fruity breath. The breath of clients with kidney disease smells of ammonia.

Abnormal Findings

Abnormal findings in the ears, nose, mouth, and throat include lesions, deformities, infectious processes, and dental problems.

EAR

Otitis Media

Otitis media is infection of the middle ear producing a red, bulging eardrum, fever, and hearing loss (Figure 8.8). The otoscopic examination reveals absent light reflex. Otitis media is more common in children, whose auditory tubes are wider, shorter, and more horizontal than those of adults, thus allowing easier access for infections ascending from the pharynx.

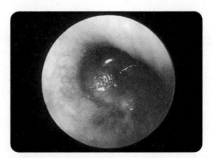

Figure 8.8 ● Otitis media.

Scarred Tympanic Membrane

A scarred tympanic membrane is a condition in which the eardrum has white patches of scar tissue due to repeated ear infections (Figure 8.9).

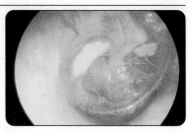

Figure 8.9 • Scarred tympanic membrane.

NOSE AND SINUSES

Rhinitis

Rhinitis is a nasal inflammation usually due to a viral infection or allergy. It is accompanied by a watery and often copious discharge, sneezing, and congestion (stuffy nose). Acute rhinitis is caused by a virus, whereas allergic rhinitis (Figure 8.10) results from contact with allergens such as pollen and dust.

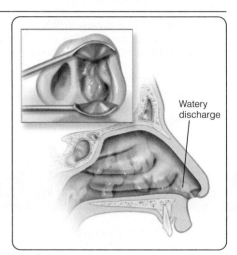

Watery discharge

Figure 8.10 • Allergic rhinitis.

Deviated Septum

A deviated septum is a slight ingrowth of the lower nasal septum (Figure 8.11). When viewed with a nasal speculum, one nasal cavity appears to have an outgrowth or shelf.

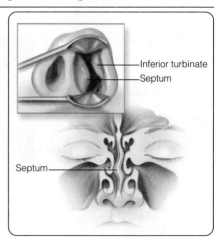

Inferior turbinate
Septum

Septum

Figure 8.11 • Deviated septum.

MOUTH AND THROAT

Ankyloglossia

Ankyloglossia is a fixation of the tip of the tongue to the floor of the mouth due to a shortened lingual frenulum (Figure 8.12). The condition is usually congenital and may be corrected surgically.

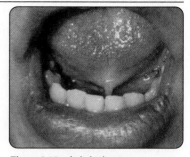

Figure 8.12 • Ankyloglossia.

Gingival Hyperplasia

Gingival hyperplasia is an enlargement of the gums (Figure 8.13) frequently seen in pregnancy, in leukemia, or after prolonged use of phenytoin (Dilantin).

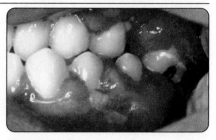

Figure 8.13 • Gingival hyperplasia.

Gingivitis

Gingivitis is inflammation of the gums (Figure 8.14). It may be caused by poor dental hygiene or a deficiency of vitamin C. If left untreated, gingivitis may progress to periodontal disease and tooth loss.

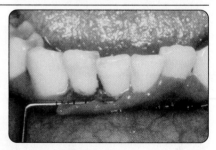

Figure 8.14 • Gingivitis.

Tonsillitis

Tonsillitis is inflammation of the tonsils. The throat is red and the tonsils are swollen and covered by white or yellow patches or exudate (Figure 8.15). Lymph nodes in the cervical chain may be enlarged. Tonsillitis may be accompanied by a high fever.

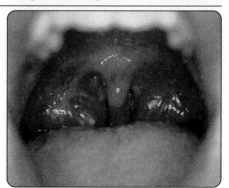

Figure 8.15 • Tonsillitis.

Herpes Simplex

Herpes simplex is a virus that is often accompanied by clear vesicles commonly called *cold sores* or *fever blisters,* usually at the junction of the skin and the lip (Figure 8.16). The vesicles erupt, then crust and heal within 2 weeks. They usually recur, especially after heavy exposure to bright sunlight (e.g., after a day at the beach).

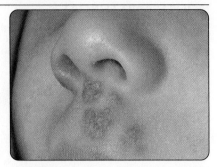

Figure 8.16 • Herpes simplex.

Carcinoma

Oral cancers are most commonly found on the lower lip or the base (underside) of the tongue (Figure 8.17). Cancer is suspected if a sore or lesion does not heal within a few weeks. Heavy smoking, especially pipe smoking, and chewing tobacco increase the risk of oral cancer, as does chronic heavy use of alcohol.

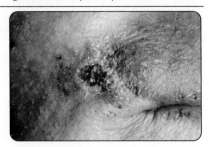

Figure 8.17 • Carcinoma.

Leukoplakia

Leukoplakia is a whitish thickening of the mucous membrane in the mouth or tongue (Figure 8.18). It cannot be scraped off. It is most often associated with heavy smoking or drinking, and can be a precancerous condition.

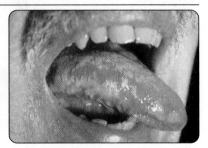

Figure 8.18 • Leukoplakia.

9

Respiratory System

The primary responsibility of the respiratory system is the exchange of gases in the body. Exchange of oxygen and carbon dioxide is essential to the homeostatic and hemodynamic process of the body.

ANATOMY AND PHYSIOLOGY REVIEW

The thorax is a closed cavity of the body, containing structures needed for respirations. The thorax has three sections: the mediastinum and the right and left pleural cavities. The **mediastinum** contains the heart, trachea, esophagus, and major blood vessels of the body. Each pleural cavity contains a lung.

TRACHEA

The trachea, located in the mediastinum, descends from the larynx in the neck to the main bronchi at the distal point, bifurcating anteriorly at about the sternal angle and posteriorly at about the vertebrae T_3 to T_5.

BRONCHI

Anteriorly, the trachea bifurcates at about the level of the sternal angle, forming the right and left main bronchi.

LUNGS

The lungs are cone-shaped, elastic, spongy, air-filled structures that are situated in the pleural cavities of the thorax on either side of the mediastinum. The apex of each lung is slightly superior to the inner third of the clavicle, and the base of each lung is at the level of the diaphragm. The left lung has two lobes (upper and lower) and tends to be longer and narrower than the right lung. The right lung has three lobes (upper, middle, and lower) and is slightly larger, wider, and shorter than the left lung.

PLEURAL MEMBRANES

The parietal membrane lines the superior aspect of the diaphragm and the thoracic wall. The visceral membrane covers the outer surface of the lung. A pleural fluid produced by these membranes acts as a lubricant, allowing the lung to glide during the respiratory cycle of inspiration and expiration.

RESPIRATORY CYCLE

Respiratory cycle, *respirations*, and *breathing* are terms used interchangeably to indicate the movement of air in and out of the body. Breathing consists of two phases: inspiration and expiration, thus the term *respiratory cycle*. The regular, even-depth, rhythmic pattern of inspiration and expiration describes **eupnea:** normal breathing. A change in this pattern, producing shortness of breath or difficulty in breathing, is **dyspnea.**

LANDMARKS

Thoracic reference points and specific anatomic structures are used as landmarks to provide an exact location for the assessment findings and an accurate orientation for documentation of findings. Figures 9.1 and 9.2 depict the bony landmarks.

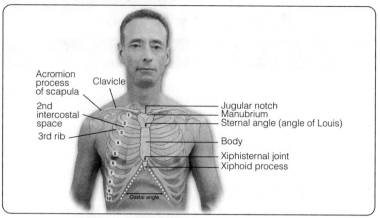

Figure 9.1 • Landmarks of the anterior thorax.

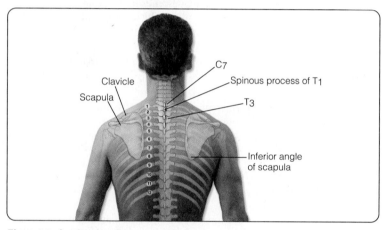

Figure 9.2 • Landmarks of the posterior thorax.

The thorax may be divided into two sections for assessment, the anterior and posterior thorax. The lateral areas are incorporated into the anterior and posterior sections. Imaginary lines are identified on the thoracic cage. These lines are depicted in Figures 9.3 and 9.4.

The apices of the lung extend 2 to 4 cm (0.78 to 1.56 in.) above the inner third of the clavicle anteriorly. Posteriorly, the apices of the lungs are located superior to the scapula between the vertebral line and midscapular line. The base of the lung has three reference points. The lung is cone shaped, and the base of the lung is located at the sixth intercostal space at the midclavicular line. At the midaxillary line the base of the lung is at the eighth intercostal space. At the scapular line on the posterior thorax, the base of the lung is at the tenth intercostal space.

SPECIAL CONSIDERATIONS

Throughout the assessment process the nurse gathers subjective and objective data reflecting the client's state of respiratory health.

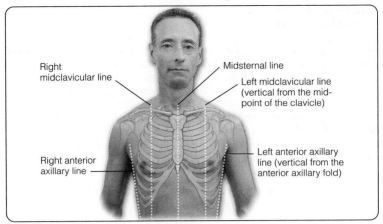

Figure 9.3 • Lines of the anterior thorax.

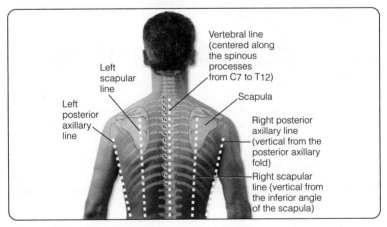

Figure 9.4 • Lines of the posterior thorax.

INFANTS AND CHILDREN

During fetal development, respirations are passive and gas exchange occurs at the placenta. At birth, rapid changes occur in the respiratory system as fetal circulation closes. Neonates have a respiratory rate and depth likely to be irregular. At this age, breathing involves use of abdominal muscles; therefore, inspection of the abdomen will yield a more accurate respiratory rate. Abdominal breathing continues during childhood until about 5 to 7 years of age. Costal (rib/chest) breathing is the expected pattern after 7 years of age.

THE PREGNANT FEMALE

The hormonal changes of pregnancy and the growing fetus produce changes in the respiratory system of the pregnant female. The ligaments of the thorax relax, the horizontal diameter expands, and the costal angle increases. At rest, the diaphragm rises into the chest to accommodate the fetus and respirations are diaphragmatic. Shortness of breath and dyspnea, especially in the last trimester, are common as the maternal and fetal demand for oxygen increases.

THE OLDER ADULT

As individuals age, body functions change. Many activities of the respiratory system demonstrate a decrease in efficiency. The lungs lose their elasticity, the skeletal muscles begin to weaken, and bones lose their density. As a result, it becomes more difficult for the older adult to expand the thoracic cage and take a deep breath. The diameters of the thoracic cage change. The appearance of a barrel chest (kyphosis) and calcification of cartilage contribute to the decrease in thoracic excursion. Weakening of the chest muscles hinders the older adult's ability to cough. Dry mucous membranes, a decreased amount of cilia in the system, and the inability to cough compromise airway clearance. Rate of respirations in the older adult is slightly higher than in the middle-aged adult. The older adult has a more shallow respiratory cycle because of the decreased vital capacity.

PSYCHOSOCIAL CONSIDERATIONS

Stress, anxiety, pain, and fatigue may exacerbate respiratory problems. Clients experiencing acute or chronic respiratory problems will have a physiologic alteration with gas exchange.

CULTURAL CONSIDERATIONS

Assessment and findings are influenced by culture. See the cultural considerations box for specific examples.

Cultural Considerations

- Chest volumes differ according to culture. Chest volume, vital capacity, and forced expiratory volume are greatest in Caucasians, followed by African Americans, Asians, and Native Americans.
- Asthma occurs more frequently in African Americans than in Caucasians.
- Obstructive sleep apnea (OSA) is twice as likely to be experienced by young African Americans compared to young Caucasians.
- Contracting TB is eight times more likely in African Americans than in Caucasians.
- African Americans are more likely to be exposed to occupational hazards that contribute to respiratory disease than are Caucasians.
- Sarcoidosis occurs more frequently and with greater severity in African Americans than in Caucasians.
- Asian, Pacific Islander, Hispanic, Native American, and migrant and farm worker populations have a higher risk for and greater incidence of TB.
- African Americans report symptoms of asthma in different terms than do Caucasians.
- Linguistic and cultural factors must be considered to avoid miscommunication and misinterpretation of information about diagnoses when caring for many immigrant populations.
- Children in urban areas and from low socioeconomic groups have a higher incidence of asthma.

Gathering the Data

FOCUSED INTERVIEW QUESTIONS

1. Describe your breathing today. Is it different from 2 months ago? From 2 years ago?

2. Have you ever been diagnosed with a respiratory disease, infection, or allergy?

3. Are you able to carry out all of your regular activities without a change in your breathing?
4. When you sleep do you lie down flat, prop yourself up with pillows, or sit up?
5. Is there anyone in your family who has had a respiratory disease or problem?
6. Do you have a cough, are you wheezing, or do you have difficulty breathing?
7. Do you now smoke or have you ever smoked tobacco or other products?
8. Have you received immunization for respiratory illnesses such as flu or pneumonia?
9. Do you use now or have you ever used medications or devices to alter or improve your respiratory function?

QUESTIONS REGARDING INFANTS AND CHILDREN

1. Is the child taking solid foods?
2. How many colds has the child had in the past 12 months?
3. Has the child been immunized against respiratory illnesses?

QUESTIONS FOR THE PREGNANT FEMALE

1. Do you experience any shortness of breath or dyspnea?

QUESTIONS FOR THE OLDER ADULT

1. Describe any changes in breathing you have experienced.

Physical Assessment

Physical assessment of the respiratory system requires the use of inspection, palpation, percussion, and auscultation. The nurse includes the anterior, posterior, and lateral aspects of the thorax when conducting each of the assessments.

EQUIPMENT

examination gown and drape
examination gloves
examination light
stethoscope

skin marker
metric ruler
tissues
face mask for the nurse

HELPFUL HINTS

- Provide an environment that is comfortable and private.
- Explain each step of the procedure.
- Provide specific instructions about what is expected of the client, for example, whether deep or regular breathing will be required.
- Tell client the purpose of each procedure and when and if discomfort will accompany any assessment.
- Pay attention to nonverbal cues that may indicate discomfort and ask client to indicate if he or she experiences any difficulties or discomforts.
- An organized and professional approach goes a long way toward putting the client at ease.
- Use Standard Precautions

TECHNIQUES AND NORMAL FINDINGS	ABNORMAL FINDINGS SPECIAL CONSIDERATIONS

ALERT! *Individuals experiencing pain and dyspnea, who are restless, anxious, and unable to follow directions, may need immediate medical assistance.*

INSPECTION OF THE ANTERIOR THORAX

1. **Observe skin color.**
   - Skin color varies among individuals, but pink undertones indicate normal oxygenation. Skin color of the thorax should be consistent with that of the rest of the body.

   ▶ Pigments and levels of oxygenation influence skin color. Pallor, cyanosis, rubor, erythema, or grayness requires further evaluation.

2. **Inspect the structures of the thorax.**
   - The clavicles should be at the same height. The sternum should be midline. The costal angle should be less than 90 degrees.

   ▶ Misalignment of clavicles may be caused by deviations in the vertebral column such as scoliosis. Increase in the costal angle in an adult may indicate chronic obstructive pulmonary disease (COPD). The thorax of children is rounder than that of adults.

3. **Inspect for symmetry.**
   - The structures of the chest and chest movement should be symmetric.

   ▶ Asymmetry may indicate postural problems or underlying respiratory dysfunction.

4. **Inspect chest configuration.**
   - The adult transverse diameter is approximately twice that of the anteroposterior diameter (AP:T = 1:2).

   ▶ A change in the ratio requires further evaluation. Remember: older adults have a decreased ratio.

5. **Count the respiratory rate.**
   - Count the number of respiratory cycles per minute. Normal adult respiratory rate is 12 to 20.
     - Observe chest movement.
     - Observe the muscles of the chest and neck, including the intercostal muscles and sternocleidomastoids.

   ▶ Intercostal muscle retraction and prominent sternocleidomastoids may be seen in respiratory distress.

TECHNIQUES AND NORMAL FINDINGS	ABNORMAL FINDINGS SPECIAL CONSIDERATIONS

INSPECTION OF THE POSTERIOR THORAX

1. **Inspect the structures of the posterior thorax.**
   - The height of the scapulae should be even; the vertebrae should be midline.

   ▶ Lateral deviation of the spine and elevation of one scapula is indicative of scoliosis.

2. **Inspect for symmetry.**
   - The structures of the chest and chest movement should be symmetric.

   ▶ Asymmetry may indicate postural problems or underlying respiratory problems.

3. **Observe respirations.**
   - Respirations should be smooth and even.

PALPATION OF THE POSTERIOR THORAX

1. **Lightly palpate the posterior thorax.**
   - Use the finger pads to lightly palpate the posterior thorax. Include the entire thorax by starting at the areas above each scapula and move from side to side to below the twelfth rib and laterally to the midaxillary line on each side (Figure 9.5).

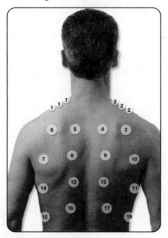

Figure 9.5 • Pattern for palpating the posterior thorax.

TECHNIQUES AND NORMAL FINDINGS

- Assess muscle mass.
- Assess for growths, nodules, and masses.
- Assess for tenderness.
- Muscle mass should be firm and underlying tissue smooth. The chest should be free of lesions or masses. The area should be nontender to palpation.

2. **Palpate and count ribs and intercostal spaces.**
   - Instruct the client to flex the neck, round the shoulders, and lean forward. Tell the client you will be applying light pressure to the spine and rib areas. Instruct the client to breathe normally and to tell you of pain or discomfort.
   - When the neck is flexed, the spinous process of C_7 is most prominent. When two spinous processes are equally prominent, they are C_7 and T_1. Use the finger pads to palpate each spinous process. The spinous processes should form a straight line. Move to the left and right to identify ribs and intercostal spaces from C_7 through T_{12}.

▶ Lateral deviation of the thoracic spinous processes indicates a scoliosis.

3. **Palpate for respiratory expansion.**
   - Explain that you will be assessing the movement of the chest during breathing by placing your hands on the lower chest and asking the client to take a deep breath.
   - Place the palmar surface of your hands, with thumbs close to the vertebrae, on the chest at the level of T_{10}. Pinch up some skin between your thumbs. Ask the client to take a deep breath.
   - The movement and pressure of the chest against your hands should feel smooth and even. Your thumbs should move away from the spine and the skin should move smoothly as the chest moves with inspiration.

▶ Unilateral decrease or delay in expansion may indicate underlying fibrotic or obstructive lung disease or may result from splinting associated with pleural pain or pneumothorax.

| **TECHNIQUES AND NORMAL FINDINGS** | **ABNORMAL FINDINGS SPECIAL CONSIDERATIONS** |

4. **Palpate for tactile fremitus.**
   - **Fremitus** is the palpable vibration on the chest wall when the client speaks. Fremitus is strongest over the trachea, diminishes over the bronchi, and becomes almost nonexistent over the alveoli of the lungs.
   - Explain that you will be feeling for vibrations on the chest while the client speaks. Tell the client you will be placing your hands on various areas of the chest while he or she repeats "ninety-nine" or "one, two, three" in a clear, loud voice.
   - Use the ulnar surface of the hand or the palmar surface of the hand at the metacarpophalangeal joints when palpating. Palpate and compare symmetric areas of the lungs by moving from side to side from apices to bases. Using one hand to palpate for fremitus is believed to increase accuracy of findings. Two-handed methods may, however, increase speed and facilitate identification of asymmetry.

▶ Decreased or absent fremitus may result from a soft voice, from a very thick chest wall, or from underlying diseases including COPD, pleural effusion, fibrosis, or tumor. Increased fremitus occurs with fluid in the lungs or in infection.

PERCUSSION OF THE POSTERIOR THORAX

1. **Recall the expected findings.**
   - Percussion allows assessment of underlying structures. The usual sound in the thorax is **resonance,** a long, low-pitched hollow sound.

▶ An unexpected finding would be hyperresonance, which is heard in conditions of overinflation of the lungs as in emphysema, or with pneumothorax.

2. **Percuss the lungs.**
   - Place the pleximeter in the intercostal space parallel to the ribs during percussion. Standing slightly to the side of the client allows the pleximeter finger to lie more firmly on the chest as you move through all thoracic areas.
   - Percuss the apex of the left lung, then the apex of the right lung. Percuss from side to side, comparing sounds, in the intercostal spaces as you percuss to the bases of the lungs and laterally to each midaxillary line using the pattern depicted in Figure 9.5.

▶ Percussion will yield dull sounds over solidified or fluid-filled areas, as may exist in pleural effusion. Percussion over bone will yield flat sounds. Be sure to check that finger placement is correct.

TECHNIQUES AND NORMAL FINDINGS	ABNORMAL FINDINGS SPECIAL CONSIDERATIONS

AUSCULTATION OF THE POSTERIOR THORAX

Auscultation of the respiratory system refers to listening to the sounds of breathing through the stethoscope. The sounds are produced by air moving through the airways. Sounds change as the airway size changes or with the presence of fluid or mucus.

The pattern for auscultation of the respiratory system is the same as that for percussion (see Figure 9.5). Use the diaphragm of the stethoscope and listen through the full respiratory cycle. When auscultating, classify each sound according to intensity, location, pitch, duration, and characteristic.

▶ Auscultation through clothing or coarse chest hair may produce deceptive sounds. Thick, coarse chest hair may be matted with a damp cloth or lotion to prevent interference with auscultation.

ALERT! *It is important to monitor the client's breathing to prevent hyperventilation.*

Four normal breath sounds are heard during respiratory auscultation. These are summarized in Table 9.1.

Table 9.1	Normal Breath Sounds		
SOUND	**LOCATION**	**RATIO INSPIRATION TO EXPIRATION**	**QUALITY**
Tracheal	Over trachea	I < E	Harsh, high-pitched
Bronchial	Next to trachea	E > I	Loud, high-pitched
Bronchovesicular	Sternal border between scapulae	I = E	Medium loudness, medium pitch
Vesicular	Remainder of lungs	I > E	Soft, low-pitched

1. **Instruct the client.**
   - Explain that you will be listening to the client's breathing with the stethoscope.
   - The client will be in the same position as during percussion. Ask the client to breathe deeply through the mouth each time the stethoscope is placed on a new spot. Tell the client to let you know if he or she is

▶ The obese client may be unable to take deep breaths due to the weight of the chest wall and the fatty deposits in the intercostal muscles and the diaphragm.

TECHNIQUES AND NORMAL FINDINGS	**ABNORMAL FINDINGS** **SPECIAL CONSIDERATIONS**

becoming tired or short of breath and if so you will stop and allow time to rest.

2. Auscultate for tracheal sounds.
- Auscultate at the vertebral line superior to C_7.

3. Auscultate for bronchial sounds.
- Start at the vertebral line at C_7 and move the stethoscope down toward T_3. The sound will be bronchial.

4. Auscultate for bronchovesicular sounds.
- The right and left primary bronchi are located at the level of T_3 and T_5. Auscultate at the right and left of the vertebrae at those levels. The breath sounds will be bronchovesicular.

▶ Auscultation of diminished but normal breath sounds in both lungs may indicate emphysema, atelectasis, bronchospasm, or shallow breathing. Breath sounds heard in just one lung indicate pleural effusion, pneumothorax, tumor, or mucous plugs in the airways in the other lung. Finding bronchial or bronchovesicular sounds in areas where one would normally hear vesicular sounds indicates that alveoli and small bronchioles are affected by fluid or exudate. Fluid and exudate decrease the movement of air through small airways and result in loss of vesicular sounds.

5. Auscultate for vesicular sounds.
- Auscultate the lungs by following the pattern used for percussion. Move the stethoscope from side to side while comparing sounds. Start at the apices and move to the bases of the lungs and laterally to the midaxillary line. The breath sounds over most of the posterior surface are vesicular.

▶ Added or adventitious sounds are superimposed on normal breath sounds and are often indicative of underlying airway problems or diseases of the cardiovascular or respiratory systems.

▶ Adventitious sounds are summarized in Table 9.2.

TECHNIQUES AND NORMAL FINDINGS	ABNORMAL FINDINGS SPECIAL CONSIDERATIONS

Table 9.2	**Adventitious Sounds**		
SOUND	**OCCURRENCE**	**QUALITY**	**CAUSES**
Rales/ Crackles			
Fine	End inspiration, do not clear with cough	High-pitched, short, crackling	Collapsed or fluid-filled alveoli open
Coarse	End inspiration, do not clear with cough	Loud, moist, low-pitched, bubbling	Collapsed or fluid-filled alveoli open
Rhonchi			
Wheezes (sibilant)	Expiration/Inspiration when severe	High-pitched, continuous	Blocked airflow as in asthma, infection, foreign body obstruction
Rhonchi (sonorous)	Expiration/inspiration Change/disappear with cough	Low-pitched, continuous, snoring, rattling	Fluid-blocked airways
Stridor	Inspiration	Loud, high-pitched crowing heard without stethoscope	Obstructed upper airway
Friction rub	Inhalation/exhalation	Low-pitched grating, rubbing	Pleural inflammation

ASSESSMENT OF THE ANTERIOR THORAX

Inspection of the anterior thorax was conducted prior to the entire assessment of the posterior thorax. That assessment included a survey and inspection of chest structures, skin color, and respiratory rate and pattern.

PALPATION OF THE ANTERIOR THORAX

1. **Position the client.**
   - The client is usually in a supine position for palpation, percussion, and auscultation of the anterior thorax. If the client is experiencing discomfort or dyspnea, a sitting position may be used, or the client may be in a Fowler's position. The breasts of female clients normally flatten when in a supine position. Large and pendulous breasts may have to be moved to perform a complete assessment. Explain this to the client and inform her that she may move and lift her own breasts if that will make her more comfortable.

▶ The obese client may be unable to lie flat during assessment of the anterior thorax.

TECHNIQUES AND NORMAL FINDINGS	ABNORMAL FINDINGS SPECIAL CONSIDERATIONS

2. Palpate the sternum, ribs, and intercostal spaces.

- Locate the suprasternal notch; palpate downward to the sternal angle (angle of Louis) where the manubrium meets the body of the sternum. Palpate laterally to the left and right to locate the second rib and second intercostal space. Continue palpating the sternum to the xiphoid process and to the left and right of the sternum to count the ribs.

- The sternum should feel flat except for the ridge of the sternal angle and should taper to the xiphoid. The ribs should feel smooth and the spacing of ribs and intercostal spaces should be symmetric.

3. Lightly palpate the anterior thorax.

- Use the finger pads to lightly palpate the anterior thorax. Include the entire thorax by starting at the areas above each clavicle and move from side to side below the costal angle and laterally to the midaxillary line.
- Assess muscle mass.
- Assess for growths, nodules, and masses.
- Assess for tenderness.
- Muscle mass should be firm and underlying tissue smooth. The chest should be free of lesions or masses. The area should be nontender to palpation.

▶ Pain may occur with inflammation of fibrous tissue or underlying structures. Crepitus may be felt if there is air in the subcutaneous tissue.

4. Palpate for respiratory expansion.

- Explain that you will be assessing movement of the chest during breathing by placing your hands on the lower chest and asking the client to take a breath.
- Place the palmar surface of your hands along each costal margin with thumbs close to the midsternal line. Pinch up some skin between your thumbs. Ask the client to take a deep breath.

TECHNIQUES AND NORMAL FINDINGS	ABNORMAL FINDINGS SPECIAL CONSIDERATIONS

- The movement of the chest beneath your hands should feel smooth and even. Your thumbs should move apart and the skin move smoothly as the chest expands with inspiration.

▶ Unilateral decrease or delay in expansion may indicate fibrotic or obstructive lung disease or may result from splinting associated with pleural pain.

PERCUSSION OF THE ANTERIOR THORAX

1. **Percuss the lungs.**
   - Begin at the apices of the lungs. Ask the client to turn the head to the opposite side of percussion to increase the size of the surface required for placing your pleximeter finger and to avoid interference from the clavicle. Move to the chest wall and place the pleximeter in the intercostal space parallel to the ribs during percussion. Percuss the anterior chest from side to side, comparing sounds, in the intercostal spaces. Percuss to the bases and laterally to the midaxillary line.

   ▶ Percussion of the anterior thorax will yield dull sounds over solidified or fluid-filled areas, as may exist in pleural effusion, consolidation, or tumor.

   - Percussion over bone or organs will yield flat or dull sounds. Avoid percussion over the clavicles, sternum, and ribs. Percussion over the heart will produce dullness to the left of the sternum from the third to fifth intercostal spaces. Percuss the left lung lateral to the midclavicular line. Percussion sounds in the lower left thorax change from resonance to tympany over the gastric air bubble. Percussion sounds in the right lower thorax change from resonance to dullness at the upper liver border.

AUSCULTATION OF THE ANTERIOR THORAX

Auscultation is used to identify and discriminate between and among normal and adventitious breath sounds. Listen to the full respiratory cycle with each placement of the stethoscope (Figure 9.6).

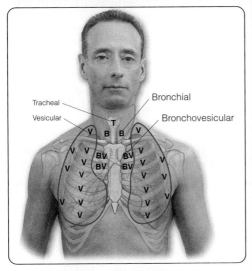

Figure 9.6 • Auscultatory sounds: Anterior thorax.

1. **Auscultate the trachea.**
   - Place the stethoscope over the trachea above the suprasternal notch. You will hear tracheal breath sounds. Move the stethoscope to the left, then the right side of the trachea, just above each sternoclavicular joint. You will hear bronchial breath sounds.

2. **Auscultate the apices.**
   - Place the stethoscope in the triangular areas just superior to each clavicle. You will hear vesicular sounds.

3. **Auscultate the bronchi.**
   - The bronchi are auscultated at the second and third intercostal spaces at the left and right sternal borders. You will hear bronchovesicular sounds.

4. **Auscultate the lungs.**
   - Auscultate the lungs by following the pattern for percussion. Move the stethoscope from side to side as you compare sounds. Move down to the sixth intercostal space and laterally to the midaxillary line. You will hear vesicular sounds.

| TECHNIQUES AND NORMAL FINDINGS | ABNORMAL FINDINGS SPECIAL CONSIDERATIONS |

5. **Interpret the findings.**
   - Refer to the descriptions and interpretations of normal and adventitious breath sounds described in auscultation of the posterior thorax.

▶ Breath sounds may be diminished in the obese client due to poor inspiratory effort resulting from the weight of the chest and fatty deposits in the respiratory musculature.

Abnormal Findings

RESPIRATORY DISORDERS

Asthma

A chronic hyperreactive condition resulting in bronchospasm, mucosal edema, and increased mucus secretion. Usually occurs in response to inhaled irritants or allergens (Figure 9.7).

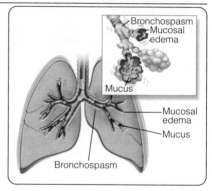

Figure 9.7 • Asthma.

Atelectasis

A condition in which there is an obstruction of airflow. The alveoli or an entire lung may collapse from airway obstruction, such as a mucous plug, lack of surfactant, or a compressed chest wall (Figure 9.8).

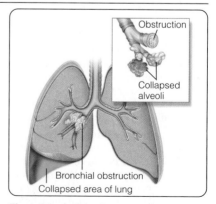

Figure 9.8 • Atelectasis.

Emphysema

A condition in which chronic inflammation of the lungs leads to destruction of alveoli and decreased elasticity of the lungs. As a result, air is trapped and lungs hyperinflate (Figure 9.9).

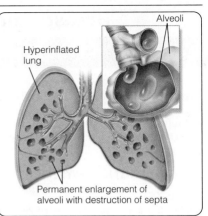

Figure 9.9 • Emphysema.

Lobar Pneumonia

An infection causes fluid, bacteria, and cellular debris to fill the alveoli (Figure 9.10).

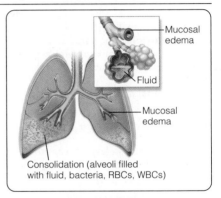

Figure 9.10 • Lobar pneumonia.

Congestive Heart Failure

Increased pressure in the pulmonary veins causes interstitial edema around the alveoli and may cause edema of the bronchial mucosa (Figure 9.11).

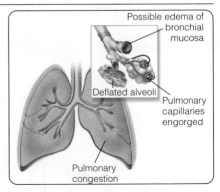

Figure 9.11 • Congestive heart failure.

10
Breasts and Axillae

The assessment of the breasts and axillae begins with a thorough health history and may be incorporated into the total body assessment along with the heart and lung assessment when the client is sitting and again when supine. It is important to incorporate assessment of the male client's breasts during the physical assessment.

ANATOMY AND PHYSIOLOGY REVIEW

BREASTS

The breasts are paired mammary glands located on the anterior chest wall and supported by major muscles of the thorax. Breast tissue extends from the second or third rib to the sixth or seventh rib and from the sternal margin to the midaxillary line, depending on body shape and size (Figure 10.1). The nipple is centrally located within a circular pigmented field of wrinkled skin called the **areola.** The surface of the areola is speckled with tiny sebaceous glands known as **Montgomery's glands** (Montgomery's tubercles). Commonly, breast tissue extends superiolaterally into the axilla as the **axillary tail** (tail of Spence).

The internal structures of the breast and the lymph nodes that drain the area are depicted in Figure 10.2.

SPECIAL CONSIDERATIONS

Age, developmental level, race, ethnicity, work history, living conditions, socioeconomics, and emotional well-being are among the factors that influence breast health.

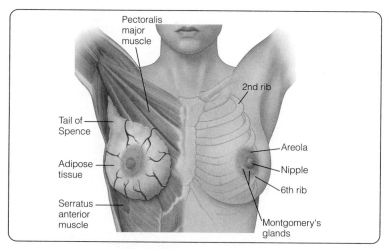

Figure 10.1 • Anatomy of the breast.

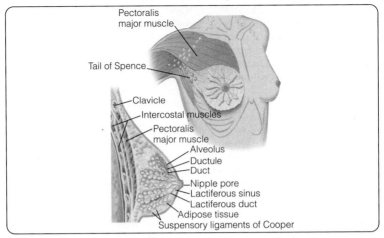

Figure 10.2 • Anterior and lateral views of breast anatomy.

INFANTS AND CHILDREN

The breast tissue of newborns is sometimes swollen because of the hyperestrogenism of pregnancy. Some infants may produce a thin discharge called "witch's milk." This secretion subsides as the infant's body eliminates maternal hormones.

Breast tissue starts to enlarge in females with the onset of puberty, usually between the ages of 9 and 13. Changes are correlated with an increased level of estrogen and progesterone in the body as sexual maturity progresses. Adolescent males may experience temporary breast enlargement, called **gynecomastia,** in one or both breasts. It is usually self-limiting and resolves spontaneously. Another concern to adolescent males is transient masses beneath one areola or both. These "breast buds" usually disappear within a year of onset.

THE PREGNANT FEMALE

During pregnancy, breast tissue enlarges as glandular and ductal tissue increases in preparation for lactation. During the second month of pregnancy, nipples and areolae darken in color and enlarge. Nipples may leak **colostrum** in the month prior to childbirth. As breast tissue enlarges, venous networks may be more pronounced.

THE OLDER ADULT

As menopause approaches, there is a decrease in glandular tissue, which is replaced by fatty tissue. The lobular texture of glandular tissue is replaced by a finer, granular texture. Breasts are less firm and tend to be more pendulous. As the suspensory ligaments relax, breast tissue hangs more loosely from the chest wall. The nipples become smaller and flatter and lose some erectile ability. The inframammary ridge thickens and can be palpated more easily.

Gynecomastia may occur in older adult males as a result of hormonal changes due to disease or medication. The nurse must be sensitive to possible embarrassment during the exam.

PSYCHOSOCIAL CONSIDERATIONS

A client's overall sense of self-esteem may be reflected in the way she feels about her breasts. Clients whose breasts are smaller or larger than average, clients with asymmetric breasts, and clients who have had a mastectomy or other breast surgery or trauma are at an increased risk for body image disturbance, self-esteem disturbance, and dysfunctional grieving.

The recommendations for early detection of breast cancer include biennial screening mammography for women between the ages of 50 and 74 years. Beginning biennial mammography before the age of 50 should be an individual decision and include cancer risk, and values regarding benefit and harm associated with mammography. Additionally, the American Cancer Society (2009) recommends annual clinical breast examination by a healthcare provider every 3 years for women from age 20 to 40 years and annually thereafter. Further, the American Cancer Society (2009) states that women should know how their breasts normally feel and report changes to their healthcare provider. Breast Self-Examination (BSE) is an option for women to consider beginning at the age of 20.

Many females do not perform BSE even after receiving instruction in the procedure. In addition, many do not seek medical attention after discovering a breast lump. These behaviors may be related to anxiety and fear of cancer or surgery, a body image change, or a change in significant relationships. The procedure for teaching BSE appears in Box 10.1

Box 10.1   **Teaching Breast Self-Examination (BSE)**

1. Teach the client to observe her breasts in front of a mirror and in good lighting. Tell her to observe her breasts in four positions:
   - With her arms relaxed and at her sides
   - With her arms lifted over her head
   - With her hands pressed against her hips
   - With her hands pressed together at the waist, leaning forward
   Instruct her to look at each breast individually, and then to compare them. She should observe for any visible abnormalities, such as lumps, dimpling, deviation, recent nipple retraction, irregular shape, edema, discharge, or asymmetry.

2. Teach the client to palpate both breasts while standing or sitting, with one hand behind her head. Tell her that many women palpate their breasts in the shower because water and soap make the skin slippery and easier to palpate. Show the client how to use the pads of her fingers to palpate all areas of her breast, using the concentric circles technique. Tell her to press the breast tissue gently against the chest wall and to be sure to palpate the axillary tail.

3. Instruct the client to palpate her breasts again while lying down, as described in step 2. Suggest that she place a folded towel under the shoulder and back on the side to be palpated. The arm on the examining side should be over her head, with the hand under the head.

4. Teach the client to palpate the areolae and nipples next. Show her how to compress the nipple to check for discharge.

5. Remind the client to use a calendar to keep a record of when she performs BSE. Teach her to perform BSE at the same time each month, usually 5 days after the onset of menses, when there is less hormonal influence on tissues.

6. Remind clients who are postmenopausal to continue monthly BSE. They should perform the exam at the same time each month.

CULTURAL CONSIDERATIONS

Assessment and findings are influenced by culture. See the cultural considerations box for specific examples.

Cultural Considerations

- Caucasian females over 40 years of age have a higher incidence of breast cancer than any other racial or ethnic group.
- African American females under 40 have a slightly higher incidence of breast cancer than Caucasians.
- Hispanics and Asians have the lowest rates of breast cancer; however, breast cancer is the leading cause of cancer deaths in Hispanic females.
- Minority females who are not well educated are more inclined to fear that a diagnosis of breast cancer means certain mortality; therefore, they avoid diagnostic procedures.
- Hispanic females put themselves last in terms of family health care. As a result, they may not seek preventive care nor seek help until symptoms appear.
- Asian females often exhibit stoicism and do not seek preventive care, but only seek help when symptoms are severe.
- Females in many immigrant cultures were raised in environments in which looking at or touching oneself is prohibited. As a result they do not conduct breast self-examinations.
- Females in immigrant cultures often distrust "medicine" and seek help from cultural healers.
- Language is a barrier for many females of immigrant cultures. Lack of information about breast health in native languages prevents them from seeking preventive services and health care for breast disease.
- Females in many cultures have concerns about disrobing and being examined by others, especially when the examiner is of the opposite sex.

Gathering the Data

FOCUSED INTERVIEW QUESTIONS

1. Describe your breasts today. How do they differ, if at all, from 3 months ago? From 3 years ago?
2. Are you still menstruating? What was the date of your last menstrual period?
3. Have you or any female family member ever had breast cancer, surgery, or diseases?
4. Have you ever had a mammogram? Do you perform breast self-examination?

QUESTIONS FOR PREADOLESCENTS

1. How do you feel about your breasts and the way they are changing?

QUESTIONS FOR THE PREGNANT FEMALE

1. What changes in your breasts have you noticed since your last examination?

QUESTIONS FOR THE OLDER ADULT

All of the preceding questions apply to the menopausal and postmenopausal client.

Physical Assessment

Physical assessment of the breasts and axillae follows an organized pattern. It begins with a client survey followed by inspection of the breasts while the client assumes a variety of positions. Palpation includes the entire surface of each breast, including the tail of Spence, and the lymph nodes of the axillae.

EQUIPMENT

examination gown and drape
clean, nonsterile examination gloves

small pillow or rolled towel
metric ruler

HELPFUL HINTS

- Provide an environment that is warm, comfortable, and private to relieve client anxiety.
- Provide specific instructions to the client; state whether the client must sit, stand, or lie down during a procedure.
- Exposure of the breasts is uncomfortable for many females. Use draping techniques to maintain the client's dignity.
- Explore cultural and language barriers at the onset of the interaction.
- In many Hispanic cultures, touching of the breasts is considered inappropriate. Explain the reasons for the examination and provide education about breast self-examination.
- Nonsterile examination gloves may be required to prevent infection when clients have lesions or drainage in and around the breasts.
- Use Standard Precautions.

TECHNIQUES AND NORMAL FINDINGS	ABNORMAL FINDINGS SPECIAL CONSIDERATIONS

INSPECTION OF THE BREAST

1. **Position the client.**
   - The client should sit comfortably and erect with the gown at the waist so both breasts are exposed (Figure 10.3).

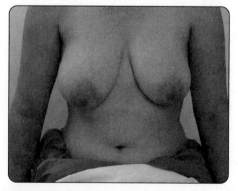

Figure 10.3 • The client is seated in the beginning of the breast examination.

TECHNIQUES AND NORMAL FINDINGS	ABNORMAL FINDINGS SPECIAL CONSIDERATIONS

2. **Inspect and compare size and symmetry of the breasts.**
   - One breast may normally be slightly larger than the other.

▶ Obvious masses, flattening of the breast in one area, dimpling, or recent increase in the size of one breast may indicate abnormal growth or inflammation.

3. **Inspect for skin color.**
   - Color should be consistent with the rest of the body. Observe for thickening, tautness, redness, rash, or ulceration.

▶ Inflamed skin is red and warm. Edema from blocked lymphatic drainage in advanced cancer causes an "orange peel" appearance called **peau d'orange.**

4. **Inspect for venous patterns.**
   - Venous patterns are the same bilaterally. Venous patterns may be more predominant in pregnancy or obesity.

▶ Pronounced unilateral venous patterns may indicate increased blood flow to a malignancy.

5. **Inspect for moles or other markings.**
   - Moles that are unchanged, nontender, and long-standing are of no concern. Striae that are present in pregnancy or recent weight loss or gain may appear purple in color. Striae become silvery white over time.

▶ Moles that have changed or appear suddenly require further evaluation. A mole along the milk line may be a supernumerary nipple.

6. **Inspect the areolae.**
   - The areolae are normally round or oval and almost equal in size. Areolae are pink in light-skinned people and brown in dark-skinned people. The areolae darken in pregnancy.

▶ Peau d'orange associated with cancer may be first seen on the areolae. Redness and fissures may develop with breast-feeding.

7. **Inspect the nipples.**
   - Nipples are normally the same color as the areolae and are equal in size and shape. Nipples are generally everted but may be flat or inverted. Nipples should point in the same direction outward and slightly upward. Nipples should be free of cracks, crust, erosions, ulcerations, pigment changes, or discharge.

▶ Recent retraction or inversion of a nipple or change in the direction of the nipple is suggestive of malignancy. Discharge requires cytologic examination. A red, scaly eczema-like area over the nipple could indicate Paget's disease, a rare type of breast cancer. The area may exude fluid, scale, or crust.

TECHNIQUES AND NORMAL FINDINGS	ABNORMAL FINDINGS SPECIAL CONSIDERATIONS

8. **Observe the breasts for shape, surface characteristics, and bilateral pull of suspensory ligaments.**
   - Ask the client to assume the following positions while you continue to inspect the breasts:
     - Inspect with the client's arms over the head, with the client's hands pressed against her waist, with the hands pressed together at the level of the waist, and with the client leaning forward from the waist.
   - The breasts normally fall freely and evenly from the chest.

   ▶ Breast cancer should be suspected if the breasts do not fall freely from the chest.

PALPATION OF THE BREAST

1. **Position the client.**
   - Ask the client to lie down. Cover the breast that is not being examined. Place a small pillow or rolled towel under the shoulder of the side to be palpated and position the client's arm over her head. This maneuver flattens the breast tissue over the chest wall.

2. **Palpate skin texture.**
   - Skin texture should be smooth with uninterrupted contour.

   ▶ Thickening of the skin suggests an underlying carcinoma.

3. **Palpate the breast.**
   - Use the finger pads of the first three fingers in a slightly rotary motion to press the breast tissue against the chest wall. Be sure to palpate the entire breast. Several patterns may be used, but the most common is the vertical strip pattern (Figure 10.4).

   ▶ The incidence of breast cancers is highest in the upper outer quadrant, including the axillary tail of Spence. Masses in the tail must be distinguished from enlarged lymph nodes.

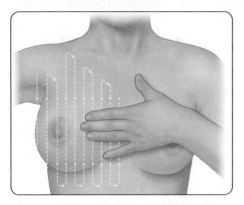

Figure 10.4 • The vertical strip method for palpation of the breast.

- An alternate pattern is concentric circles. Start at the periphery and palpate into a small circle until you reach the nipple (Figure 10.5).

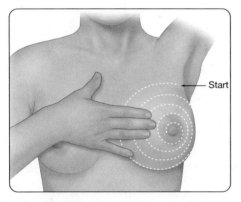

Figure 10.5 • The concentric circle pattern for palpation of the breast.

- In female clients with pendulous breasts, palpate with one hand under the breast to support it and the other hand pushing against breast tissue in a downward motion.

TECHNIQUES AND NORMAL FINDINGS	ABNORMAL FINDINGS SPECIAL CONSIDERATIONS

4. **Palpate the nipple and areolae.**
   - Compress the tissue between the thumb and forefinger to observe for drainage. Confirm that the nipple is free of discharge, that it is nontender, and that the areola is free of masses.
   - Repeat steps 1 through 5 on the other breast.

▶ Lactation not associated with childbearing is called **galactorrhea.** It occurs most commonly with endocrine disorders or medications including some antidepressants and antihypertensives.

Unilateral discharge from the nipple is suggestive of benign breast disease, an intraductal papilloma, or cancer.

EXAMINATION OF THE AXILLAE

1. **Instruct the client.**
   - Explain that you will be examining the axillae by looking and palpating. Tell the client that she will sit for this examination and you will support the arm while palpating with the other hand. Explain that relaxation will make the examination more comfortable. Tell the client to inform you of any discomfort.

2. **Position the client.**
   - Ask the client or assist the client to assume a sitting position. Flex the arm at the elbow and support it on your arm. Note the presence of axillary hair. Confirm that the axilla is free of redness, rashes, lumps, or lesions. With the palmar surface of your fingers, reach deep into the axilla. Gently palpate the anterior border of the axilla (anterior or subpectoral nodes), the central aspect along the rib cage (central nodes), the posterior border (subscapular/posterior nodes), and along the inner aspect of the upper arm (lateral nodes).

▶ Infections of the breast, arm, and hand cause enlargement and tenderness of the axillary lymph nodes. Hard, fixed nodes are suggestive of cancer or lymphoma. Clients who have had a wide local excision (removal of tumor and narrow margin of normal tissue) or mastectomy (removal of tumor and extensive areas of surrounding tissue) need to be examined carefully. The remaining tissue on the chest wall should be palpated as it would be for nonsurgical clients.

TECHNIQUES AND NORMAL FINDINGS	ABNORMAL FINDINGS SPECIAL CONSIDERATIONS

INSPECTION OF THE MALE BREAST

1. **Instruct the client.**
   - Explain all aspects of the procedure and the purpose for each part of the examination.

2. **Position the client.**
   - The client is in the sitting position with the gown at the waist.

3. **Inspect the male breasts.**
   - Observe that breasts are flat and free of lumps or lesions.

PALPATION OF THE MALE BREAST AND AXILLAE

1. **Position the client.**
   - Place the client in a supine position.

2. **Instruct the client.**
   - Explain that you will be using the pads of your fingers to gently palpate the breast area. Instruct the client to report any discomfort.

3. **Palpate the male breasts.**
   - Using the finger pads of the first three fingers, gently palpate the breast tissue, using concentric circles until you reach the nipple. The male breast feels like a thin disk of tissue under a flat nipple and areola.

▶ Gynecomastia (breast enlargement in males) is a temporary condition seen in infants, at puberty, and in older males. In older males it may accompany hormonal treatment for prostate cancer. Breast cancer in the male is usually identified as a hard nodule fixed to the nipple and underlying tissue. Nipple discharge may be present.

4. **Palpate the nipple.**
   - Compress the nipple between your thumb and forefinger.
   - The nipple should be free of discharge.

5. **Repeat on the other breast.**

6. **Palpate the axillae.**
   - Palpate axillary nodes in the male as you would for the female.

Abnormal Findings

Some of the problems identified during the physical assessment are entirely within the realm of nursing and are addressed with appropriate nursing interventions. Some problems, however, require collaborative management. Benign breast disease, fibroadenoma, intraductal papilloma, mammary duct ectasia, and breast cancer are the most common breast conditions that will challenge the nurse and the rest of the healthcare team.

COMMON ABNORMALITIES OF THE MALE BREAST

Male breast tissue is similar to that of the female. Therefore, changes in relation to hormone secretion and disease occur. Gynecomastia and carcinoma are the two common abnormalities in the male breast.

11

Cardiovascular System

The cardiovascular system circulates blood continuously throughout the body to deliver oxygen and nutrients to the body's organs and tissues and to dispose of their excreted wastes.

ANATOMY AND PHYSIOLOGY REVIEW

The **heart** lies behind the sternum in a thin sac called the pericardium. The heart extends from the second rib to the fifth intercostal space. It sits obliquely within the thoracic cavity between the lungs and above the diaphragm in the **mediastinal space.** The heartbeat is most easily palpated over the apex, a point referred to as the point of maximum impulse (PMI).

The heart wall is composed of three layers—**epicardium, myocardium,** and **endocardium.**

The heart is composed of four chambers, the right and left atria and the right and left ventricles (Figure 11.1). The right side of the heart receives deoxygenated blood from the body and sends it to the lungs. The left side of the heart receives the oxygenated blood from the lungs and pumps it to the body.

The **atrioventricular (AV) valves** separate the atria from the ventricles. The tricuspid valve lies between the right atrium and the right ventricle, whereas the thicker mitral (bicuspid) valve lies between the left atrium and left ventricle.

The **semilunar valves** separate the ventricles from the vascular system. The pulmonary semilunar valve separates the right ventricle from the trunk of the pulmonary arteries, whereas the aortic semilunar valve separates the left ventricle from the aorta.

HEART SOUNDS

Closure of the valves of the heart gives rise to heart sounds (see Table 11.1). Normal heart sounds include S_1 and S_2. These are heard as the *lub-dub* of the heart when auscultated over the precordium, the area of the chest that lies over the heart. The first heart sound, S_1 (*lub*), is heard when the AV valves close. The second heart sound, S_2 (*dub*), occurs when the aortic and pulmonic valves close. The heart sounds are associated with the contraction and relaxation phases of the heart.

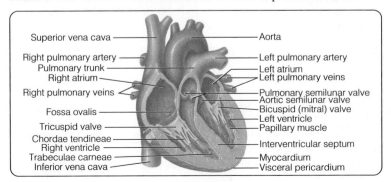

Figure 11.1 • Structural components of the heart.

141

Table 11.1 Characteristics of Heart Sounds

HEART SOUNDS		CARDIAC CYCLE TIMING	AUSCULTATION SITE	POSITION	PITCH
S_1 S_2 LUB — dub		Start of systole	Best at apex with diaphragm	Position does not affect the sound	High
S_1 S_2 lub — DUB		End of systole	Both at 2nd ICS; pulmonary component best at LSB; aortic component best at RSB with diaphragm	Sitting or supine	High
S_1 S_2 S_3		Early diastole right after S2	Apex with the bell	Auscultated better in left lateral position or supine	Low
S_1 S_2 S_4		Late diastole right before S1	Apex with the bell	Auscultated in almost a left lateral position or supine	Low

Two other heart sounds that may be present in some healthy individuals are S_3 and S_4. S_3 is heard after S_2 and is termed a *ventricular gallop*. The S_4 is heard before S_1 and is termed an *atrial gallop*.

Heart sounds are interpreted according to the characteristics of pitch, duration, intensity, phase, and location on the precordium. Table 11.1 provides information about the characteristics of heart sounds.

Heart murmurs are harsh, blowing sounds caused by disruption of blood flow into the heart, between the chambers of the heart, or from the heart into the pulmonary or aortic systems. (See Table 11.2.)

CARDIAC CONDUCTION SYSTEM

The **sinoatrial (SA) node** initiates the electrical impulse. The SA node is located at the junction of the superior vena cava and right atrium. The autonomic nervous system feeds into the SA node.

Table 11.2 Distinguishing Heart Murmurs

Murmurs are graded on a rather subjective scale of 1–6:

- Grade 1: Barely audible with stethoscope, often considered physiologic not pathologic. Requires concentration and a quiet environment.
- Grade 2: Very soft but distinctly audible.
- Grade 3: Moderately loud; there is no thrill or thrusting motion associated with the murmur.
- Grade 4: Distinctly loud, in addition to a palpable thrill.
- Grade 5: Very loud, can actually hear with part of the diaphragm of the stethoscope off the chest; palpable thrust and thrill present.
- Grade 6: Loudest, can hear with the diaphragm off the chest; visible thrill and thrust.

The **intra-atrial conduction pathway,** loosely organized conducting fibers, assist in the propagation of the electrical current emitted from the SA node through the right and left atrium.

The **atrioventricular (AV) node** and **bundle of His** function to receive the current that spread throughout the atria. Here the impulse is slowed for about 0.1 second before it passes onto the bundle branches. The AV node is also capable of initiating electrical impulses in the event of SA node failure.

The right and left **bundle branches** spread the electrical current through the ventricular myocardial tissue. Arising from bundle branches are the **Purkinje fibers.** These fibers fan out and penetrate into the myocardial tissue to spread the current into the tissues themselves. Both sympathetic nervous fibers and parasympathetic nervous fibers interact with the myocardial tissue.

LANDMARKS FOR CARDIOVASCULAR ASSESSMENT

Landmarks for assessing the cardiovascular system include the sternum, clavicles, and ribs. These are depicted in Figure 11.2.

CARDIAC CYCLE

The **cardiac cycle** describes the events of one complete heartbeat—that is, the contraction and relaxation of the atria and ventricles. The cardiac cycle can be divided into three periods: ventricular filling, ventricular systole, and isovolumetric relaxation. Electrical representations of the cardiac cycle are documented by deflections on recording paper. The terms describing the electrical deflections are P wave, PR interval, QRS interval, and T wave. They are recorded as an **electrocardiogram (ECG)** (Figure 11.3).

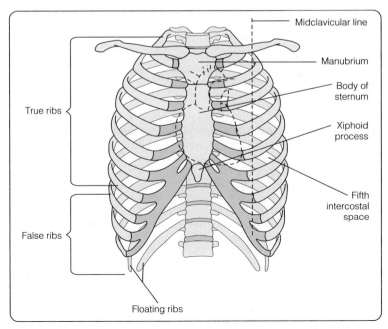

Figure 11.2 • Landmarks for cardiovascular assessment.

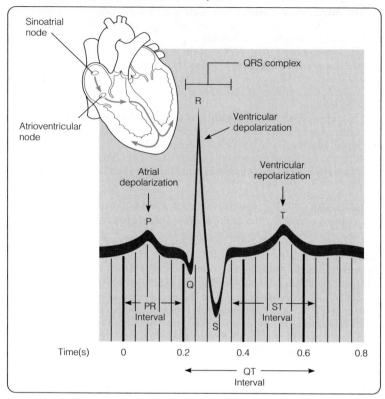

Figure 11.3 • Electrocardiogram wave.

SPECIAL CONSIDERATIONS

INFANTS AND CHILDREN

During fetal development the lungs are nonfunctional, and oxygen is carried in blood from the placenta to the right side of the heart. The majority of this blood passes through the foramen ovale to the left side of the heart, then into the aorta to enter the systemic circulation. The *foramen ovale* is a passageway for blood between the right and left atria. The rest of the blood passes through the pulmonary artery and ductus arteriosus and enters the aorta. The *ductus arteriosus* is an opening between the pulmonary artery and the descending aorta.

Inflation of the lungs at birth causes the pulmonary vasculature to dilate. Oxygenation occurs for the first time within the newborn's lungs. The foramen ovale closes shortly after birth. The ductus arteriosus closes within 24 to 46 hours in response to multiple physiologic events. The nurse should use a small diaphragm and bell with an infant or child for optimal auscultation of heart sounds.

PREGNANT FEMALE

During pregnancy the heart is displaced to the left and upward, and the apex is pushed laterally and to the left. Dilation of surface veins, together with the low resistance of the uteroplacental circulation, increases the venous return to the heart. Preexisting murmurs may become louder.

OLDER ADULT

During normal aging in the absence of disease, the heart walls may thicken to some extent. The left atrium may increase in size over time. Significant enlargement of the left ventricle can be attributed to the influence of hypertension. Aging can also contribute to the loss of ventricular compliance as the cardiac valves and large vessels become more rigid. The aorta may dilate and lengthen.

Systolic murmurs become more common as people age, especially because of aortic stenosis. These murmurs are usually best auscultated in the aortic area or base of the heart. Nonphysiologic murmurs are not normal findings. However, an S_4 sound is a common finding in older adults who do not have identified cardiovascular disease.

PSYCHOSOCIAL CONSIDERATIONS

Stress causes an individual to experience longer periods of sympathetic stimulation, which increases the workload on the heart. Systemic vascular resistance may be elevated for longer periods of time, especially in situations of excessive stress.

CULTURAL CONSIDERATIONS

Assessment and findings are influenced by culture. See the cultural considerations box for specific examples.

Cultural Considerations

- Hypertension is a risk factor for coronary heart disease. Hypertension occurs more frequently in African Americans and Hispanics than in other cultural groups.
- Obesity contributes to cardiovascular disease. Obesity is increasing in all populations in the United States but is seen in greatest numbers in Hispanic females and African American youths.
- Diabetes is a risk factor for cardiovascular disease and is increasing in incidence in Native Americans, Hispanics, and African Americans.
- Smoking contributes to cardiovascular disease. Smoking is most prevalent in African American and Hispanic males.

- Native Americans under the age of 35 have twice the heart disease mortality of other groups.
- African American females between the ages of 25 and 54 have greater risk for coronary heart disease than other groups of the same age.
- Caucasian females between the ages of 65 and 74 years have a higher incidence of cardiovascular disease than African American females.
- African Americans with heart failure have higher mortality rates than Caucasians.
- High serum cholesterol levels increase the risk for heart disease. Caucasians have higher serum cholesterol levels than African Americans.

Gathering the Data

Cardiovascular assessment includes gathering subjective and objective data. Subjective data collection occurs during the client interview, before the actual physical assessment.

FOCUSED INTERVIEW QUESTIONS

1. Describe how you are feeling. Has your sense of well-being changed in the last 2 months? Is your sense of well-being different than it was 2 years ago?
2. Are you able to perform all of the activities needed to meet your personal and work-related responsibilities?
3. Is there anyone in your family who has had a cardiovascular problem or disease?
4. Have you ever been diagnosed with a cardiovascular disease, infection, or experienced any symptoms that may suggest the presence of cardiovascular disease: activity intolerance, loss of appetite, bloody sputum (mucus), changes in sexual activities or performance, confusion or difficulty with thinking or concentrating, chest discomfort, coughing, dizziness, dyspnea (difficulty breathing), fatigue, fever, hoarseness, frequent urination at night, leg pains after activity, sleeping pattern alteration, syncope (fainting), palpitations, or swelling?
5. Have you ever had a diagnostic test, such as an electrocardiogram, stress test, or echocardiogram, or a surgical procedure for a cardiovascular problem?
6. Do you smoke or are you frequently exposed to secondhand smoke?
7. Do you take any drugs such as cocaine?
8. How would you describe your personality?

QUESTIONS REGARDING INFANTS AND CHILDREN

1. What is the child's energy level?
2. Does the infant take a long time to feed?
3. Does the infant or child favor squatting rather than sitting up straight?

QUESTIONS FOR THE PREGNANT FEMALE

1. Do you have any history of heart disease?
2. Has hypertension been apparent during this pregnancy?

QUESTIONS FOR THE OLDER ADULT

1. Have you noticed any change— no matter how subtle—in your ability to concentrate, to remember things, or to perform simple mental tasks such as writing a letter or balancing your checkbook?

Physical Assessment

Physical assessment of the cardiovascular system requires gathering objective data related to the function of the heart as determined by the heart rate and the quality and characteristics of the heart sounds. The techniques for assessment include inspection, palpation, and auscultation.

EQUIPMENT

examination gown
Doppler ultrasonic stethoscope
metric rulers

stethoscope
examination drape
lamp

HELPFUL HINTS

- Provide specific instructions throughout the assessment. Explain what is expected of the client and state that he or she will be able to breathe regularly throughout the examination.
- Assessment of the heart will require several position changes; the nurse should assist the client if necessary; allow time for movement if the client is uncomfortable; and explain the purpose of the position change.
- The nurse's hands and the stethoscope should be warmed before beginning the examination.
- The room should be quiet so that subtle sounds may be heard.
- Provide adequate draping to prevent unnecessary exposure of the female breasts.
- Use Standard Precautions.

TECHNIQUES AND NORMAL FINDINGS	ABNORMAL FINDINGS SPECIAL CONSIDERATIONS

INSPECTION

1. **Inspect the client's face, lips, ears, and scalp.**
   - These structures can provide valuable clues to the client's cardiovascular health.

   ▶ Flushed skin may indicate rheumatic heart disease or presence of a fever. Grayish undertones are often seen in clients with coronary artery disease or those in shock. A ruddy color may indicate polycythemia.

2. **Inspect the jugular veins.**
   - With the client sitting upright, adjust the gooseneck lamp to cast shadows on the client's neck. Tangential lighting is effective in visualizing the jugular vessels.
   - Note that the jugular veins are not normally visible when the client sits upright. The external jugular vein is located over the sternocleidomastoid muscle. The internal jugular vein, which is the best indicator of central venous pressure, is located behind this muscle, medial to the external jugular and lateral to the carotid artery.

TECHNIQUES AND NORMAL FINDINGS	ABNORMAL FINDINGS SPECIAL CONSIDERATIONS

- If you are able to visualize the jugular veins, measure their distance superior to the clavicle. (Be sure not to confuse the carotid pulse with pulsations of the jugular veins.) The carotid pulse is lateral to the trachea. If jugular vein pulsations are visible, palpate the client's radial pulse and determine if these pulsations coincide with the palpated radial pulse.
- Next, have the client lie at a 45-degree angle if the client can tolerate this position without pain and is able to breathe comfortably.
- Place the first of the metric rulers vertically at the angle of Louis. Place the second metric ruler horizontally at a 90-degree angle to the first ruler. One end of this ruler should be at the angle of Louis and the other end in the jugular area on the lateral aspect of the neck (Figure 11.4).

▶ Obvious pulsations that are present during inspiration and expiration and coincide with the arterial pulse are commonly seen with severe congestive heart failure.

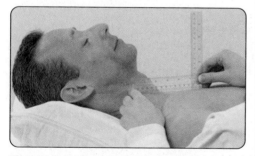

Figure 11.4 • Assessment of central venous pressure.

- Inspect the neck for distention of the jugular veins. Raise the lateral portion of the horizontal ruler until it is at the top of the height of the distention and assess the height in centimeters of the elevation from the vertical ruler.
- The jugular veins normally distend only 3 cm (1.17 in.) above the sternal angle when the client is lying at a 45-degree angle. You need to measure the distention only on one side.

▶ Distention of the neck veins indicates elevation of central venous pressure commonly seen with congestive heart failure, fluid overload, or pressure on the superior vena cava.

TECHNIQUES AND NORMAL FINDINGS	ABNORMAL FINDINGS SPECIAL CONSIDERATIONS

3. Inspect the carotid arteries.

- The carotid arteries are located lateral to the client's trachea in a groove that is medial to the sternocleidomastoid muscle.

- With the client still lying at a 45-degree angle, using tangential lighting, inspect the carotid arteries for pulsations. Pulsations should be visible bilaterally.

▶ Bounding pulses are not normal findings and may indicate fever. The absence of a pulsation may indicate an obstruction either internal or external to the artery.

4. Inspect the client's chest.

- Inspect the entire chest for pulsations. Observe the client first in an upright position and then at a 30-degree angle, which is a low- to mid-Fowler's position. In particular, observe for pulsations over the five key landmarks (Figure 11.5).

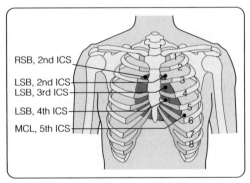

RSB, 2nd ICS
LSB, 2nd ICS
LSB, 3rd ICS
LSB, 4th ICS
MCL, 5th ICS

Figure 11.5 • Landmarks in precordial assessments.

- Inspect the entire chest for heaves or lifts while the client is sitting upright and again with the client at a 30-degree angle.

PALPATION

1. Palpate the chest in five areas. You should not feel any pulsation, heave, or vibratory sensation against your palm except when palpating over the MCL, fifth ICS, when you should feel a soft vibration, a tapping sensation, with each heartbeat.

▶ Pulsations or heaves are associated with valvular disease, increased pressure or enlargement of the heart.

▶ **Thrills** are soft vibratory sensations best assessed with either the fingertips or the palm flattened on the chest.

TECHNIQUES AND NORMAL FINDINGS	ABNORMAL FINDINGS SPECIAL CONSIDERATIONS

2. **Palpate the client's carotid pulses.**
   Palpate each carotid pulse separately.
   Normal findings bilaterally should
   demonstrate equality in intensity and
   regular pattern. The pulses should be
   strong but not bounding. If the pulse is
   difficult to palpate, ask the client to turn
   the head slightly to the examining side.

▶ Diminished or absent
carotid pulses may be found
in clients with carotid disease or dissecting ascending
aneurysm. Absence of both
pulses indicates asystole
(absent heart rate). If the
client is in critical care and
has an arterial line, a print-
out of the arterial wave-
form should be obtained.

ALERT! *The carotid pulses must never be
palpated simultaneously since this may obstruct
blood flow to the brain, resulting in severe bradycar-
dia (slow heart rate) or asystole (absent heart rate).*

AUSCULTATION

1. **Auscultate the client's chest with the
   diaphragm of the stethoscope.**
   * Start the auscultation with the client
     sitting upright.
   * Inch the stethoscope slowly across
     the chest and listen over each of
     the five key landmarks (see
     Figure 11.5).
   * Listen over the RSB, second ICS.
   * In this location, the S_2 sound should be
     louder than the S_1 sound, because this
     site is over the aortic valve.
   * Listen over the LSB, second ICS.
   * Also in this location the S_2 sound should
     be louder than the S_1 sound, because
     this site is over the pulmonic valve.
   * Listen over the LSB, third ICS, also
     called Erb's point.
   * You should hear both the S_1 and S_2
     heart tones, relatively equal in intensity.
   * Listen at the LSB at the fourth ICS.
   * In this location the S_1 sound should be
     louder than the S_2 sound, because the
     closure of the tricuspid valve is best
     auscultated here.

▶ In obese clients, heart
sounds are best heard at
the apical area with the
client in the left lateral
position and at the aortic
and pulmonic areas.

TECHNIQUES AND NORMAL FINDINGS	**ABNORMAL FINDINGS SPECIAL CONSIDERATIONS**

- Listen over the apex: fifth ICS, LMCL.
- In this location the S_1 sound should also be louder than the S_2 sound, because the closure of the mitral valve is best auscultated here.

2. **Auscultate the client's chest with the bell of the stethoscope.**
   - Place the bell of the stethoscope lightly on each of the five key landmark positions shown with step 1.
   - Listen for softer sounds over the five key landmarks. Start with the bell and listen for the S_3 and S_4 sounds. Then listen for murmurs.

   ▶ Low-pitched sounds are best auscultated with light application of the bell. Sounds such as S3, S4, murmurs (originating from stenotic valves), and gallops are best heard with the bell.

3. **Auscultate the carotid arteries.**
   - Listen with the diaphragm and bell of the stethoscope. Have the client hold the breath briefly. You may hear heart tones. This finding is normal.
   - You should not hear any turbulent sounds like murmurs.

   ▶ A **bruit,** a loud blowing sound, is an abnormal finding. It is most often associated with a narrowing or stricture of the carotid artery usually associated with atherosclerotic plaque.

4. **Compare the apical pulse to a carotid pulse.**
   - Auscultate the apical pulse.
   - Simultaneously palpate a carotid pulse.
   - Compare the findings. The two pulses should be synchronous. The carotid artery is used because it is closest to the heart and most accessible.

   ▶ An apical pulse greater than the carotid rate indicates a pulse deficit. The rate, rhythm, and regularity must be evaluated.

Abnormal Findings

Ventricle Tachycardia

Ventricle tachycardia is rapid, regular heartbeat as high as 200 beats/min (Figure 11.6).

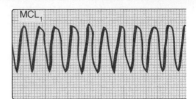

Figure 11.6 • Ventricle tachycardia.

Ventricular Fibrillation

Ventricular fibrillation is total absence of regular heart rhythm (Figure 11.7).

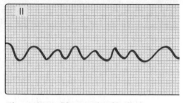

Figure 11.7 • Ventricular fibrillation.

Heart Block

Slow heart rate can be as low as 20 to 40 beats/min (Figure 11.8). Conduction between the atria and ventricles is disrupted.

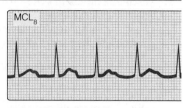

Figure 11.8 • Heart block.

Atrial Flutter

The atrial rate can be as high as 200 beats/min and exceeds the ventricular response and rate (Figure 11.9).

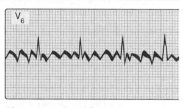

Figure 11.9 • Atrial flutter.

Atrial Fibrillation

Atrial fibrillation is dysrhythmic atrial contraction with no regularity or pattern (Figure 11.10).

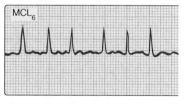

Figure 11.10 • Atrial fibrillation.

12
Peripheral Vascular System

The **peripheral vascular system** is made up of the blood vessels of the body. Together with the heart and the lymphatic vessels, they make up the body's circulatory system, which transports blood and lymph throughout the body.

ANATOMY AND PHYSIOLOGY REVIEW

The peripheral vascular system is composed of arteries, veins, and lymphatics. The parts of the peripheral vascular and lymphatic systems are depicted in Figure 12.1, Figure 12.2, Figure 12.3, Figure 12.4, and Figure 12.5.

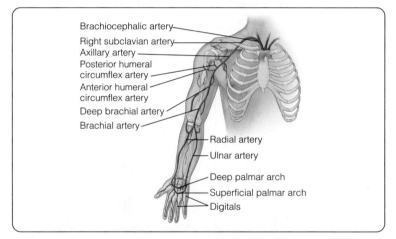

Brachiocephalic artery
Right subclavian artery
Axillary artery
Posterior humeral circumflex artery
Anterior humeral circumflex artery
Deep brachial artery
Brachial artery
Radial artery
Ulnar artery
Deep palmar arch
Superficial palmar arch
Digitals

Figure 12.1 • Main arteries of the arm.

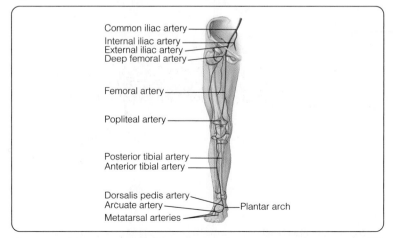

Common iliac artery
Internal iliac artery
External iliac artery
Deep femoral artery
Femoral artery
Popliteal artery
Posterior tibial artery
Anterior tibial artery
Dorsalis pedis artery
Arcuate artery
Plantar arch
Metatarsal arteries

Figure 12.2 • Main arteries of the leg.

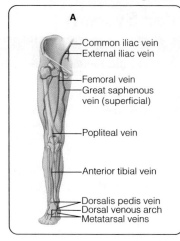

Common iliac vein
External iliac vein
Femoral vein
Great saphenous vein (superficial)
Popliteal vein
Anterior tibial vein
Dorsalis pedis vein
Dorsal venous arch
Metatarsal veins

Figure 12.3(A) • The main veins of the leg. Anterior view.

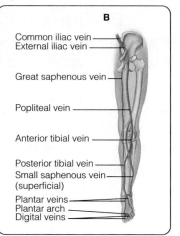

Common iliac vein
External iliac vein
Great saphenous vein
Popliteal vein
Anterior tibial vein
Posterior tibial vein
Small saphenous vein (superficial)
Plantar veins
Plantar arch
Digital veins

Figure 12.3(B) • The main veins of the leg. Posterior view.

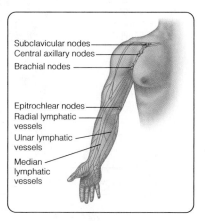

Subclavicular nodes
Central axillary nodes
Brachial nodes
Epitrochlear nodes
Radial lymphatic vessels
Ulnar lymphatic vessels
Median lymphatic vessels

Figure 12.4 • Main lymph nodes of the arm.

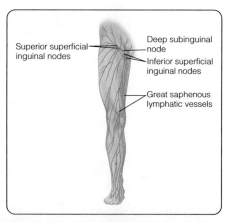

Superior superficial inguinal nodes
Deep subinguinal node
Inferior superficial inguinal nodes
Great saphenous lymphatic vessels

Figure 12.5 • Main lymph nodes of the leg.

SPECIAL CONSIDERATIONS

INFANTS AND CHILDREN

Assessing the blood pressure of an infant less than 1 year of age is difficult without special equipment. In young children, the blood pressure should be measured on the thigh. The pulse increases if the child has a fever. For every degree of fever, the pulse may increase 8 to 10 beats per minute (beats/min). The lymphatic system develops rapidly from birth until puberty and then subsides in adulthood. The presence of enlarged lymph nodes in a child may not indicate illness.

THE PREGNANT FEMALE

Blood pressure should be monitored throughout the pregnancy to test for pregnancy-induced hypertension. Pressure from the uterus on the lower extremities can obstruct venous return and lead to hypotension when the client is lying on her back, or it can cause edema, varicosities of the leg, and hemorrhoids.

THE OLDER ADULT

The aging process causes arteriosclerosis or calcification of the walls of the blood vessels. The arterial walls lose elasticity and become more rigid. This increase in peripheral vascular resistance results in increased blood pressure. The enlargement of calf veins can pose the risk of blood clots in leg veins. When evaluating the various arterial pulses, the nurse should keep in mind that the heart rate slows with the aging process. It is common for older clients to manifest irregular pulses often with occasional pauses or extra beats.

PSYCHOSOCIAL CONSIDERATIONS

Stress is among the factors that contribute to development of hypertension. An individual's ability to cope can determine the risk of developing hypertension in response to stress.

CULTURAL CONSIDERATIONS

Assessment and findings are influenced by culture. See the cultural considerations box for specific examples.

Cultural Considerations

- Skin color variations across ethnic groups may affect assessment of circulation. The nurse must use skin temperature, capillary refill, and pulse characteristics when pink undertones are not easily detected.
- African Americans have a higher incidence of hypertension than other groups.
- Diabetes increases the risk for peripheral vascular disease and is increasing in prevalence in Native Americans and Hispanics.

- Obesity is a risk factor for hypertension and peripheral vascular disease. Obesity is increasing in all groups at all ages but occurs most frequently in Hispanic females and African American children.
- Smoking increases the risk for hypertension and peripheral vascular disease. Smoking is most prevalent in African American and Hispanic males.

Gathering the Data

Health assessment of the peripheral vascular system includes gathering subjective and objective data. In physical assessment of the peripheral vascular system, the techniques of inspection, palpation, and auscultation will be used.

FOCUSED INTERVIEW QUESTIONS

1. Describe your circulation. Have you ever been diagnosed with a disease of your circulatory or lymphatic system?
2. Have you or any member of your family ever had heart problems, respiratory disease, diabetes, varicose veins, or blood clots?
3. Have you noticed any swelling or shiny skin, particularly on your legs? If yes, is the swelling in one leg or both legs?
4. Have you noticed any changes in temperature, sensation, or hair growth in your arms or legs?
5. Do you have any swollen glands? If so, where are they in your body?
6. For male clients: Have you experienced any difficulty in achieving an erection?
7. Do you ever have pains in your legs, or leg cramps? If so, please describe the pain or cramp, the location, and the time it most often occurs.
8. Do you smoke?

QUESTIONS REGARDING INFANTS AND CHILDREN

1. Has the infant become lethargic?
2. Has the child had blood pressure screening?
3. Does the child have any enlarged lymph nodes?

QUESTIONS FOR THE PREGNANT FEMALE

1. Have you had your blood pressure monitored?
2. Are you experiencing swelling of the face, hands, or legs?

QUESTIONS FOR THE OLDER ADULT

No additional questions for the older adult are required.

Physical Assessment

Physical assessment of the peripheral vascular and lymphatic systems requires the use of inspection, palpation, auscultation, and assessment of blood pressure.

EQUIPMENT

examination gown
sphygmomanometer

stethoscope
Doppler ultrasonic stethoscope

HELPFUL HINTS

- The client should don an examination gown, but undergarments may remain in place.
- The client should remove watches and jewelry that may interfere with assessment.
- Socks and stockings should be removed.
- The client will sit, stand, and lie in a supine position during various aspects of the assessment. The nurse should provide assistance and support when required and ensure that the client's respiratory effort will not be affected by moving about or when lying flat.
- Use Standard Precautions.

TECHNIQUES AND NORMAL FINDINGS	ABNORMAL FINDINGS SPECIAL CONSIDERATIONS

BLOOD PRESSURE

1. Position the client.

- Place the client in a sitting position on the examination table.

  ▶ Be sure to select the correct cuff size, especially for obese clients. Inappropriate cuff size can alter the blood pressure reading.

- Take the blood pressure in both arms. Assess the palpable systolic pressure.
- Auscultate the blood pressure.

  ▶ Assessing the palpable systolic pressure helps to avoid an inaccuracy due to auscultatory gap when auscultating blood pressure.

- The blood pressure normally does not vary more than 5 to 10 mmHg in each arm.

  ▶ A difference of 10 mmHg or more between the arms may indicate an obstruction of arterial flow to one arm.

- Table 12.1 includes current guidelines regarding interpretation of blood pressure readings for adults.

  ▶ A systolic reading below 90 or a diastolic reading under 60 may be an early indication of shock, which requires immediate medical attention.

Table 12.1	National Institutes of Health (NIH) Blood Pressure Guidelines	
BP CLASSIFICATION	**SYSTOLIC BP mmHg**	**DIASTOLIC BP mmHg**
Normal	<120	and <80
Prehypertension	120–139	or 80–89
Stage 1 Hypertension	140–159	or 90–99
Stage 2 Hypertension	≥160	or ≥100

TECHNIQUES AND NORMAL FINDINGS	ABNORMAL FINDINGS SPECIAL CONSIDERATIONS

CAROTID ARTERIES

1. Inspect the neck for carotid pulsations.

- With the client in a supine position, inspect the neck from the hyoid bone to the clavicles. Bilateral pulsations will be seen between the trachea and sternocleidomastoid muscle.

▶ The absence of pulsation may indicate internal or external obstruction.

2. Palpate the carotid pulses.

- Place the pads of your first two or three fingers on the client's neck between the trachea and the sternocleidomastoid muscle, just below the angle of the jaw.

▶ Assessment of the carotid pulses may be difficult in obese clients with short, thick necks.

- Ask the client to turn the head slightly toward your hand to relax the sternocleidomastoid muscle.

- Palpate one side of the neck at a time. If you are having difficulty finding the pulse, try varying the pressure of your fingers, feeling carefully below the angle of the jaw.

▶ A rate over 90 beats/min is considered abnormal unless the client is anxious or has recently been exercising or smoking. A rate below 60 is also considered abnormal.

- Note the rate, rhythm, amplitude, and symmetry of the carotid pulses. Compare this rate to the apical pulse.

▶ However, some athletes have a resting pulse as low as 50 beats/min. An irregular rhythm, or a pulse with extra beats or missed beats is considered abnormal. An exaggerated pulse or a weak, thready pulse is abnormal. A discrepancy between the two carotid pulses is abnormal.

3. Auscultate the carotid pulses.

- Using the diaphragm of the stethoscope, auscultate each carotid artery high in the neck, inferior to the angle of the jaw, and medial to the sternocleidomastoid muscle. Ask the client to hold his or her breath for several seconds to decrease tracheal sounds. You may need to have the client turn the head slightly to the side not being examined.

- Repeat the procedure using the bell of the stethoscope.

- While auscultating, you should hear a very quiet sound. Normal heart sounds could be transmitted to the neck, but there should be no swishing sounds.

▶ A swishing sound indicates the presence of a **bruit,** an obstruction causing turbulence, such as a narrowing of the vessel due to the buildup of cholesterol.

▶ An increased cardiac output such as that seen in hyperthyroidism or anemia also will produce a bruit.

ARMS

1. Assess the hands.
- Take the client's hands in your hands. Note the color of skin and nail beds, the temperature and texture of the skin, and the presence of any lesions or swelling. Look at the fingers and nails from the side and observe the angle of the nail base. The angle should be about 160 degrees.

2. Observe for capillary refill in both hands.
- Holding one of the client's hands in your hand, apply pressure to one of the client's fingernails for 5 seconds.
- The area under pressure should turn pale. Release the pressure and note how rapidly the normal color returns.
- In a healthy client, the color should return in less than 1 to 2 seconds.
- Repeat the procedure for the other hand.

▶ A delayed capillary refill could indicate decreased cardiac output or constriction of the peripheral vessels. However, cigarette smoking, anemia, or cold temperatures can also cause delayed capillary refill.

3. Palpate the radial pulse.
- The radial pulses are found on the ventral and medial side of each wrist. Ask the client to extend one hand, palm up.
- Palpate with two fingers over the radial bone.
- Repeat the procedure for the other arm. Note the rate, rhythm, amplitude, and symmetry of the pulses.
- Characteristics of peripheral pulse are included in Box 12.1.

▶ It is not necessary to palpate the ulnar pulses, located medial to the ulna on the flexor surface of the wrist. They are deeper than the radial pulses and are difficult to palpate.

TECHNIQUES AND NORMAL FINDINGS	ABNORMAL FINDINGS SPECIAL CONSIDERATIONS

Box 12.1 Assessing Peripheral Pulses

Assess peripheral pulses by palpating with gentle pressure over the artery. Use the pads of your first three fingers.

Note the following characteristics:

- Rate—the number of beats per minute
- Rhythm—the regularity of the beats
- Symmetry—pulses on both sides of body should be similar
- Amplitude—the strength of the beat, assessed on a scale of 0 to 4:

4 = Bounding
3 = Increased
2 = Normal
1 = Weak
0 = Absent or nonpalpable

4. Palpate both brachial pulses.

- The brachial pulses are found just medial to the biceps tendon.
- Ask the client to extend the arm.
- Palpate over the brachial artery just superior to the antecubital region.
- Repeat the procedure for the other arm.

▶ If any pulses are difficult to palpate, a Doppler flowmeter should be used. When positioned over a patent artery, this device emits sound waves as the blood moves through the artery.

5. Perform Allen's test.

- If you suspect an obstruction or insufficiency of an artery in the arm, Allen's test may determine the patency of the radial and ulnar arteries.
- Ask the client to place the hands on the knees with palms up.
- Compress the radial arteries of both wrists with your thumbs.
- Ask the client to open and close his or her fist several times.
- While you are still compressing the radial arteries, ask the client to open his or her hands.
- The palms should become pink immediately, indicating patent ulnar arteries.
- Next, occlude the ulnar arteries and repeat the same procedure to test the patency of the radial arteries.

▶ If normal color does not return, the ulnar arteries may be occluded.

▶ If normal color does not return, the radial arteries may be occluded.

| TECHNIQUES AND NORMAL FINDINGS | ABNORMAL FINDINGS SPECIAL CONSIDERATIONS |

6. **Palpate the epitrochlear lymph node in each arm.**
   - The epitrochlear node drains the forearm and the third, fourth, and fifth fingers.
   - Hold the client's right hand in your right hand. With your left hand, reach behind the elbow to the groove between the biceps and triceps muscles.
   - Note the size and consistency of the node. Normally, it is not palpable or is barely palpable.
   - Repeat the procedure for the left arm.

   ▶ An enlarged node may indicate an infection in the hand or forearm.

7. **Palpate the axillary lymph nodes.**
   - With the palmar surface of your fingers, reach deep into the axilla. Gently palpate the anterior border of the axilla (anterior or subpectoral nodes), the central aspect along the rib cage (central nodes), the posterior border (subscapular/posterior nodes), and along the inner aspect of the upper arm (lateral nodes).

LEGS

1. **Inspect both legs.**
   - Observe skin color, hair distribution, and any skin lesions.
     Hair growth should be symmetric.
     The skin should be intact with no lesions.

   ▶ If peripheral vessels are constricted, the skin will be paler than the rest of the body. If the vessels are dilated, the skin will have a reddish tone.

2. **Palpate the legs for temperature.**
   - Palpate from the feet up the legs, using the dorsal surface of your hands.
   - Note any discrepancies.
   - The skin should be the same temperature on both legs.

   ▶ If the peripheral vessels are constricted, the skin will feel cool. If the peripheral vessels are dilated, the skin will feel warm. A difference in the temperature of the feet may be a sign of arterial insufficiency.

3. **Assess the legs for the presence of superficial veins.**
   - With the client in a sitting position and legs dangling from the examination table, inspect the legs.

TECHNIQUES AND NORMAL FINDINGS	ABNORMAL FINDINGS SPECIAL CONSIDERATIONS

- Now ask the client to elevate the legs.
- The veins may appear as nodular bulges when the legs are in the dependent position, but any bulges should disappear when the legs are elevated.
- Palpate the veins for tenderness or inflammation (phlebitis).

▶ **Varicosities** (distended veins) frequently occur in the anterolateral aspect of the thigh and lower leg or on the posterolateral aspect of the calf. These bulging veins do not disappear when legs are elevated. Varicose veins are dilated but have a diminished blood flow and an increased intravenous pressure. An incompetent valve, a weakness in the vein wall, or an obstruction in a proximal vein causes varicosities.

4. **Perform the manual compression test.**
- If varicose veins are present, you can determine the length of the varicose vein and the competency of its valves with the manual compression test.
- Ask the client to stand.
- With the fingers of one hand, palpate the lower part of the varicose vein.
- Keeping that hand on the vein, compress the vein firmly at least 15 to 20 cm higher with the fingers of your other hand.
- You will not feel any pulsation beneath your lower fingers if the valves of the varicose vein are still competent.

▶ If the valves are incompetent, an impulse in the vein will be felt between your two hands.

5. **Perform Trendelenburg's test.**
- A second test to evaluate valve competence in the presence of varicosities is Trendelenburg's test.
- Assist the client to a supine position.
- Elevate the leg to 90 degrees until the venous blood has drained from the leg.
- Place a tourniquet around the upper thigh.
- Help the client to stand.
- Watch for filling of the venous system.
- The saphenous vein should fill from below in about 30 to 35 seconds.

▶ A rapid filling of the superficial veins from above indicates incompetent valves.

- After the client has been standing for 20 to 30 seconds, remove the tourniquet and note whether the varicose veins fill from above.
- Competent valves prevent sudden retrograde filling.

▶ A sudden filling of superficial veins after removing the tourniquet indicates backward filling past incompetent valves.

TECHNIQUES AND NORMAL FINDINGS

ABNORMAL FINDINGS
SPECIAL CONSIDERATIONS

6. **Test for Homans' sign.**
   - Assist the client to a supine position.
   - Flex the client's knee about 5 degrees.
   - Now sharply dorsiflex the client's foot.
   - Ask whether the client feels calf pain.
   - This maneuver exerts pressure on the posterior tibial vein and should not cause pain.

   ▶ A positive **Homans' sign** could indicate a blood clot in one of the deep veins of the leg. However, a positive Homans' sign could also indicate an inflammation of one of the superficial leg veins or an inflammation of one of the tendons of the leg. The reliability of Homans' sign in indicating disease has been shown to be inconsistent. Follow-up studies such as a venous Doppler examination may be required to identify the presence of a clot in the deep veins of the leg.

7. **Palpate the inguinal lymph nodes.**
   - Move the client's gown aside over the inguinal region. Palpate over the top of the medial thigh.
   - If the nodes can be palpated, they should be movable and not tender.
   - Repeat the procedure for the other leg.

   ▶ Lymph nodes that are larger than 1 cm or tender may be an indication of an infection in the legs.

8. **Palpate both femoral pulses.**
   - The femoral pulses are inferior and medial to the inguinal ligament.
   - Ask the client to flex the knee and externally rotate the hip. Palpate over the femoral artery.
   - The femoral artery is deep, and you may need to place one hand on top of the other to locate the pulse. Repeat the procedure for the other leg.

   ▶ If it is not possible to palpate the femoral pulse, an artery may be occluded.

9. **Palpate both popliteal pulses.**
   - The pulsations of the popliteal artery can be palpated deep in the popliteal fossa lateral to the midline.
   - Ask the client to flex the knee and relax the leg.
   - Palpate the popliteal pulse.
   - If you cannot locate the pulse, ask the client to roll onto the abdomen and flex the knee.
   - Palpate deeply for the pulse.

   ▶ If the popliteal pulse cannot be palpated, an artery may be occluded.

TECHNIQUES AND NORMAL FINDINGS	ABNORMAL FINDINGS SPECIAL CONSIDERATIONS

10. Palpate both dorsalis pedis pulses.

- The dorsalis pedis pulses may be felt on the medial side of the dorsum of the foot.
- Palpate the pulse lateral to the extensor tendon of the great toe.
- Use light pressure.

▶ The absence of a dorsalis pedis pulse may not be indicative of occlusion because another artery may be supplying blood to this area of the foot. Edema in the foot will make palpation difficult.

11. Palpate both posterior tibial pulses.

- The posterior tibial pulses may be palpated behind and slightly inferior to the medial malleolus of the ankle, in the groove between the malleolus and the Achilles tendon.
- Palpate the pulse by curving your fingers around the medial malleolus.

▶ If it is not possible to palpate the posterior tibial pulse, an artery may be occluded. If the client has edematous ankles, this pulse may be difficult to palpate.

12. Assess for arterial supply to the lower legs and feet.

- If you suspect an arterial deficiency, test for arterial supply to the lower extremities. Ask the client to remain supine.
- Elevate the client's legs 12 inches above the heart.
- Ask the client to move the feet up and down at the ankles for 60 seconds to drain the venous blood.
- The skin will be blanched in color because only arterial blood is present.
- Now ask the client to sit up and dangle the feet.
- Compare the color of both feet.
- The original color should return in about 10 seconds.
- The superficial veins in the feet should fill in about 15 seconds.
- The feet of a dark-skinned person may be difficult to evaluate, but the soles of the feet should reflect a change in color.

▶ Marked pallor of the elevated extremities may indicate arterial insufficiency.

TECHNIQUES AND NORMAL FINDINGS

ABNORMAL FINDINGS
SPECIAL CONSIDERATIONS

13. **Check for edema of the legs.**
    - Press the skin for at least 5 seconds over the tibia, behind the medial malleolus, and over the dorsum of each foot.
    - Look for a depression in the skin (called pitting edema) caused by the pressure of your fingers.
    - If edema is present, you should grade it on a scale of 1+ (mild) to 4+ (severe) (Figure 12.6).

▶ Pitting edema can be related to a failure of the right side of the heart or an obstruction of the lymphatic system. Edema in only one leg may indicate an occlusion of a large vein in the leg. Diminished arterial flow thickens toenails, which often become yellow and loosely attached to the nail bed. Clients with diabetes often acquire fungal and bacterial infections of the nail because of increased glucose collecting in the skin under the nail.

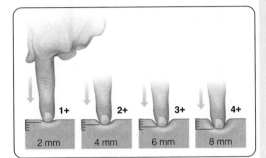

Figure 12.6 • Grading pitting edema.

14. **Inspect the toenails for color and thickness.**
    - Nails should be pink and not thickened. Clubbing should not be present.

Abnormal Findings

Findings from physical assessment of the peripheral vascular and lymphatic systems include normal and abnormal pulses (Table 12.2) and common alterations of the peripheral vascular and lymphatic systems including arterial and venous insufficiency, aneurysms, varicosities, Raynaud's disease, deep vein thrombosis, and lymphedema.

Table 12.2	Normal and Abnormal Pulses		
NAME OF PULSE	CHARACTERISTICS	ARTERIAL WAVEFORM PATTERN	CONTRIBUTING CONDITIONS
Normal	• Regular, even in intensity		• Normal
Absent	• No palpable pulse, no waveform		• Arterial line disconnected • Cardiac arrest
Weak/thready	• Intensity of pulse is +1 • May wax and wane • May be difficult to find		• Shock • Severe peripheral vascular disease
Bounding	• Intensity of pulse is +4 • Very easy to observe in arterial locations near surface of skin • Very easy to palpate and difficult to obliterate with pressure from fingertips		• Hyperdynamic states such as seen with hyperthyroidism, exercise, anxiety, vasodilation seen in high cardiac output syndromes • May be due to normal aging secondary to arterial wall stiffening • Aortic regurgitation • Anemia
Biferiens	• Has two systolic peaks with a dip in between • Easier to detect in the carotid location • In the case of hypertrophic obstructive cardiomyopathy only one systolic peak palpated, but waveform demonstrates double systolic peak		• Aortic regurgitation • Combination of aortic regurgitation and stenosis • Hypertrophic obstructive cardiomyopathy

Pulsus Alternans	• Alternating strong and weak pulses • Equal interval between each pulse		• Aortic regurgitation • Terminal left ventricular heart failure • Systemic hypertension
Pulsus Bigeminus	• Alternating strong and weak pulses, but the weak pulse comes in early after the strong pulse		• Regular bigeminal dysrhythmias such as PVCs and PACs
Pulsus Paradoxus	• Reduced intensity of pulse during inspiration versus expiration	 Expiration Inspiration	• Cardiac tamponade • Acute pulmonary embolus • Pericarditis • May be present in clients with chronic lung disease • Hypovolemic shock • Pregnancy
Water-hammer, Corrigan's Pulse	• Rapid systolic upstroke and no dicrotic notch secondary to rapid collapse		• Aortic regurgitation
Unequal	• Difference in intensity or amplitude between right and left pulses	 Right femoral Left femoral	• Dissecting aneurysm (location of aneurysm determines where the difference in amplitude is felt)

13
Abdomen

The **abdomen** is not a system unto itself. It is the largest cavity of the body and contains many organs and structures that belong to various systems of the body.

ANATOMY AND PHYSIOLOGY REVIEW

The abdomen is composed of the alimentary canal, the intestines, accessory digestive organs, the urinary system, the spleen, and reproductive organs (Figure 13.1). It is situated in the anterior region of the body, inferior to the diaphragm of the respiratory system and superior to the pelvic floor. The abdominal muscles, the intercostal margins, and the pelvis form the anterior borders of the abdomen. The vertebral column and the lumbar muscles form the posterior borders of the abdomen.

The alimentary canal is the continuous hollow tube extending from the mouth to the anus, and includes the esophagus, stomach, small intestine, and large intestine. The accessory digestive organs contribute to the digestive process of foods. These structures connect to the alimentary canal by ducts and include the liver, gallbladder, and pancreas.

Other structures to consider in the abdominal assessment include the peritoneum, muscles, aorta, kidneys, ureters, bladder, spleen, and the reproductive organs.

LANDMARKS

Landmarks for the abdomen include the xiphoid process, umbilicus, costal margin, iliac crests, and pubic bone. **Mapping** is the process of dividing the abdomen into quadrants for the purpose of examination. The identification of organs within each of the four equal quadrants of the abdomen is depicted in Figure 13.2.

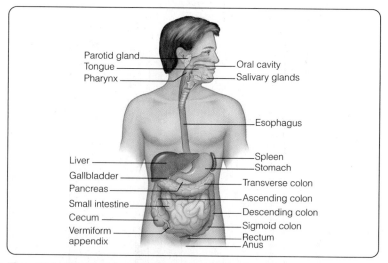

Parotid gland
Tongue
Pharynx
Oral cavity
Salivary glands
Esophagus
Liver
Gallbladder
Pancreas
Small intestine
Cecum
Vermiform appendix
Spleen
Stomach
Transverse colon
Ascending colon
Descending colon
Sigmoid colon
Rectum
Anus

Figure 13.1 • Organs of the alimentary canal and related accessory organs.

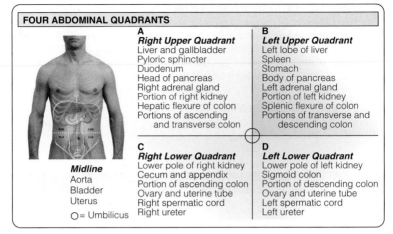

FOUR ABDOMINAL QUADRANTS

A
Right Upper Quadrant
Liver and gallbladder
Pyloric sphincter
Duodenum
Head of pancreas
Right adrenal gland
Portion of right kidney
Hepatic flexure of colon
Portions of ascending
    and transverse colon

B
Left Upper Quadrant
Left lobe of liver
Spleen
Stomach
Body of pancreas
Left adrenal gland
Portion of left kidney
Splenic flexure of colon
Portions of transverse and
    descending colon

C
Right Lower Quadrant
Lower pole of right kidney
Cecum and appendix
Portion of ascending colon
Ovary and uterine tube
Right spermatic cord
Right ureter

D
Left Lower Quadrant
Lower pole of left kidney
Sigmoid colon
Portion of descending colon
Ovary and uterine tube
Left spermatic cord
Left ureter

Midline
Aorta
Bladder
Uterus
O = Umbilicus

Figure 13.2 • Upper torso: Organs of the four abdominal quadrants.

SPECIAL CONSIDERATIONS

A variety of factors may influence health and include age, developmental level, race, ethnicity, work history, living conditions, socioeconomics, and emotional well-being.

INFANTS AND CHILDREN
The abdomen of the newborn and infant is round. The umbilical cord, containing two arteries and one vein, is ligated at the time of delivery. The stump dries and ultimately forms the umbilicus. The toddler has a characteristic "pot-belly" appearance. Respirations are abdominal; therefore, movement of the abdomen is seen with breathing. Children have the tendency to swallow more air than adults when eating, thus creating a greater sound of tympany when percussion is performed. The area of tympany on the right side of the abdomen is smaller because the liver is larger in children.

THE PREGNANT FEMALE
As the pregnancy progresses, the uterus enlarges and moves into the abdominal cavity. By the 14th week of the pregnancy, the fundus should be above the pubic bone and easily palpable. By the 36th week, the fundus is high in the abdomen, close to the diaphragm, and compresses many abdominal structures.

THE OLDER ADULT
In the older adult, the abdomen may be more rounded or protuberant due to increased adipose tissue distribution, decreased muscle tone, and reduced fibroconnective tissue. The abdomen tends to be softer and more relaxed than in the younger adult. There is a gradual decrease in secretion of saliva, digestive enzymes, peristalsis, intestinal absorption, and intestinal activity. The loss of teeth makes chewing and swallowing of food difficult. Ill-fitting, broken, or lost dentures also alter nutritional status.

PSYCHOSOCIAL CONSIDERATIONS

High stress levels may cause or aggravate abdominal problems. Self-perception may have a subtle influence on the client's weight. Clients who perceive themselves as naturally thin may show greater dedication to restricting their caloric intake and exercising to maintain that self-image. Conversely, clients who perceive themselves as naturally fat may overeat and avoid exercise, feeling that there is nothing they can do to alter their weight. Surgical scars may alter an individual's body image.

CULTURAL CONSIDERATIONS

Assessment and findings are influenced by culture. See the cultural considerations box for specific examples.

Cultural Considerations

- Chronic hepatitis C occurs more commonly in African Americans and Hispanics.
- Alcoholic and drug abuse liver disease occurs more frequently in Native Americans and African Americans.
- Gallstones and gallbladder cancer occur more frequently in Mexican Americans and Native Americans.
- African Americans have a greater incidence of colorectal cancer than Caucasians.
- *Helicobacter pylori,* a major cause of peptic ulcer disease, occurs more frequently in African Americans and Hispanics.
- Obesity is a risk factor for gastrointestinal diseases and is on the rise in the United States. Currently, 54% of adults and 25% of children in the United States are overweight.

- Adult obesity is seen more frequently in African American and Hispanic females.
- Japanese individuals are at greater risk of gastric cancer.
- Lactose intolerance occurs with greatest frequency in non-Caucasian Americans and Jewish Americans.
- Linguistic and cultural factors must be considered to avoid miscommunication and misinterpretation of information about diagnoses when caring for many immigrant populations.
- The nurse must be sensitive to cultural issues about disrobing for an abdominal assessment.
- Females may require the presence of another female during physical assessment of the abdomen, especially when the examiner is not of the same sex.

Gathering the Data

Health assessment of the abdomen includes the gathering of subjective and objective data. Subjective data collection occurs during the client interview, before the actual physical assessment.

FOCUSED INTERVIEW QUESTIONS

1. Describe your appetite and weight. Has either changed in the last 48 hours? In the last month? In the last year?

2. Describe your bowel habits. Describe the color and consistency of your stool. Do you have control of your bowels?

3. Have you or any member of your family ever been diagnosed with an abdominal disease or infection?
4. Do you have nausea, difficulty chewing or swallowing your food?
5. Are you having any abdominal pain at this time? If yes, describe the pain in relation to location, onset, duration, severity.
6. Have you recently done any traveling? Where did you travel?

QUESTIONS REGARDING INFANTS AND CHILDREN

1. Is the baby breast-fed or bottle-fed?
2. Does the baby tolerate the feeding? Is the baby colicky? What do you do to relieve the colic?
3. How much water does the baby drink?

QUESTIONS FOR THE PREGNANT FEMALE

1. Are you experiencing any nausea, vomiting, heartburn, or flatulence?
2. Are you experiencing any elimination problems such as constipation?

Physical Assessment

Physical assessment of the abdomen requires the use of inspection, auscultation, percussion, and palpation. This order differs from that of physical assessment of other systems. The nurse should remember to auscultate after inspection. Delaying percussion and palpation prevents disturbance of the normal bowel sounds.

EQUIPMENT

examination gown and drape
skin marker
clean, nonsterile examination gloves
metric ruler

examination light
tissues
stethoscope
tape measure

HELPFUL HINTS

- Provide an environment that is warm and comfortable.
- Encourage the client to void prior to the examination.
- Provide instructions about what is expected of the client, for example, taking several deep breaths to relax abdominal muscles.
- Pay attention to nonverbal cues that may indicate discomfort. Facial gestures, legs flexed at the knees, and abdominal guarding with the hands are all indices of discomfort.
- When a client is experiencing abdominal pain, examine that area last.
- Stand on the right side of the client, unless otherwise indicated, because the liver and right kidney are in the right side of the abdomen.
- Maintain the dignity of the client through appropriate draping techniques.
- Use Standard Precautions.

TECHNIQUES AND NORMAL FINDINGS	ABNORMAL FINDINGS SPECIAL CONSIDERATIONS

INSPECTION OF THE ABDOMEN

1. **Determine the contour of the abdomen.**
   - Observe the profile of the abdomen between the costal margins and the symphysis pubis.
   - The abdominal profile should be viewed at eye level. You may need to sit or kneel to observe the abdominal profile.
   - Normal findings include flat, rounded, or scaphoid contours.

   ▶ A protuberant abdomen is normal in pregnancy. It may indicate obesity or ascites in a nonpregnant client.

2. **Observe the position of the umbilicus.**
   - The umbilicus is normally in the center of the abdomen. It may be inverted or protruding. The umbilicus should be clean and free of inflammation or drainage.

   ▶ A protruding or displaced umbilicus is a normal variation in pregnant females. In the nonpregnant adult, it could indicate an abdominal mass or distended urinary bladder. Inflammation or drainage may indicate an infection or complication from recent laparoscopic surgery. A displaced or protruding umbilicus may be a sign of a hernia in a child.

   ALERT! *A client with drainage from the umbilicus following laparoscopic surgery should be referred to the physician immediately.*

3. **Observe skin color.**
   - The abdominal skin should be consistent in color and luster with the skin of the rest of the body. The skin is smooth, moist, and free of lesions.

   ▶ Taut, glistening skin could indicate ascites.

4. **Observe the location and characteristics of lesions, scars, and abdominal markings.**
   - Lesions such as macules, moles, and freckles are considered normal findings.

   ▶ **Striae,** commonly called stretch marks, are silvery, shiny, irregular markings on the skin. These are seen in obesity, pregnancy, and ascites.
   ▶ Scars indicate previous surgery or trauma and the possibility of underlying adhesions. The location of all lesions must be documented as baseline data and for determination of change in future assessment.

TECHNIQUES AND NORMAL FINDINGS	ABNORMAL FINDINGS SPECIAL CONSIDERATIONS

5. **Observe the abdomen for symmetry, bulging, or masses.**
   - First observe the abdomen while standing at the client's side. Second, observe the abdomen while standing at the foot of the examination table. Compare the right and left sides. The sides should appear symmetric in shape, size, and contour.

▶ Asymmetry may indicate masses, adhesions, or strictures of underlying structures.

6. **Observe the abdominal wall for movement.**
   - Movements can include pulsations or peristaltic waves. In thin clients it is normal to observe a pulsation of the abdominal aorta below the xiphoid process. The observation of peristaltic waves in thin clients is normal.

▶ Marked pulsations could indicate aortic aneurysm or increased pulse pressure. Increased peristaltic activity could indicate gastroenteritis or an obstructive process.

AUSCULTATION OF THE ABDOMEN

ALERT! *It is important to auscultate before percussing and palpating, because the latter techniques could alter peristaltic action.*

The pattern for auscultation of bowel sounds is to begin in the RLQ and then proceed through each of the remaining quadrants.

1. **Auscultate for bowel sounds.**
   - Use the diaphragm of the stethoscope. Start in the RLQ and move through the other quadrants. Note the character and frequency of the sounds. Count the sounds for at least 60 seconds.

▶ Hyperactive sounds are common in gastroenteritis and diarrhea. Hypoactive sounds are common following abdominal surgery and occur in end-stage intestinal obstruction. Absence of bowel sounds may indicate paralytic ileus. Bowel sounds may be difficult to hear in obese clients with large amounts of adipose tissue in the abdomen.

   - Normal bowel sounds are irregular, gurgling, and high-pitched. They occur from 5 to 320 times per minute. Borborygmi are a normal finding.

▶ Clients with paralytic ileus or intestinal obstruction require immediate attention.

| TECHNIQUES AND NORMAL FINDINGS | ABNORMAL FINDINGS SPECIAL CONSIDERATIONS |

2. **Auscultate for vascular sounds.**
   - Use the bell of the stethoscope. Listen at the midline below the xiphoid process for aortic sounds. Move the stethoscope from side to side as you listen over the renal, iliac, and femoral arteries.

▶ Bruits heard during systole and diastole may indicate arterial occlusion.

   A venous hum usually indicates increased portal tension.

3. **Auscultate for friction rubs.**
   - Auscultate the abdomen, listening for a coarse, grating sound. Listen carefully over the liver and spleen. Friction rubs are not normally heard.

PERCUSSION OF THE ABDOMEN

1. **Percuss the abdomen.**
   - Place your pleximeter finger on the abdomen during the examination. Review the technique of percussion in chapter 2. Start in the RLQ and percuss through all of the remaining quadrants.
   - Percussion over the abdomen produces tympany. Tympany is more pronounced over the gastric bubble. Dullness is heard over the liver and spleen.

▶ Dullness may indicate an enlarged uterus, distended urinary bladder, or ascites. Dullness in the LLQ may indicate the presence of stool in the colon. It is important to ask when the client last had a bowel movement.

PERCUSSION OF THE LIVER

Percuss the liver to determine the upper and lower borders at the anterior axillary line, mid-clavicular line, and midsternal line. Measure the distance between marks drawn to identify the borders.

1. **Percuss the liver.**
   - Begin percussion at the level of the umbilicus and move toward the rib cage along the extended right MCL.
   - The first sound you should hear is tympany. When the sound changes to dullness, you have identified the lower border of the liver. Mark the point with a skin-marking pen. The lower border is normally at the costal margin.
   - Percuss downward from the fourth intercostal space along the right MCL. The first sound you should hear is resonance because you are over the lung. Percuss downward until the sound changes to dullness. This is the upper border of the liver. Mark the

▶ Dullness below the costal margin suggests liver enlargement or downward displacement due to respiratory disease. Dullness above the fifth or sixth intercostal space could indicate an enlarged liver (hepatomegaly) or displacement upward due to ascites or a mass.

TECHNIQUES AND NORMAL FINDINGS	**ABNORMAL FINDINGS** **SPECIAL CONSIDERATIONS**

point with a pen. The upper border should be at the level of the sixth intercostal space.

- Measure the distance between the two points. The distance should be approximately 5 to 10 cm (2 to 4 in.). This distance is called the *liver span.*
- Percuss along the midsternal line, using the same technique as before. The liver size at the midsternal line should be approximately 4 to 8 cm (1.5 to 3 in.).
- To determine the movement of the liver with breathing, ask the client to take a deep breath and hold it. Percuss upward along the extended MCL.

▶ Movement of the liver is diminished when atelectasis or pneumothorax of the right lung exists.

- The lower liver border should descend about 1 inch. Remember, liver size is influenced by age, gender, height, and disease process.

PERCUSSION OF THE SPLEEN

The spleen is located in the left side of the abdomen. Percussion is conducted to identify enlargement of the organ.

1. **Instruct the client.**
   - Explain that you will be tapping on the left side of the client's abdomen to examine the spleen. Tell the client to continue to relax, taking deep breaths if required.

2. **Percuss the spleen.**
   - Percuss the abdomen on the left side posterior to the midaxillary line.
   - A small area of splenic dullness will usually be heard from the sixth to tenth intercostal spaces.

▶ Splenic dullness at the left anterior axillary line indicates splenomegaly, an enlarged spleen. The dull percussion sound is identifiable before an enlarged spleen is palpable. The spleen enlarges anteriorly and inferiorly.

TECHNIQUES AND NORMAL FINDINGS	ABNORMAL FINDINGS SPECIAL CONSIDERATIONS

PERCUSSION OF THE GASTRIC BUBBLE

Percussion of the gastric bubble is conducted to determine the area occupied by the stomach.

1. **Instruct the client.**
   - Explain that you will be tapping on the client's abdomen over the stomach area. Repeat the explanation about relaxation if required.

2. **Percuss the gastric bubble.**
   - Percuss the abdomen in the area between the left costal margin and the midsternal line extended below the xiphoid process.
   - The percussion sound will be tympany.

▶ A dull percussion sound suggests a stomach mass. Dull percussion sounds may occur after a meal.
▶ A very loud sound and an increased area suggest gastric dilation.

PALPATION OF THE ABDOMEN

ALERT! *Palpation of the abdomen is contraindicated in the following conditions: suspected appendicitis, dissecting abdominal aortic aneurysm, polycystic kidneys, and transplanted organs.*

1. **Lightly palpate the abdomen.**
   - Place the palmar surface of your hand on the abdomen and extend your fingers. Lightly press into the abdomen with your fingers (Figure 13.3).

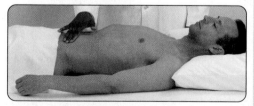

Figure 13.3 • Light palpation of abdomen.

TECHNIQUES AND NORMAL FINDINGS	ABNORMAL FINDINGS SPECIAL CONSIDERATIONS

- Move your hand over the four quadrants by lifting your hand and then placing it in another area. Do not drag or slide your hand over the surface of the skin.
- The abdomen should be soft, smooth, nontender, and pain-free.

2. Deeply palpate the abdomen.

- Proceed as for light palpation, described in the previous step. Exert pressure with your hand to depress the abdomen about 0.78 cm (2 in.).
- Palpate all four quadrants in an organized sequence.

▶ Masses, tumors, or obstructions may be palpated.

- In an obese client or a client with an enlarged abdomen, use a bimanual technique. Place the fingers of your nondominant hand over your dominant hand (Figure 13.4).

▶ In the pregnant female the uterus is palpable. The height of the fundus varies according to the week of gestation.

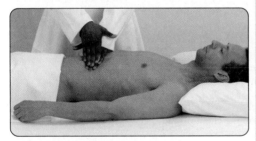

Figure 13.4 • Deep palpation of abdomen.

- Identify the size of the underlying organs and any masses for tenderness. The pancreas is nonpalpable because of its size and location.

▶ A mass in the LLQ may be stool in the colon.
▶ A vaguely palpable sensation of fullness in the epigastric region may be pancreatic in origin.

ADDITIONAL PROCEDURES

1. Palpate the aorta for pulsations.

- Using your fingertips, press deeply and firmly in the upper abdomen to the left of midline below the xiphoid process.
- The average adult aorta is 3 cm (1.17 in.) wide.

▶ Obesity and masses make palpation of the aorta difficult.
▶ The widened aorta may indicate aneurysm.

TECHNIQUES AND NORMAL FINDINGS	ABNORMAL FINDINGS SPECIAL CONSIDERATIONS

2. Palpate for rebound tenderness.

- With the client in a supine position, hold your hand at a 90-degree angle to the abdominal wall in an area of no pain or discomfort. Press deeply into the abdomen, using a slow steady movement.
- Rapidly remove your fingers from the client's abdomen.
- Ask if the client feels any pain. Normally, the client feels the pressure but no pain.

▶ The experience of sharp stabbing pain as the compressed area returns to a noncompressed state is known as **Blumberg's sign.** This finding occurs in peritoneal irritation and requires immediate medical attention. Pain referred to McBurney's point 0.39 to 0.78 cm (I to 2 in.), above the anterosuperior iliac spine, on a line between the ileum and the umbilicus) on palpation of the left lower abdomen is Rovsing's sign, suggestive of peritoneal irritation in appendicitis.

3. Percuss the abdomen for ascites.

- **Ascites** is an abnormal collection of fluid in the peritoneal cavity. With the client in a supine position, percuss at the midline to elicit tympany. Continue to percuss in lateral directions away from the midline and listen for dullness.
- Mark the skin, identifying possible levels of fluid.
- An alternative method, called *shifting dullness,* is to position the client on the right or left side. Percuss the abdomen. Because fluid settles, anticipate tympany at a superior level and dullness at lower levels.
- If ascites is suspected, measure the abdominal girth with a tape measure.

▶ Ascites is found in congestive heart failure, cirrhosis, and renal failure, and in many types of cancer.
▶ Ascites may occur in morbid obesity due to portal hypertension resulting from pressure on the abdominal blood vessels.

4. Test for psoas sign.

- Perform this test when lower abdominal pain is present and you suspect appendicitis.
- With the client in a supine position, place your left hand just above the level of the client's right knee. Ask the client to raise the leg to meet your hand. Flexion of the hip causes contraction of the psoas muscle (Figure 13.5).

▶ Pain during this maneuver is indicative of irritation of the psoas muscle associated with the peritoneal inflammation or appendicitis.

TECHNIQUES AND NORMAL FINDINGS	ABNORMAL FINDINGS SPECIAL CONSIDERATIONS

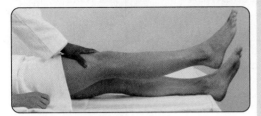

Figure 13.5 • Psoas sign.

- Normally there is no abdominal pain associated with this maneuver.

5. Test for Murphy's sign.
  - While palpating the liver, ask the client to take a deep breath. The diaphragm descends, pushing the liver and gallbladder toward your hand. In a healthy client, liver palpation is painless.

▶ Sharp abdominal pain and the need to halt the examination is a positive Murphy's sign. This occurs in clients with cholecystitis.

Abnormal Findings

ABNORMAL ABDOMINAL SOUNDS

When conducting an abdominal assessment, the nurse auscultates for bowel sounds and for vascular sounds. Table 13.1 includes information for interpretation of abnormal abdominal sounds.

ABDOMINAL PAIN

Pain is associated with acute and chronic conditions that affect the digestive organs and abdominal structures. Table 13.2 provides information about several disorders that cause abdominal pain. Disruption of function of the abdominal structures may result in referred pain. **Referred pain** is located where the development of structures occurred in the fetus.

Table 13.1	Abnormal Abdominal Sounds	
SOUND	**LOCATION**	**CAUSATIVE FACTORS**
Bowel Sounds		
Hyperactive sounds	Any quadrant	Gastroenteritis, diarrhea
Hyperactive sounds followed by absence of sound	Any quadrant	Paralytic ileus
High-pitched sounds with cramping	Any quadrant	Intestinal obstruction
Vascular Sounds		
Systolic bruit (blowing)	Midline below xiphoid	Aortic arterial obstruction
	Left and right lower costal borders at clavicular line	Stenosis of renal arteries
	Left and right abdomen at clavicular line between umbilicus and anterior iliac spine	Stenosis of iliac arteries
Venous hum (continuous tone)	Epigastrium and around umbilicus	Portal hypertension
Rubbing		
Friction rub (harsh, grating)	Left and right upper quadrants, over liver and spleen	Tumor or inflammation of organ

ABDOMINAL HERNIAS

A **hernia,** commonly called a rupture, is a protrusion of an organ or structure through an abnormal opening or weakened area in a body wall. The abdominal wall is the most common site of hernias. This weakening could be congenital or acquired. If the protruding or displaced abdominal contents return to their normal position when the client relaxes, the hernia is said to be reducible or reduced. When the displaced or protruding structures do not return to their normal position, the hernia is said to be incarcerated or nonreducible. An incarcerated hernia can become strangulated. In strangulated hernias, the blood supply to the displaced abdominal contents is compromised. The strangulated visceral contents can become gangrenous. Overstretched rectus muscles with weakened fascia cause an umbilical hernia.

Table 13.2 Pain in Common Abdominal Disorders

DISORDER	DEFINITION	PAIN CHARACTERISTICS	PRECIPITATING FACTORS
Appendicitis	Acute inflammation of vermiform appendix	Epigastric and periumbilical Localizes to RLQ Sudden onset	Obstruction (fecal stone, adhesions)
Cholecystitis	Acute or chronic inflammation of wall of gallbladder	RUQ, radiates to right scapula Sudden onset	Fatty meals, obstruction of duct in cholelithiasis
Diverticulitis	Inflammation of diverticula (outpouches of mucosa through intestinal wall)	Cramping LLQ Radiates to back	Ingestion of fiber-rich diet, stress
Duodenal Ulcer	Breaks in mucosa of duodenum	Aching, gnawing, epigastric	Stress, use of NSAIDs
Ectopic Pregnancy	Implantation of blastocyte outside of the uterus, generally in the fallopian tube	Fullness in the rectal area Abdominal cramping, unilateral pain	Tubal damage, pelvic infection, hormonal disorders, lifting, bowel movements
Gastritis	Inflammation of mucosal lining of the stomach (acute and chronic)	Epigastric pain	Acute: NSAIDs, alcohol abuse, stress, infection Chronic: *H. pylori* Autoimmune responses
Gastroesophageal Reflux Disorder (GERD)	Backflow of gastric acid to the esophagus	Heartburn, chest pain	Food intake, lying down after meals
Intestinal Obstruction	Blockage of normal movement of bowel contents	Small intestine: aching Large intestine: spasmodic pain Neurogenic: diffuse abdominal discomfort Mechanical: colicky pain associated with distention	Mechanical: physical block from impaction, hernia, volvulus Neurogenic: manipulation of bowel during surgery, peritoneal irritation
Irritable Bowel Syndrome (Spastic Colon)	Problems with GI motility	LLQ accompanied by diarrhea and/or constipation Pain increases after eating and decreases after bowel movement	Stress, intolerated foods, caffeine, lactose intolerance, alcohol, familial linkage
Pancreatitis	Inflammation of the pancreas	Upper abdominal, knifelike, deep epigastric or umbilical area pain	Ductal obstruction, alcohol abuse, use of acetaminophen, infection

Umbilical Hernia

An *umbilical hernia* occurs at the umbilicus. The abdominal rectus muscle separates or weakens, allowing abdominal structures, usually the intestines, to push through and come closer to the skin. Umbilical hernias are more common in children than in adults.

Ventral (Incisional) Hernias

A *ventral hernia* is also known as an incisional hernia because it occurs at the site of an incision. The incision weakens the muscle, and the abdominal structures move closer to the skin. Causes include obesity, repeated surgeries, infection during the postoperative period, impaired wound healing, and poor nutrition.

Hiatal Hernia

A *hiatal hernia* is due to a weakening in the diaphragm that allows a portion of the stomach and the esophagus to move into the thoracic cavity. This hernia is classified as sliding or rolling and is more common in adults than children.

ALTERATIONS OF THE GASTROINTESTINAL TRACT

Alterations of the gastrointestinal tract include nutritional problems, eating disorders, cancers, and inflammatory diseases.

Ulcerative colitis is a recurrent inflammatory process causing ulcer formation in the lower portions of the large intestine and rectum. This condition is common in adolescents and young adults. The distribution of the inflammatory process is diffuse. The ulcerative areas abscess and later become necrotic. Diarrhea, abdominal pain, and cramping with weight loss are common symptoms of the disease process.

Esophagitis is an inflammatory process of the esophagus. It is caused by a variety of irritants. The more common causes include smoking, alcohol abuse, reflux of gastric contents, and ingestion of extremely hot or cold foods and liquids.

Peritonitis is a local or generalized inflammatory process of the peritoneal membrane of the abdomen. The precipitant can be an infectious process (pelvic inflammatory disease), perforation of an organ (ruptured duodenal ulcer), internal bleeding (ruptured ectopic pregnancy), or trauma (stab wound to abdomen).

Hepatitis is an inflammatory process of the liver. Its causes include viruses, bacteria, chemicals, and drugs. Types of hepatitis include the following.

Hepatitis A virus (HAV) infectious hepatitis is transmitted via enteric routes (feces or oral routes).

Hepatitis B virus (HBV) is transmitted parenterally, sexually, or perinatally.

Hepatitis C virus (HCV) is transmitted via blood and blood products, parenterally, and through unknown factors.

Hepatitis D virus (HDV) is the same as HBV and requires HBV to replicate.

Hepatitis E virus (HEV) is a non-A, non-B type transmitted enterically. HEV is most common in those who travel to India, Africa, Asia, and Central America.

Crohn's disease is a chronic inflammatory process of the ileum. It is sometimes called regional ileitis, which is a misnomer because it can involve any part of the lower intestinal tract. Crohn's disease is characterized by "skipped" sections of involvement. It is most common in young adults and usually has an insidious onset. The inflammation involves all layers of the intestinal mucosa. Transverse fissures develop in the bowel, producing a characteristic cobblestone appearance.

14

Urinary System

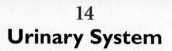

The urinary system consists of the kidneys, ureters, bladder, and urethra.

ANATOMY AND PHYSIOLOGY REVIEW

The structures of the urinary system are depicted in Figure 14.1.

LANDMARKS

During assessment of the urinary system the landmarks are the costovertebral angle, the rectus abdominis muscle, and the symphysis pubis. The **costovertebral angle (CVA)** is the area on the lower back formed by the vertebral column and the downward curve of the last posterior rib. The rectus abdominis muscles are a longitudinal pair of muscles that extend from the pubis to the rib cage on either side of the midline. The symphysis pubis is the joint formed by the union of the two pubic bones by cartilage at the midline of the body.

SPECIAL CONSIDERATIONS

The client's urinary health status is influenced by a number of factors, including age, developmental level, race, ethnicity, work history, living conditions, socioeconomics, and emotional health.

INFANTS AND CHILDREN

Renal blood flow increases with a significant allotment to the renal medulla at birth. The glomerular filtration rate also increases at birth and continues to increase until the first or second year of life.

It is important to consider the health practices of the family when the genital areas are unclean in infants or children of any age. Presence of a diaper rash

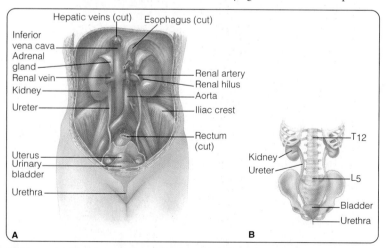

Figure 14.1 • The urinary system. A. Anterior view of the urinary organs of a female. B. Relationship of the kidneys to the vertebrae.

is a clue that the nurse should explore the family's hygiene practices; however, diaper rash is often difficult to control, and supportive teaching is indicated.

THE PREGNANT FEMALE

During the first trimester, the enlarging uterus presses against the bladder, increasing the frequency of urination. Frequency decreases during the second trimester and then recurs during the third trimester as the presenting part of the fetus descends into the pelvis and again presses on the bladder.

During pregnancy, the amount of urine produced increases, causing the client to feel the need to urinate more frequently. There is also a tendency for the urine to test positive for sugar.

THE OLDER ADULT

Renal blood flow and perfusion gradually decrease. The older adult has a reduced capacity to produce ammonia, which interacts with acids. Reduced ability to clear medications and acids, along with reduced ability to resorb bicarbonate and glucose, makes the older client more susceptible to toxicity related to medications, the effects of respiratory or metabolic acidosis, increased concentrations of glucose in the urine, and the loss of fluids.

Major changes in both males and females include urinary retention leading to increased urinary infections; involuntary bladder contractions resulting in urgency, frequency, and incontinence; decreased bladder capacity causing frequent voiding; and weakening of the urinary sphincters causing urgency and incontinence.

Nocturia (nighttime urination) is another major concern of older persons, especially males. Benign prostatic hypertrophy (hyperplasia) is a common cause of urinary retention and obstruction in males. As males age, the prostate gland enlarges, encroaching upon the urethra. Postmenopausal females experience a decrease in estrogen that affects the strength of the pubic muscles and may lead to urine leakage, reduced acidity in the lower urinary tract, and urinary tract infection (UTI).

PSYCHOSOCIAL CONSIDERATIONS

Clients suffering from incontinence are at increased risk for social isolation, self-esteem disturbance, and other psychosocial problems. Increasing BMI has been associated with stress and urge incontinence. In addition, the increased weight of adipose tissue in obesity impacts the function of the muscles of the bladder and rectal sphincters, resulting in incontinence. Incontinence in combination with decreased mobility in obese clients may result in problems with perineal and rectal hygiene leading to odor, greater risk of urinary infection, and skin irritation.

CULTURAL CONSIDERATIONS

Assessment and findings are influenced by culture. See the cultural considerations box for specific examples.

Cultural Considerations

- African Americans have a higher incidence of hypertension, which is a risk factor for chronic renal disease.
- The incidence of diabetes is increasing with highest rates in Hispanic females. Diabetes is a risk factor for urinary tract infection and chronic renal disease.
- Hygiene practices differ across cultures. Hygiene can influence the development of urinary tract infections.
- The functions of the urinary system are considered private in many cultures.

Gathering the Data

Assessment of the health of the urinary system includes gathering subjective and objective data. Subjective data collection occurs during the client interview, before the actual physical assessment.

FOCUSED INTERVIEW QUESTIONS

1. What are your normal patterns when you urinate; have you noticed any change?
2. When you urinate, do you feel you are able to empty your bladder completely?
3. Are you always able to control when you are going to urinate?
4. Do you ever have to get up at night to urinate?
5. Have you or any family member ever been diagnosed with a disease or infection of the kidney or bladder?
6. Do you have any of these problems: high blood pressure, diabetes, frequent bladder infections, kidney stones?
7. Do you ever have any pain, burning, or other discomfort before, during, or after urination in your back, sides, or abdomen?

QUESTIONS REGARDING INFANTS AND CHILDREN

1. Has the child ever been diagnosed with a kidney disorder?
2. Have you ever observed any unusual shape or structure in the child's genital anatomy?
3. Have you started toilet training with the child?

QUESTIONS FOR THE PREGNANT FEMALE

1. Have you noticed any changes in your urinary pattern?
2. Have you noticed unusual swelling in your ankles, feet, fingers, or wrists?

QUESTIONS FOR THE OLDER ADULT

1. Have you noticed any unusual swelling in your ankles, feet, fingers, or wrists?
2. *For male clients:* Have you noticed difficulty initiating the stream of urine, voiding in small amounts, and feeling the need to void more frequently than in the past?

Physical Assessment

Physical assessment of the urinary system includes the use of inspection, palpation, percussion, and auscultation.

EQUIPMENT

examination gown and drape
clean, nonsterile examination gloves

stethoscope
specimen container

HELPFUL HINTS

- Have the client empty the bladder before the examination and collect a urine specimen at that time.
- Provide clear instructions for specimen collection and provide privacy.
- Males and females respond in a variety of ways when exposed for examination of private areas. Use appropriate draping to maintain the dignity of the client.
- Explain each step of the procedures and tell the client to report any discomfort or difficulty.
- Use Standard Precautions.

TECHNIQUES AND NORMAL FINDINGS	ABNORMAL FINDINGS SPECIAL CONSIDERATIONS

1. **Assess the general appearance.**
   - Assess general appearance and inspect the client's skin for color, hydration status, scales, masses, indentations, or scars.
   - The client should not show signs of acute distress and should be mentally alert and oriented.

   ▶ Clients with kidney disorders frequently look tired and complain of fatigue. If a kidney disorder is suspected, it is important to look for signs of circulatory overload (pulmonary edema) or peripheral edema (puffy face or fingers), or indications of pruritus (scratch marks on the skin).

2. **Inspect the abdomen for color, contour, symmetry, and distention.**

   - It may be helpful to stand at the foot of the exam table and inspect the abdomen from there.

   ▶ Elevated nitrogenous wastes (azotemia) in the blood contribute to mental confusion.
   ▶ A distended bladder may be visible in the suprapubic area, indicating the need to void and perhaps the inability to do so.

TECHNIQUES AND NORMAL FINDINGS

ABNORMAL FINDINGS
SPECIAL CONSIDERATIONS

- Note that visual inspection of the suprapubic area may confirm the presence or absence of a distended bladder.
- Normally, the client's abdomen is not distended, is relatively symmetric, and is free of bruises, masses, and swellings.

3. **Auscultate the right and left renal arteries to assess circulatory sounds.**
   - Gently place the bell of the stethoscope over the extended midclavicular line (MCL) on either side of the abdominal aorta, which is located above the level of the umbilicus.
   - Be sure to auscultate both the right and left sides, and over the epigastric and umbilical areas.
   - In most cases, no sounds are heard; however, an upper abdominal bruit is occasionally heard in young adults and is considered normal. On a thin adult, renal artery pulsation may be auscultated.

THE KIDNEYS AND FLANKS

1. **Inspect the left and right costoverte-bral angles for color and symmetry.**
   - The color should be consistent with the rest of the back.

2. **Inspect the flanks (the side areas be-tween the hips and the ribs) for color and symmetry.**
   - The costovertebral angles and flanks should be symmetric and even in color.

ALERT! *Do not percuss or palpate the client who reports pain or discomfort in the pelvic region. Do not percuss or palpate the kidney if a tumor of the kidney is suspected, such as a neuroblastoma or Wilms' tumor. Palpation increases intra-abdominal pressure, which may contribute to intraperitoneal spreading of this neuroblastoma. Deep palpation should be performed only by experienced practitioners.*

▶ Many diseases may contribute to abdominal distention. These include renal conditions such as polycystic kidney disease; enlarged kidneys, as seen in acute pyelonephritis; ascites (accumulation of fluid) due to hepatic disease; and displacement of abdominal organs. Pressure from the abdominal contents on the diaphragm may alter the client's breathing pattern.

▶ A protrusion or elevation over a costovertebral angle occurs when the kidney is grossly enlarged or when a mass is present.

▶ This finding must be carefully correlated to other diagnostic cues as the assessment proceeds. If ecchymosis is present (Grey Turner's sign), there may be other signs of trauma such as blunt, penetrating wounds or lacerations.

| **TECHNIQUES AND NORMAL FINDINGS** | **ABNORMAL FINDINGS SPECIAL CONSIDERATIONS** |

3. Gently palpate the area over the left costovertebral angle.

- Watch the reaction and ask the client to describe any sensation the palpation causes. Normally, the client expresses no discomfort.

4. Use blunt or indirect percussion to further assess the kidneys.

- Place your left palm flat over the left costovertebral angle.
- Thump the back of your left hand with the ulnar surface of your right fist, causing a gentle thud over the costovertebral angle (Figure 14.2).

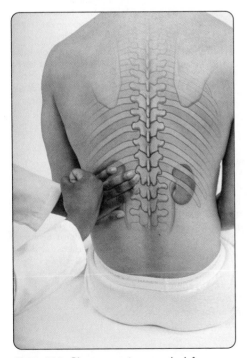

Figure 14.2 • Blunt percussion over the left costovertebral angle.

▶ Pain, discomfort, or tenderness from an enlarged or diseased kidney may occur over the costovertebral angle, flank, and abdomen. When questioned, the client complains of a dull, steady ache. This type of pain is associated with polycystic formation, pyelonephritis, and other disorders that cause kidney enlargement. In the client with polycystic kidney disease, a sharp, sudden, intermittent pain may mean that a cyst in the kidney has ruptured. If the costovertebral angle is tender, red, and warm, and the client is experiencing chills, fever, nausea, and vomiting, the underlying kidney could be inflamed or infected.

▶ The pain caused by calculi (stones) in the kidney or upper ureter is unique and different in character, severity, and duration than that caused by kidney enlargement. This pain occurs as calculi travel from the kidney to the ureters and the urinary bladder.

▶ Some clients experience no pain, and others feel excruciating pain. A stationary stone causes a dull, aching pain. As stones travel down the urinary tract, spasms occur. These spasms produce sharp, intermittent, colicky pain (often accompanied by chills, fever, nausea, and vomiting) that radiates from the flanks to the lower quadrants of the abdomen, and in some cases, the upper thigh and scrotum or labium.

TECHNIQUES AND NORMAL FINDINGS	ABNORMAL FINDINGS SPECIAL CONSIDERATIONS

▶ If the client reports severe pain, **hematuria** (blood in the urine) or **oliguria** (diminished volume of urine), and nausea and vomiting, it is important to be alert for hydroureter, a frequent complication that occurs when a renal calculus moves into the ureter. The calculus blocks and dilates the ureter, causing spasms and severe pain. Hydroureter can lead to shock, infection, and impaired renal function. If the nurse suspects hydroureter or obstruction at any point in the urinary tract, medical collaboration must be sought immediately.

- Repeat the procedure on the right side. Ask the client to describe the sensation as you examine each side.
- The client should feel no pain or tenderness with pressure or percussion.

▶ Pain or discomfort during and after blunt percussion suggests kidney disease. This finding is correlated with other assessment findings.

THE LEFT KIDNEY

1. **Attempt to palpate the lower pole of the left kidney.**
   - Although it is not usually palpable, attempt to palpate the lower pole of the kidney for size, contour, consistency, and sensation. Note that the rib cage obscures the upper poles.

▶ When enlargement occurs in the presence of conditions such as neoplasms and polycystic disease, the kidneys may be palpable. Otherwise, they are rarely palpable.

ALERT! *Because deep kidney palpation can cause tissue trauma, novice nurses should not attempt either deep palpation or capture of the kidney unless supervised by an experienced nurse or nurse practitioner. Deep kidney palpation should not be done in clients who have had a recent kidney transplant or an abdominal aortic aneurysm.*

TECHNIQUES AND NORMAL FINDINGS	ABNORMAL FINDINGS SPECIAL CONSIDERATIONS

- Position the client in a supine position. All palpation should be performed from the client's right side.
- While standing on the client's right side, reach over the client and place your left hand between the posterior rib cage and the iliac crest (the left flank).
- Place your right hand on the left upper quadrant of the abdomen lateral and parallel to the left rectus muscle just below the costal margin.
- Instruct the client to take a deep breath. As the client inhales, lift the client's left flank with your left hand and press deeply with your right hand (approximately 4 cm) to attempt to palpate the lower pole of the kidney.

▶ Care must be taken not to mistake an enlarged spleen for an enlarged left kidney. An enlarged kidney feels smooth and rounded, whereas an enlarged spleen feels sharper, with a more delineated edge.

2. **Attempt to capture the left kidney.**
- Because of its position deep in the retroperitoneal space, the left kidney is not normally palpable. The capture maneuver may enable you to palpate it. This maneuver is possible because the kidneys descend during inspiration and slide back into their normal position during exhalation.
- Standing on the client's right side, place your left hand under the client's back to elevate the flank as before. Place your right hand on the left upper quadrant of the abdomen lateral and parallel to the left rectus muscle with the fingertips just below the left costal margin. Instruct the client to take a deep breath and hold it. As the client inhales, attempt to capture the kidney between your two hands. Ask the client to exhale slowly and then to briefly hold the breath. At the same time, slowly release the pressure of your fingers.
- As the client exhales, you will feel the captured kidney move back into its previous position. The kidney surface should be rounded, smooth, firm, and nontender.

▶ An enlarged palpable kidney could be painful for the client. This suggests tumor, cyst, or hydronephrosis.

TECHNIQUES AND NORMAL FINDINGS	ABNORMAL FINDINGS SPECIAL CONSIDERATIONS

THE RIGHT KIDNEY

1. **Attempt to palpate the lower pole of the right kidney.**
   - Standing on the client's right side, place your left hand under the back parallel to the right twelfth rib (about halfway between the costal margin and iliac crest) with your fingertips reaching for the costovertebral angle. Place your right hand on the right upper quadrant of the abdomen lateral to the right rectus muscle and just below the right costal margin.
   - Instruct the client to take a deep breath. As the client inhales, lift the flank with your left hand and use deep palpation to feel for the lower pole of the kidney.

2. **Attempt to capture the right kidney.**
   - Place your left hand under the client's right flank.
   - Place your right hand on the right upper quadrant of the abdomen with the fingertips lateral and parallel to the right rectus muscle just below the right costal margin.
   - Instruct the client to take a deep breath and hold it. As the client inhales, attempt to capture the kidney between your two hands.
   - Ask the client to exhale slowly and then to briefly hold the breath. At the same time, slowly release the pressure of your fingers.
   - As the client exhales you will feel the captured kidney move back into its previous position. The kidney surface should be rounded, smooth, firm, and nontender.
   - The lower pole of the right kidney is palpable in some individuals, especially in thin, relaxed females. If palpable, the lower pole of the kidney has a smooth, firm, uninterrupted surface.
   - During the capture maneuver, some clients describe a nonpainful sensation as the kidney slides between the nurse's fingers back into its normal position.

▶ It is important not to mistake an enlarged liver for an enlarged right kidney. An enlarged kidney feels smooth and rounded, whereas an enlarged liver is closer to the midline and has a more distinct border. Polycystic kidney disease or carcinoma should be suspected when there is gross enlargement of the kidney. The kidneys may be two or three times their normal size in clients with polycystic disease.

TECHNIQUES AND NORMAL FINDINGS	ABNORMAL FINDINGS SPECIAL CONSIDERATIONS

THE URINARY BLADDER

1. **Palpate the bladder to determine symmetry, location, size, and sensation.**
   - Use light palpation over the lower portion of the abdomen. The abdomen should be soft.
   - Use deep palpation to locate the fundus (base) of the bladder, approximately 5 to 7 cm (2 to 2.5 in.) below the umbilicus in the lower abdomen. Once you have located the fundus of the bladder, continue to palpate, outlining the shape and contour.
   - Slide your fingers over the surface of the bladder and continue palpating to determine smoothness and continuity.
   - The surface of the bladder should feel smooth and uninterrupted. An empty bladder is usually not palpable. When the bladder is moderately full, it should be firm, smooth, symmetric, and nontender. As the bladder fills, the fundus can reach the level of the umbilicus. A full bladder is firm and buoyant.

▶ A distended bladder feels smooth, round, and taut. An asymmetric contour or nodular surface suggests abnormal growth that should be correlated with other findings. In males with urethral obstruction due to hypertrophy or hyperplasia of the prostate, the bladder is enlarged.

2. **Percuss the bladder to determine its location and degree of fullness.**
   - Begin with direct percussion of the bladder over the suprapubic area.
   - Move your fingers upward toward the umbilicus as you continue to percuss. A full bladder produces a dull tone upon percussion. Continue percussing upward toward the umbilicus until no more dull tones are heard. The point at which dull tones cease is the upper margin of the bladder.
   - Some practitioners conclude the assessment of the urinary system with the inspection and palpation of the penis and urethral meatus in the male client or the inspection of the urethral meatus in the female client. Other practitioners consider these structures with the assessment of the genitalia.

▶ Bedside bladder ultrasonography, bladder scanning, has become the preferred method to assess urinary retention.

Abnormal Findings

Common alterations of the urinary system include bladder cancer, kidney and urinary tract infections, calculi, tumors, renal failure, and changes in urinary elimination. Each of these alterations are discussed in the following sections.

Bladder Cancer

Seen later in life, bladder cancer occurs more frequently in males than in females. Smoking has been linked to this disease. The client may be totally asymptomatic or have hematuria, flank pain, and frequent urination.

Glomerulonephritis

This entity is an inflammation of the glomerulus. The key clinical manifestations are hematuria with red blood cell casts and proteinuria.

Renal Calculi

Calculi are stones that block the urinary tract. They are usually composed of calcium, struvite, or a combination of magnesium, ammonium, phosphate, and uric acid. Pain is the primary symptom. The pain may radiate and is variable in location and severity. Other symptoms include spasms, nausea, vomiting, pain on urination, frequency and urgency of urination, and gross hematuria.

Renal Tumor

Renal tumors may be either benign or malignant, with malignant being more common. Research has shown that there is an association with renal tumors and smoking. The key manifestations of renal tumors are hematuria, flank pain, weight loss, and palpable mass in the flank.

Renal Failure

Renal failure may be acute or it may progress to a chronic state. Acute renal failure that does not progress to a chronic state includes three stages: oliguria, diuresis, and recovery. Other symptoms include fluid retention, hyperkalemia, hyperphosphatemia, nausea, and vomiting. Uremia is the classic hallmark of chronic renal failure. Anorexia, nausea, vomiting, mentation changes, uremic frost, pruritus, weight loss, fatigue, and edema are common symptoms of uremia.

Urinary Tract Infection

Bacteria cause urinary tract infections. The bladder is the most common site of the infection, which results in inflammation of the bladder called cystitis; however, infection may include the kidneys. Clients may be asymptomatic, but the classic symptoms include urgency, frequency, dribbling, pain upon urination, and suprapubic or lower back pain. Hematuria, as well as cloudy and foul-smelling urine, may accompany the other signs.

Changes in Urinary Elimination

The following are examples of alterations in urinary elimination:

Dysreflexia affects clients with spinal cord injuries at level T_7 or higher. Bladder distention causes a sympathetic response that can trigger a potentially life-threatening hypertensive crisis.

Incontinence is the inability to retain urine. If this is the client's problem, the nurse must determine which of the five types of incontinence is present.

- **Functional incontinence** occurs when the client is unable to reach the toilet in time because of environmental, psychosocial, or physical factors.
- **Reflex incontinence** occurs in clients with spinal cord damage when urine is involuntarily lost.

- **Stress incontinence**, involuntary urination, occurs when intra-abdominal pressure is increased during coughing, sneezing, or straining. Aging changes may also contribute to stress incontinence.
- **Urge incontinence** may be caused by consuming a significant volume of fluids over a relatively short period of time. Urge incontinence may also be due to diminished bladder capacity.
- **Total incontinence** is related to a neurologic condition.

Urinary retention is a chronic state in which the client cannot empty the bladder. In most cases, the client voids small amounts of overflow urine when the bladder reaches its greatest capacity.

15
Male Reproductive System

The male reproductive system produces hormones, which impact physical development and sexual behavior. Some of the male reproductive organs serve dual roles as part of the reproductive system and the urinary system.

ANATOMY AND PHYSIOLOGY REVIEW

The male reproductive system is divided anatomically into external and internal genital organs. The penis and scrotum, the two external organs, are easily inspected and palpated. Only some of the internal structures are palpable. Figure 15.1 illustrates the gross anatomy of the male reproductive system.

The **scrotum** is a loosely hanging, pliable, pear-shaped pouch of darkly pigmented skin that is located behind the penis. It houses the testes, which produce sperm.

The **testes** are two firm, rubbery, olive-shaped structures that manufacture sperm and are the primary male sex organs. The **spermatic cord** is composed of fibrous connective tissue and forms a protective sheath around the nerves, blood vessels, lymphatic structures, and muscle fibers associated with the scrotum.

Positioned on top of and just posterior to each testicle is the **epididymis,** which is palpable upon physical examination. It forms the beginning of the male duct system.

The ductus deferens (vas deferens) is a tubular structure that stretches from the end of the epididymis to the ejaculatory duct. It runs through the inguinal

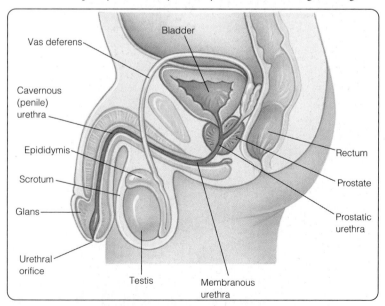

Figure 15.1 • Gross anatomy of the male reproductive organs.

canal, on the backside of the bladder, and to the ejaculatory duct as it enters into the prostate gland. The **urethra** serves as a conduit for the transportation of both urine and semen to the outside of the body. It is composed of three sections: the prostatic urethra, the membranous urethra, and the spongy (penile) urethra.

The **seminal vesicles** are a pair of saclike glands located between the bladder and rectum.

The **prostate gland** borders the urethra near the lower part of the bladder. It is partially palpable through the front wall of the rectum because it lies just anterior to the rectum (see Figure 15.1). Cowper's glands or **bulbourethral glands** are located below the prostate within the urethral sphincter.

PENIS

Internally, the penile shaft consists of the penile urethra and three columns of highly vascular, erectile tissue: the two dorsolateral columns (corpora cavernosa) and the midventral column surrounding or encasing the urethra. The penis contracts and elongates during sexual arousal when its vasculature dilates as it fills with blood. The distal end of the urethra (the external meatus) appears as a small opening centrally located on the glans of the penis, the cone-shaped distal end of the organ. In uncircumcised males, the glans is covered by a layer of skin called the foreskin.

INGUINAL AREAS

The inguinal areas are located laterally to the pubic region over the iliac region or the upper part of the hip bone. Within this area are the inguinal ligaments and the inguinal canals, which lie above the inguinal ligaments. The inguinal canals are associated with the abdominal muscles and actually represent a potential weak link in the abdominopelvic wall. When a separation of the abdominal muscle exists, the weak points of these canals afford an area for the protrusion of the intestine into the groin region. This is called an **inguinal hernia.**

PERIANAL AREA

The **anus,** the terminal end of the gastrointestinal system, opens onto the perineum at the midpoint of the gluteal folds, and has internal and external muscles. The external muscles are skeletal muscles, which form the part of the anal sphincter that voluntarily controls evacuation of stool. Above the anus is the rectum with the prostate gland in close proximity to the anterior surface of the rectum. Mucosa of the anus is moist, darkly pigmented, and hairless. Lying between the scrotum and the anus is the **perineum,** which has a smooth surface and is free of lesions.

SPECIAL CONSIDERATIONS

Reproductive health status is influenced by a number of factors including age, developmental level, race, ethnicity, work history, living conditions, socioeconomics, and emotional well-being.

INFANTS AND CHILDREN

The male newborn's genitals should be clearly evident and not ambiguous. The penis may vary in size but averages about 2.5 cm (0.98 in.) in length and is slender. The urethral meatus should be in the center of the glans. The foreskin may be somewhat tight and not retractable until 2 or 3 years of age.

The onset of puberty in the male child occurs between 10 and 15 years of age. At this time, under the influence of elevating levels of testosterone, the male child begins to develop adult male characteristics.

A summary of the changes is presented in Table 15.1.

THE OLDER ADULT

The older male client experiences the following changes. Pubic hair thins and grays, the prostate gland enlarges, the size of the penis and testes may diminish,

Table 15.1 Maturation Stages in the Male

Stage 1.

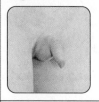

Preadolescent, hair present is no different than that on abdomen. Testes, scrotum, and penis are the same size and shape as young child.

Stage 2.

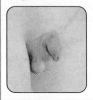

Pubic hair slightly pigmented, longer, straight hair, often still downy usually at base of penis, sometimes on scrotum; enlargment of scrotum and testes.

Stage 3.

Pubic hair dark, definitely pigmented, curly pubic hair around base of penis; enlargement of penis, especially in length, further enlargement of testes, descent of scrotum.

Stage 4.

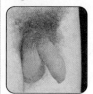

Pubic hair definitely adult in type but not in extent, spread no further than inguinal fold. Continued enlargement of penis and sculpturing of glans, increased pigmentation of scrotum.

Stage 5.

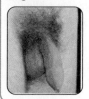

Hair spread to medial surface of thighs in adult distribution. Adult stage, scrotum ample, penis reaching nearly to bottom of scrotum.

the scrotum hangs lower, and the testes are softer to palpation. Testosterone production decreases, resulting in diminished libido.

PSYCHOSOCIAL CONSIDERATIONS

Fatigue, depression, and stress can decrease sexual desire in a client of any age. A male's body image may be affected by his perception of his penis size in relation to that of other males. Some males fear that they are "too small" to

| Box 15.1 | Testicular Self-Examination |

Testicular cancer has no early warning signs. Thus, males should perform a testicular self-exam monthly, beginning in adolescence. Describe to the client how to perform the exam:

- The best time to perform the exam is in the shower or bath, since the heat and steam will warm your hands and the water will help your hands to glide over the skin surface. If your hands are cold, a reflex response will occur, causing your testicles to move up against your body. They will then be more difficult for you to feel.
- Feel each testicle by applying gentle pressure with your thumb, index, and middle fingers. If your testicle hurts while you feel it, you are pressing too hard.
- The contour of the testicle should be smooth, rounded, and firm.
- You will feel the epididymis on top of and behind each testicle.
- You should not feel any distinct lumps or areas of hardness, nor should your testicle be enlarged. If any of these signs are present, make an appointment with your physician immediately.

satisfy a female sexually. Testicular cancer is the most common type of cancer in males between ages of 20 and 35, thus the need to perform self-examination. See Box 15.1.

Due to the uncertainty related to the benefits of treating prostate cancer detected by prostatic specific antigen (PSA) in men younger than 75 years of age, it is recommended that the test not be conducted until the client has been apprised of the potential but uncertain benefits and known harms of screening and treatment, including erectile dysfunction, urinary incontinence, bowel dysfunction, and death. Males should be assisted to consider the evidence and their personal preferences before a decision to be tested is made. PSA screening in males 75 years of age and older is not recommended.

CULTURAL CONSIDERATIONS
Assessment and findings are influenced by culture. See the cultural considerations box for specific examples.

Cultural Considerations

- Penile cancer is rare in the United States; however, it accounts for almost 10% of male cancers in Africa and South America.
- Prostate cancer occurs more frequently in African Americans than in Caucasians.
- Testicular cancer occurs more frequently in Caucasians than in any other ethnic group.
- Bladder cancer occurs twice as frequently in Caucasians as in African Americans.
- The rates for STDs are higher in African American and Hispanic populations than in Caucasians.
- Circumcision of the male is required in some religions (Judaism, Islam) and preferred in many cultures to promote hygiene. It is seen with the least frequency in Hispanics.
- In many cultures, physical assessment is limited to same-sex examiners.

Gathering the Data

Health assessment of the male reproductive system includes gathering subjective and objective data. Subjective data collection occurs during the client interview, before the actual physical assessment.

FOCUSED INTERVIEW QUESTIONS

1. Are you sexually active? Do you have any concerns about your sexual health?
2. Do you have or have you ever tried to have children?
3. Have you ever been diagnosed with an illness, infection, or disease of the reproductive organs? Have you ever been diagnosed with mumps, benign prostatic hypertrophy, erectile dysfunction, cancer of the system, or a sexually transmitted disease?
4. Have you ever been tested for, exposed to, or had HIV, discharge from the penis, or any unusual itching in your genital or rectal areas?
5. Do you perform testicular self-examination?

QUESTIONS REGARDING INFANTS AND CHILDREN

1. Have you noticed any redness, swelling, discharge that is discolored or foul smelling, asymmetry, lumps, or masses in the child's genital areas?
2. Has the child complained of itching, burning, or swelling in the genital area?

The nurse should ask the preschool child, school-age child, or adolescent the following questions:

1. Has anyone ever touched you when you didn't want him or her to? Where? (The nurse may want to have the child point to a picture.)
2. Has anyone ever asked you to touch him or her when you didn't want to? (If the child answers yes, the child may be sexually abused. The nurse should try to obtain additional information by asking the following questions but remember to be sensitive.) Where did he or she ask you to touch him or her? Who touched you? How many times did this happen? Who knows about this?

QUESTIONS FOR THE OLDER ADULT

The questions for older male adults are the same as those for younger male adults. In addition, the nurse should explore whether older clients perceive any changes in their sexuality related to advancing age.

Physical Assessment

Physical assessment of the male reproductive system follows an organized pattern. It begins with inspection and palpation of the external genitalia. This is followed by inspection of the perianal area, palpation of the bulbourethral and prostate glands via rectal examination, and examination of stool for occult blood.

EQUIPMENT

examination gown and drape
clean, nonsterile examination gloves
examination light
flashlight

lubricant
slides and swabs to obtain a
    specimen of abnormal discharge

HELPFUL HINTS

- Provide an environment that is warm and private.
- Explain each step in the procedure and provide specific instructions about what is expected of the client. For example, the nurse should state whether the client will be expected to sit, stand, or bear down during an assessment.
- Males from puberty through adulthood respond in a variety of ways when the genitals are exposed for examination. It is imperative to maintain the client's dignity throughout the assessment.
- Explore cultural issues and seek remedies for concerns at the onset of the interaction.
- Use Standard Precautions.

TECHNIQUES AND NORMAL FINDINGS	ABNORMAL FINDINGS SPECIAL CONSIDERATIONS

INSPECTION

1. Position the client.
- The client stands in front of the examiner for the first part of the assessment.

2. Position yourself on a stool sitting in front of the client.

3. Inspect the pubic hair.
- Observe the pubic hair for normal distribution, amount, texture, and cleanliness.
- Confirm that pubic hair is distributed heavily at the symphysis pubis in a diamond- or triangular-shaped pattern, thinning out as it extends toward the umbilicus. The hair will thin as it reaches the inner thigh area and over the scrotum. Hair should be absent on the penis.
- If the client has complained of itching in his pubic area, comb through the pubic hair with two or three fingers.
- Confirm the absence of small bluish gray spots, or nits (eggs), at the base of the pubic hairs.

▶ The amount, distribution, and texture of pubic hair vary according to the client's age and race. Absent or extremely sparse hair in the pubic area may be indicative of sexual underdevelopment. The pubic hair of elderly males may be gray and thinning (see Table 15.1).

▶ These signs indicate the presence of pubic lice (crabs). Marks may be visible from persistent scratching to relieve the intense itching crabs cause.

4. Inspect the penis.
- Inspect the penis size, pigmentation, glans, location of the dorsal vein, and the urethral meatus.
- Start by confirming that the penis size is appropriate for the stage of development of the client. In adult males, penis size varies.
- Note the pigmentation of the penis.

▶ Penis size varies according to the developmental stage of the client (see Table 15.1).

▶ The penis may appear small in obese males because obese men develop a pad of fat in the pubic area and the flaccid penis becomes buried in it.

TECHNIQUES AND NORMAL FINDINGS	ABNORMAL FINDINGS SPECIAL CONSIDERATIONS

- Pigmentation should be evenly distributed over the penis. The color depends on the client's race but will be slightly darker than the color of the skin over the rest of his body.
- Assess the looseness of the skin over the shaft of the penis. The skin should be loose over the flaccid penis.
- Confirm that the dorsal vein is midline on the shaft.
- Inspect the glans penis. It should be smooth and free of lesions or discharge. No redness or inflammation should be present. **Smegma,** a white, cheesy substance, may be present. This finding is considered normal.

- If the client is uncircumcised, either ask the client to pull the foreskin back or do so yourself. To retract the foreskin, gently pull the skin down over the penile shaft from the side of the glans using the thumb and first two fingers or forefinger.

- Gently move the foreskin back into place over the glans. The foreskin should move smoothly.

▶ Pigmentation of the penis of males with lighter complexions ranges from pink to light brown. In dark-skinned clients, the penis is light to dark brown.

▶ Discharge or lesions may indicate the presence of infective diseases such as *herpes, genital warts,* or *syphilis,* or may indicate cancer. If discharge is present, the substance should be cultured. Consistency, color, and odor are noted.
▶ Phimosis is a condition in which the foreskin is so tight that it cannot be retracted.
▶ Paraphimosis describes a condition in which the foreskin, once retracted, becomes so tight that it cannot be moved back over the glans.
▶ Immediate assistance must be sought if the foreskin cannot be retracted. Prolonged constriction of the vessels can obstruct blood flow and lead to tissue damage or necrosis.

5. **Assess the position of the urinary meatus.**
   - The meatus should be located in the center of the tip of the penis (Figure 15.2).

▶ In rare cases, the urinary meatus is located on the upper side of the glans (*epispadias*) or the under side of the glans (*hypospadias*). These conditions are usually corrected surgically shortly after birth.
▶ A pinpoint appearance of the urinary meatus is indicative of **urethral stricture.**

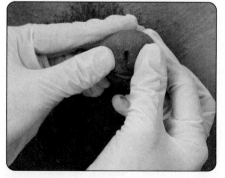

Figure 15.2 • Assessing the position of the urinary meatus.

TECHNIQUES AND NORMAL FINDINGS	ABNORMAL FINDINGS SPECIAL CONSIDERATIONS

6. **Inspect the scrotum.**
   - Ask the client to hold his penis up so that the scrotum is fully exposed. Optionally, you may hold the penis up by letting it rest on the back of your nondominant hand.
   - Observe the shape of the scrotum and how it hangs. It should be pear shaped, with the left side hanging lower than the right.

     ▶ An appearance of flatness could suggest testicular abnormality. Elderly males may have a pendulous, sagging scrotal sac.

   - Inspect the front and back of the scrotum. The skin should be wrinkled, loosely fitting over its internal structures. Note any swelling, redness, distended veins, and lesions. If swelling is present, note if it is unilateral or bilateral.

     ▶ Scrotal swelling and inflammation could suggest problems such as orchitis (inflammation of the testicles), *epididymitis* (inflammation of the epididymis), *scrotal edema* (an accumulation of fluid in the scrotum), *scrotal hernia,* or *testicular torsion* (twisting of the testicle onto the spermatic cord). Swelling and inflammation may also be seen in renal, cardiovascular, and other systemic disorders.

   - If you detect a mass, you may want to perform transillumination.
   - In a darkened room, place a lighted flashlight behind the area in which the abnormal mass was palpated.
   - Note that the light shines through the scrotum with a red glow. The testicle shows up as a nontransparent oval structure.
   - Repeat these steps on the other side and compare the results.

     ▶ Note any area where the light does not transilluminate. Light will not penetrate a mass. Masses may indicate *testicular tumor,* **spermatocele** (a cyst located in the epididymis), or other conditions.

7. **Inspect the inguinal area.**
   - The inguinal area should be flat. This may be difficult to confirm if the client is overweight. Even in the presence of adipose tissue, the contour of the inguinal area should be consistent with the rest of the body. Lymph nodes are present in this location, but not normally visible.

TECHNIQUES AND NORMAL FINDINGS	**ABNORMAL FINDINGS** **SPECIAL CONSIDERATIONS**

- Inspect both the right and left inguinal areas with the client breathing normally.
- Have the client hold his breath and bear down as if having a bowel movement.
- Observe for any evidence of lumps or masses. The contour of the inguinal areas should remain even.

▶ Masses or lumps may be related to the presence of an inguinal hernia or cancer within the reproductive, abdominal, urinary, lymphatic, and other systems.

PALPATION

1. **Palpate the penis.**
   - Place the glans between your thumb and forefinger.
   - Gently compress the glans, allowing the meatus to gape open (Figure 15.3).
     The meatus should be pink, patent, and free of discharge.

▶ The client may be hesitant to verbalize pain when palpation is performed. It is important to watch for nonverbal facial and body gestures.

▶ A *urethral stricture* is suspected if the meatus is only about the size of a pinpoint.

▶ Signs of *urethritis* include redness and edema around the glans and foreskin, eversion of urethral mucosa, and drainage. If urethritis is suspected, the client should be asked if he experiences itching and tenderness around the meatus and painful urination. If drainage is present, observe for color, consistency, odor, and amount. Obtain a specimen if indicated. Suspect a gonococcal infection (gonorrhea) if the drainage is profuse and thick, purulent, and greenish yellow.

▶ Consider inflammation or infection higher up in the urinary tract if redness, edema, and discharge are visible around the urethral opening, because the mucous membrane in the urethra is continuous with the mucous membrane in the rest of the tract.

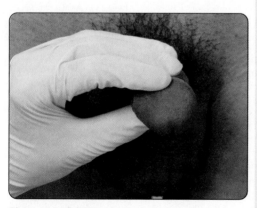

Figure 15.3 • Palpating the penis.

TECHNIQUES AND NORMAL FINDINGS	ABNORMAL FINDINGS SPECIAL CONSIDERATIONS

- Note any discharge or tenderness.

- Continue gentle palpation and compression up the entire shaft of the penis.

2. **Palpate the scrotum.**
   - Ask the client to hold his penis up to expose the scrotum.
   - Gently palpate the left and then the right scrotal sacs. Each scrotal sac should be nontender, soft, and boggy. The structures within the sacs should move easily with your palpation.
   - Note any tenderness, swelling, masses, lesions, or nodules.

▶ Be alert for any lesions, masses, swelling, or nodules.
▶ Note characteristics of any abnormal findings. Culture any discharge.

▶ Assess shape, size, consistency, location, and mobility of any masses. If the client expresses pain, lift the scrotum. If the pain is relieved, the client may have epididymitis, inflammation of the epididymis.

ALERT! *If you cannot insert your finger with gentle pressure, do not force your finger into the opening.*

3. **Palpate the testes.**
   - Be sure that your hands are warm.
   - Approach each testis from the bottom of the scrotal sac and gently rotate it between your thumb and fingertips. Each testis should be nontender, oval shaped, walnut-sized, smooth, elastic, and solid.

▶ The cremasteric reflex may cause the testicles to migrate upward temporarily. Cold hands, a cold room, or the stimulus of touch could cause this response. To prevent this reflexive action when examining a child, have him sit tailor style. Gentle pressure over the canal with the nondominant hand can reduce this response.

4. **Palpate the epididymis.**
   - Slide your fingertips around to the posterior side of each testicle to find the epididymis, a small, crescent-shaped structure.

▶ In some clients, the epididymis may be palpated on the front surface of each testis.

5. **Palpate the spermatic cord.**
   - Slide your fingers up just above the testicle, feeling for a vertical, ropelike structure about 3 mm wide.
   - Gently grasp the cord between your thumb and index finger.

▶ A cord that is hard, beaded, or nodular could indicate the presence of a varicosity or varicocele. A **varicocele** is a distended cord and is a common cause of male infertility. Upon palpation, it may feel like a "bag of worms."

TECHNIQUES AND NORMAL FINDINGS

- Do not squeeze or pinch. Trace the cord up to the external inguinal ring using a gentle rotating motion.
- The cord should feel thin, smooth, nontender to palpation, and resilient.

6. **Palpate the inguinal region.**
   - Start by preparing the client for palpation in the right inguinal area.
   - Ask the client to shift his balance so that his weight is on his left leg.
   - Place your right index finger in the upper corner of the right scrotum.
   - Slowly palpate the spermatic cord up and slightly to the client's left.
   - Allow the client's scrotal skin to fold over your index finger as you palpate.
   - Proceed until you feel an opening that feels like a triangular slit. This is the external ring of the inguinal canal. Attempt to gently glide your finger into this opening (Figure 15.4).

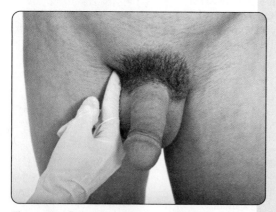

Figure 15.4 • Palpating the inguinal canal.

- If the opening has admitted your finger, ask the client to either cough or bear down.
- Palpate for masses or lumps.

▶ An *inguinal hernia* feels like a bulge or mass.

▶ A *direct inguinal hernia* can be palpated in the area of the external ring of the inguinal ligament. It will be felt either right at the external ring opening or just behind it.

TECHNIQUES AND NORMAL FINDINGS	ABNORMAL FINDINGS SPECIAL CONSIDERATIONS

▶ An *indirect inguinal hernia* is more common, especially in younger males. It is located deeper in the inguinal canal than the direct inguinal hernia. It can pass into the scrotum, whereas a direct inguinal hernia rarely protrudes into the scrotum.

▶ It is also possible that a *femoral hernia* may be present. It is more commonly found in the right inguinal area and near the inguinal ligament. If the client displays an acute bulge with tenderness, pain, nausea, or vomiting, he may have a strangulated hernia. Help him to lie down and request immediate medical assistance.

- Repeat this procedure by palpating the client's left inguinal area. Use your left index finger when performing the palpation.

ALERT! *Do not pinch or squeeze any mass, lesion, or other structure.*

7. Palpate the inguinal lymph chain.
- Using the pads of your first three fingers, palpate the inguinal lymph nodes.
- Confirm that nodes are nonpalpable and the area is nontender.
- Occasionally some of the inguinal lymph nodes are palpable. They are usually less than 0.5 cm in size, spongy, movable, and nontender.

▶ It is important to assess if a node is larger than 0.5 cm or if multiple nodes are present. Tenderness in this area suggests infection of the scrotum, penis, or groin area.

8. Inspect the perianal area.
- Reposition the client. Ask the client to turn and face the table and bend over at the waist. The client can rest his arms on the table.
- If the client is unable to tolerate this position, he may lie on his left side on the examination table with both knees flexed.
- Inspect the sacrococcygeal and perianal areas. The skin should be smooth and without lesions.

▶ Tufts of hair or dimpling at the sacrococcygeal area are associated with pilonidal cysts. Rashes, redness, excoriation, or inflammation in the perianal area can signal infection or parasitic infestation.

9. Palpate the sacrococcygeal and perianal areas.
- The areas should be nontender and without palpable masses.

▶ Tenderness, mass, or inflammation may indicate pilonidal cyst, anal abscess, fissure, or pruritus.

TECHNIQUES AND NORMAL FINDINGS	ABNORMAL FINDINGS SPECIAL CONSIDERATIONS

10. Inspect the anus.

- Spread the buttocks apart. Visualize the anus. The skin is darker and coarse. The area should be free of lesions.

▶ Lesions may include skin tags, warts, hemorrhoids, or fissures.

▶ Obese males may have fecal incontinence due to pressure of the enlarged abdomen on the bowel and sphincter. This may result in rashes, excoriation, or lesions.

- Ask the client to bear down. The tissue stretches, but there are no bulges or discharge.

▶ Fistulas, fissures, internal hemorrhoids, or rectal prolapse are more easily detected when the client bears down.

11. Palpate the bulbourethral gland and the prostate gland.

- Lubricate your right index finger with lubricating gel.
- Tell the client that you are going to insert your finger into his rectum in order to palpate his prostate gland. Explain that the insertion may cause him to feel as if he needs to have a bowel movement. Tell him that this technique should not cause pain but to inform you immediately if it does.
- Place the index finger of your dominant hand against the anal opening. Be sure that your finger is slightly bent and not forming a right angle to the buttocks. If you insert your index finger at a right angle to the buttocks, the client may experience pain.
- Apply gentle pressure as you insert your bent finger into the anus.
- As the sphincter muscle tightens, stop inserting your finger.
- Resume as the sphincter muscle relaxes.
- Press your right thumb gently against the perianal area.
- Palpate the bulbourethral gland by pressing your index finger gently toward your thumb. This should not cause the client to feel pain or tenderness. No swelling or masses should be felt.

▶ If the bulbourethral gland is inflamed, the client may feel pain upon palpation. Referral for further examination is warranted.

| **TECHNIQUES AND NORMAL FINDINGS** | **ABNORMAL FINDINGS SPECIAL CONSIDERATIONS** |

- Release the pressure between your index finger and thumb. Continue to insert your index finger gently.
- Palpate the posterior surface of the prostate gland.
- Confirm that it is smooth, firm, even somewhat rubbery, nontender, and extends out no more than 1 cm into the rectal area.

▶ Note tenderness, masses, nodules, hardness, or softness. Nodules are characteristic of *prostate cancer.* Tenderness indicates inflammation.

- Remove your finger slowly and gently.
- Remove your gloves.
- Help the client to a standing position.
- Wash your hands.
- Give the client tissues to wipe the perianal area.

12. **Stool examination**
    - Inspect feces remaining on the gloved finger. Feces are normally brown and soft.
    - Test feces for occult blood. Normally, the test is negative. A positive test may signal the presence of occult blood but may occur if red meat was eaten within 3 days of the test.

▶ Rectal bleeding is suspected when bright red blood is on the surface of the stool. Feces mixed with bright red blood are associated with bleeding above the rectum. Black, tarry stool is associated with upper gastrointestinal tract bleeding.

Abnormal Findings

Abnormal findings of the male reproductive system include inguinal hernias, disorders of the penis, abnormalities of the scrotum, and problems in the perianal area. Table 15.2 describes the three types of inguinal hernias.

Table 15.2   Inguinal Hernias

TYPE OF HERNIA	CHARACTERISTICS	SIGNS AND SYMPTOMS
Direct Hernia	Extrusion of abdominal intestine into inguinal ring. Bulging occurs in the area around the pubis. Abdominal intestine may remain within the inguinal canal or extrude past the external ring.	Most often is painless. Appears as a swelling. During palpation, have the client cough. You will feel pressure against the side of your finger.
Indirect Hernia	Abdominal intestine may remain within the inguinal canal or extrude past the external ring. Most common type of hernia. Located within the femoral canal.	Appears as a swelling. During palpation, have the client cough. You will feel pressure against your fingertip. Palpate soft mass.
Femoral Hernia	Bulge occurs over the area of the femoral artery. The right femoral artery is affected more frequently than the left. Lowest incidence of all three hernias.	May not be painful; however, once strangulation occurs, pain is severe.

16
Female Reproductive System

The female reproductive system provides for both human reproduction and sexual gratification. Many factors influence the female client's reproductive health on both physiologic and psychologic levels. The nurse should approach the client in as nonthreatening a manner as possible and assure the client that the information provided and the results of the physical assessment will remain confidential.

ANATOMY AND PHYSIOLOGY REVIEW

The female reproductive system is unique in that it experiences cyclic changes in direct response to hormonal levels of estrogen and progesterone during the childbearing years.

EXTERNAL GENITALIA
Female external genitalia include the mons pubis, labia, glands, clitoris, and perianal area. These are depicted in Figure 16.1.

INTERNAL REPRODUCTIVE ORGANS
The internal female reproductive organs are the vagina, uterus, cervix, fallopian tubes, and ovaries. These organs are depicted in Figure 16.2.

SPECIAL CONSIDERATIONS

The subjective and objective data gathered throughout the assessment process inform the nurse about the client's state of health. A variety of factors including age, developmental level, race, ethnicity, work history, living conditions, socio-economics, and emotional well-being influence health and must be considered during assessment.

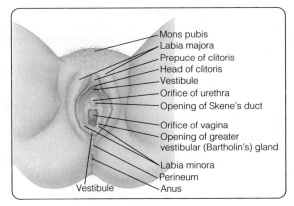

Figure 16.1 • External female genitalia.

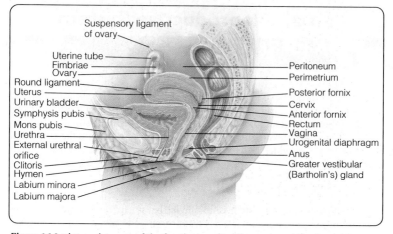

Figure 16.2 • Internal organs of the female reproductive system within the pelvis.

Anatomy and physiology change with growth and development. The nurse must be aware of expected changes as data are gathered and findings are interpreted. The following sections describe specific variations in the female reproductive system across the age span.

INFANTS AND CHILDREN

The female infant's labia majora will be enlarged at birth in response to maternal hormones. The urinary meatus and vaginal orifice should be visible. Bloody and mucoid discharge (false menses) is commonly seen in newborns due to exposure to maternal hormones in utero.

The female child reaches puberty a few years before the male. Changes begin to occur at any time from 8 to 13 years of age; most commonly, breast changes begin at age 9 and menstruation at age 12. Table 16.1 describes Tanner's stages of maturation in girls.

Adolescents often express interest in the changes related to puberty. The desire to explore sexual relationships and sexual contact, from kissing and fondling to intercourse, may be intense. Adolescents may need counseling on relationship issues, birth control, protection against sexually transmitted diseases (STDs), and delaying sexual activity. A history of human papillomavirus (HPV) and more than four sexual partners in a lifetime increases a female client's risk for cervical cancer. Gardasil, a vaccine, can protect against most cervical cancers related to HPV. The Centers for Disease Control and Prevention (CDC) Advisory Committee on Immunization Practices recommended routine 3-dose vaccination of girls aged 11 and 12 years. The vaccine is also recommended for girls and women ages 13 through 26 years who have not yet been vaccinated or who have not received all 3 doses. A female adolescent may be concerned about or confused by an attraction to individuals of the same sex.

Table 16.1	**Maturation Stages in the Female**

Stage 1.

Preadolescent, no growth of pubic hair.

Stage 2.

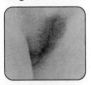

Initial, scarcely pigmented straight hair, especially along medial border of the labia.

Stage 3.

Sparse, dark, visibly pigmented curly pubic hair on labia.

Stage 4.

Hair coarse and curly, abundant but less than adults.

Stage 5.

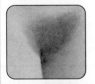

Lateral spreading in triangle shape to medial surface of thighs.

Stage 6.

Further extension laterally and upward.

THE PREGNANT FEMALE

Pregnancy brings a multitude of changes to the female reproductive organs. The uterus, cervix, ovaries, and vagina undergo significant structural changes related to the pregnancy and the influence of hormones. The uterus enlarges, moves high into the abdominal cavity, and irregular contractions occur. The cervical and vaginal changes are in preparation for the delivery of the fetus. Goodell's sign and Chadwick's sign are noted.

THE OLDER ADULT

Between the ages of 46 and 55, menstrual periods become shorter and less frequent until they stop entirely. Menopause is said to have occurred when the female has not experienced a menstrual period in over a year.

PSYCHOSOCIAL CONSIDERATIONS

Fatigue, depression, and stress can decrease sexual desire in a female client of any age. Grief over the loss of a relationship, whether because of separation, divorce, or death, can have long-term effects on a client's willingness to seek new relationships.

CULTURAL CONSIDERATIONS

Assessment and findings are influenced by culture. See the cultural considerations box for specific examples.

Cultural Considerations

- Female circumcision or female genital mutilation (FGM) is a traditional or cultural practice in Africa, Asia, and Middle Eastern countries.
- FGM is increasingly found in the United States and Canada among immigrants from Africa, Asia, and the Middle East.
- The death rate from cervical cancer is higher than average in African Americans, Hispanics, and Native Americans.
- Leiomyosarcoma, one form of uterine cancer, occurs with greater frequency in African Americans than in other groups.
- In many cultures and religions, physical examination by a healthcare provider of the opposite sex is prohibited.
- Discussion of sexual activity and reproductive function is unacceptable in many cultures.
- Language barriers often prevent females from seeking or obtaining information or actual care associated with female reproductive issues.

Gathering the Data

Health assessment of the female reproductive system includes gathering subjective and objective data. Collection of subjective data occurs during the client interview, before the physical assessment.

FOCUSED INTERVIEW QUESTIONS

1. Do you have any concerns about your reproductive health? Have you had concerns in the past? If so, please tell me about those concerns.

2. Describe your menstrual periods including onset, duration, frequency, and problems.

3. Have you ever been pregnant? If so, how many times, did you

have any problems during pregnancy, the delivery, or postpartum? *If the client answers yes:* Describe the problem(s). Was delivery vaginal or by cesarean section? Have you ever had a miscarriage?

4. Have you ever sought professional help for fertility problems? If so, describe this experience.

5. Are you sexually active? Are there any obstacles to your ability to achieve sexual satisfaction? Have you noticed a change in your sex drive recently? Do you use contraceptives? Which type?

6. Do you now have or have you ever had an illness or infection associated with the female reproductive system such as dysmenorrhea; uterine fibroids; uterine, ovarian, or vulvar cancer; vaginitis; pelvic inflammatory disease?

7. Have you ever had an abnormal Pap smear?

8. Have you ever had or been exposed to a sexually transmitted disease such as herpes, gonorrhea, syphilis, HPV, HIV, or chlamydia?

9. Have you had any problems in and around your rectal area, such as pain, itching, burning, or bleeding?

QUESTIONS REGARDING INFANTS AND CHILDREN

1. Have you noticed any redness, swelling, or discharge that is discolored or foul smelling in the child's genital areas?

2. Has the child complained of itching, burning, or swelling in the genital area?

For the preschool or school-age child: Has anyone ever touched you when you didn't want him or her to?

For the adolescent: Are you having sex with anyone now?

QUESTIONS FOR THE PREGNANT FEMALE

Questions for the pregnant female would include menstrual, obstetric, gynecologic, family, and partner histories.

QUESTIONS FOR THE OLDER ADULT

1. When did menopause begin for you?

2. Tell me about physical changes you have noticed since menopause.

3. Have you had any vaginal bleeding since starting menopause?

Physical Assessment

Physical assessment of the female reproductive system includes the techniques of inspection and palpation. In addition, the speculum is used to visualize the vagina and cervix.

EQUIPMENT

examination gown and examination drape
clean, nonsterile examination gloves
lubricant

Pap smear equipment
speculum
handheld mirror

• Provide a warm, private environment.
• Have the client void and empty bowels before the examination.
• Use appropriate draping to maintain the client's dignity.
• Determine if the client has had this kind of assessment before. If not, booklets with diagrams are helpful before proceeding.
• It is helpful to show the client pictures of equipment, slides, and the bimanual examination.
• Use an unhurried, deliberate manner and ask the client how she is doing as the examination proceeds.
• Explore and remedy cultural or language issues at the onset of the interaction.
• Use Standard Precautions.

TECHNIQUES AND NORMAL FINDINGS	ABNORMAL FINDINGS SPECIAL CONSIDERATIONS

INSPECTION

1. Position the client.
• Ask the client to lie down on the examination table.
• Assist her into the lithotomy position (supine with knees and hips flexed so that feet rest flat on the examination table), and then have her slide her hips as close to the end of the table as possible.
• Place her feet in the stirrups.

▶ In the obese client, the presence of large thighs and extra adipose tissue in the perineal area may require having an assistant to hold thighs apart or to move extra tissue during the examination. It may be necessary to raise the hips and increase flexion of the hips to visualize genital structures.

2. Inspect the pubic hair.
• Confirm that the hair grows in an inverted triangle and is scattered heavily over the mons pubis. It should become sparse over the labia majora, perineum, and inner thighs.

▶ A sparse hair pattern may be indicative of delayed puberty. It is also a common and normal finding in females of Asian ancestry. The elderly client's pubic hair will become sparse, scattered, and gray. Table 16.1 depicts Tanner's stages of female development.

• If the client has complained of itching in the pubic area, comb through the pubic hair with two or three fingers.
• Confirm the absence of small, bluish gray spots, or nits (eggs), at the base of the pubic hairs.

▶ These signs indicate pubic lice (crabs). Marks may be visible from persistent scratching to relieve the intense itching caused by the lice.

TECHNIQUES AND NORMAL FINDINGS	ABNORMAL FINDINGS SPECIAL CONSIDERATIONS

3. **Inspect the labia majora.**
   - Confirm that the labia majora are fuller and rounder in the center of the structure and that the skin is smooth and intact.
   - Compare the right and left labia majora for symmetry.
   - Observe for any lesions, warts, vesicles, rashes, or ulcerations. If you notice drainage, note the color, distribution, location, and characteristics.
   - Remember to change gloves as needed during the exam to prevent cross-contamination. Also remember to culture any abnormal discharge.
   - Confirm the absence of any swelling or inflammation in the area of the labia majora.

▶ The labia majora of older females may be thinner and wrinkled.

▶ These findings may signal a variety of conditions. *Contact dermatitis* appears as a red rash with associated lesions that are weepy and crusty. There often are scratches due to intense itching.

▶ **Genital warts** are raised, moist, cauliflower-shaped papules.

▶ Red, painful vesicles accompanied by localized swelling are seen in *herpes infection.*

▶ Swelling over red, inflamed skin that is tender and warm to palpation may indicate an abscess in the Bartholin's gland. The abscess may be caused by gonorrhea.

4. **Inspect the labia minora.**
   - Confirm that the labia minora are smooth, pink, and moist.
   - Observe for any redness or swelling. Note any bruising or tearing of the skin.

5. **Inspect the clitoris.**
   - Place your right or left hand over the labia majora and separate these structures with your thumb and index finger.
   - The clitoris should be midline, about 1 cm in length, with more fullness in the center. It should be smooth (Figure 16.3).

▶ The older female may have drier, thinner labia minora.

▶ Redness and swelling indicate the presence of an infective or inflammatory process. Bruising or tearing of the skin may suggest forceful intercourse or sexual abuse, especially in the case of adolescents and children.

▶ An elongated clitoris may signal elevated levels of testosterone and warrants further investigation and referral to a physician.

TECHNIQUES AND NORMAL FINDINGS	ABNORMAL FINDINGS SPECIAL CONSIDERATIONS

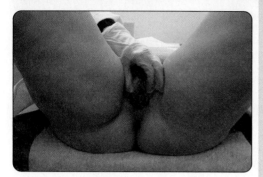

Figure 16.3 • Inspection of the clitoris.

- Observe for any redness, lesions, or tears in the tissue.

6. Inspect the urethral orifice.
- Confirm that the urethral opening is midline, pink, smooth, slitlike, and patent.
- Ask the client to cough. No urine should leak from the urethral opening.
- Inspect for any redness, inflammation, or discharge.

▶ Urine leakage indicates stress incontinence and weakening of the pelvic musculature.
▶ These symptoms indicate urinary tract infection.
▶ Pressure of the enlarged abdomen in the obese client may lead to urinary incontinence resulting in redness, and excoriation.

7. Inspect the vaginal opening, perineum, and anal area.
- Confirm that the vaginal opening or introitus is pink and round. It may be either smooth or irregular.
- Locate the **hymen,** which is a thin layer of skin within the vagina. It may be present in females who have never had sexual intercourse.
- Inspect for tears, bruising, or lacerations.
- The **perineum,** the space between the vaginal opening and anal area, should be smooth and firm.
- Scars from episiotomy procedures may be observed in parous females. These are normal.
- The anus should be intact, moist, and darkly pigmented. There should be no lesions.
- Have the client bear down.

▶ Tears, bruising, or lacerations could be due to forceful, consensual sex or rape. Additional follow-up is needed after examination. It is important not to ask any questions that the client may interpret as probing or threatening during the physical assessment.
▶ Thin, fragile perineal tissues indicate atrophy. Tears and fissures may indicate trauma.

TECHNIQUES AND NORMAL FINDINGS	**ABNORMAL FINDINGS SPECIAL CONSIDERATIONS**

- Inspect for any protrusions from the vagina.

▶ A **prolapsed uterus** may protrude right at the vaginal wall with straining, or it may hang outside of the vaginal wall without any straining.

PALPATION

1. **Palpate the vaginal walls.**
   - Explain to the client that you are going to palpate the vaginal walls. Tell her that she will feel you insert a finger into the vagina.
   - Place your left hand above the labia majora and spread the labia minora apart with your thumb and index finger.
   - With your right palm facing toward the ceiling, gently place your right index finger at the vaginal opening.
   - Insert your right index finger gently into the vagina.
   - Gently rotate the right index finger counterclockwise. The vaginal wall should feel rugated, consistent in texture, and soft.
   - Ask the client to bear down or cough.
   - Note any bulging in this area.

▶ A **cystocele** is a hernia that is formed when the urinary bladder is pushed into the anterior vaginal wall.
▶ A **rectocele** is a hernia that is formed when the rectum pushes into the posterior vaginal wall.

2. **Palpate the urethra and Skene's glands.**
   - Explain to the client that you are going to palpate her urethra. Tell her that she will again feel pressure against her vaginal wall.
   - Your left hand should still be above the labia majora and you should still be spreading the labia minora apart with your thumb and index finger.
   - Your right index finger should still be inserted in the client's vagina.
   - With your right index finger, apply very gentle pressure upward against the vaginal wall.
   - Milk the Skene's glands by stroking outward.
   - Now apply the same upward and outward pressure on both sides of the urethra.

▶ Bulging may occur with uterine prolapse, cystocele, or rectocele.

TECHNIQUES AND NORMAL FINDINGS	ABNORMAL FINDINGS SPECIAL CONSIDERATIONS

- No pain or discharge should be elicited.

3. **Palpate the Bartholin's glands.**
   - With your right index finger still inserted in the client's vagina, gently squeeze the posterior region of the labia majora between your right index finger and right thumb (Figure 16.4).

▶ Discharge from the urethra or Skene's glands may indicate an infection such as gonorrhea. A culture must be obtained.

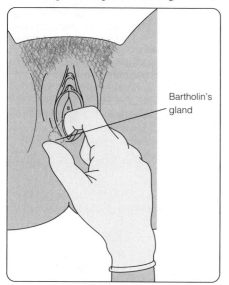

Bartholin's gland

Figure 16.4 • Palpating Bartholin's glands.

- Perform this maneuver bilaterally, palpating both Bartholin's glands.
- No lump or hardness should be felt. No pain response should be elicited. No discharge should be produced.

▶ Lumps, hardness, pain, or discharge suggest the presence of an abscess and infective process. Often the source is a gonorrheal infection. A culture should be obtained of any discharge.

INSPECTION WITH A SPECULUM

Be sure that the client has not douched within 24 hours before obtaining cervical and vaginal specimens. Otherwise, the results of the test may be inaccurate.

▶ If the client has vaginitis, the speculum examination should be delayed until the problem has been treated unless this is the client's chief complaint and the reason for her visit.

TECHNIQUES AND NORMAL FINDINGS	ABNORMAL FINDINGS SPECIAL CONSIDERATIONS

1. **Select the speculum.**
   - The speculum should be the proper size for the client.
   - Use a speculum that has been prewarmed with a heating pad. Do not prewarm a speculum with warm water, because it is not desirable to introduce water into the vagina. Do not use gel lubricant, as it may distort the cells in your specimens.

2. **Hold the speculum in your dominant hand.**
   - Place the index finger on top of the blades, the third finger on the bottom of the blades, and be sure to move the thumb just underneath the thumbscrew before inserting.

3. **Insert the speculum.**
   - Tell the client that you are going to examine her cervix, and that to do so, you are going to insert a speculum. If this is the client's first vaginal examination, show her the speculum, and briefly demonstrate how you will use it to visualize her cervix. Have a mirror available to share findings with the client. Also explain that she will feel pressure, first of your fingers, and then of the speculum. You may also want to show her a booklet with a picture demonstrating the technique.
   - With your nondominant hand, place your index and middle fingers on the posterior vaginal opening and apply pressure gently downward.
   - Turn the speculum blades obliquely.
   - Place the blades over your fingers at the vaginal opening and slowly insert the closed speculum at a 45-degree downward angle (Figure 16.5). This angle matches the downward slope of the vagina when the client is in the lithotomy position.

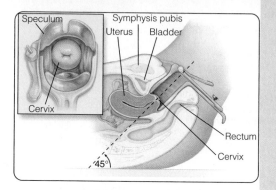

Speculum

Symphysis pubis

Uterus Bladder

Cervix

Rectum

Cervix

45°

Figure 16.5 • Speculum inserted into vagina.

- Ask the client to bear down as you insert the speculum. It is normal for the client to tense as the speculum is inserted, and bearing down helps to relax the muscles.
- Once the speculum is inserted, withdraw your fingers and turn the speculum clockwise until the blades are in a horizontal plane.
- Advance the blades at a downward 45-degree angle until they are completely inserted.
- This maneuver should not cause the client pain.
- Avoid pinching the labia or pulling on the client's pubic hair. If insertion of the speculum causes the client pain, stop immediately and reevaluate your technique.
- To open the speculum blades, squeeze the speculum handle.
- Sweep the speculum blades upward until the cervix comes into view.
- Adjust the speculum blades as needed until the cervix is fully exposed between them.
- Tighten the thumbscrew to stabilize the spread of the blades.

4. **Visualize the cervix.**
   - Confirm that the cervix is pink, moist, round, and centrally positioned, and that it has a small opening in the center called the os.

TECHNIQUES AND NORMAL FINDINGS	ABNORMAL FINDINGS SPECIAL CONSIDERATIONS

- Note any bluish coloring.

▶ A bluish coloring is seen during the second month of pregnancy and is called *Chadwick's sign*. Otherwise, a bluish color is indicative of cyanosis.

- Confirm that any secretions are clear or white and without odor.

▶ Green discharge that has a foul smell is associated with gonorrhea. Thick discharge is seen in *candidiasis*. Frothy, yellow-green discharge is seen in *trichomoniasis*. A yellow discharge can also be visualized in chlamydial infection. *Bacterial vaginitis* presents with a creamy-gray to white discharge that has a fishy odor.

- Confirm that the cervix is free from erosions, ulcerations, lacerations, and polyps.

▶ Erosions are associated with carcinoma or infections. Ulcerations can be due to carcinoma, syphilis, and tuberculosis. Yellow cysts or nodules are *nabothian cysts*, benign cysts that may appear after childbirth.

OBTAINING THE PAP SMEAR AND GONORRHEA CULTURE

The Pap (Papanicolaou) smear consists of three specimens: an endocervical swab, a cervical scrape, and a vaginal pool sample.

Have ready prelabeled slides for specimens, either (a) one labeled *endocervical*, one labeled *vaginal*, and one labeled *cervical* or (b) one slide that has sections for each sample.

1. **Perform an endocervical swab.**
   - Carefully insert a saline-moistened, cotton-tipped applicator or Cytobrush® GT into the vagina and into the cervical os.

▶ Moistening the applicator with saline prevents the cells from being absorbed into the cotton.

The cytobrush is recommended over the cotton-tipped applicator because more endocervical cells adhere to it, thus yielding more accurate results.

TECHNIQUES AND NORMAL FINDINGS	ABNORMAL FINDINGS SPECIAL CONSIDERATIONS

- Do not force insertion of the applicator.

▶ If the applicator cannot be slipped into the cervical os, a tumor may be blocking the opening.

- Rotate the applicator in a complete circle.
- Roll a thin coat across the slide labeled *endocervical.*
- Spray fixative on the slide immediately or place it in a container filled with fixative.

▶ A thin coat is preferred because a thick coat may be difficult to assess under the microscope.

2. **Obtain a cervical scrape.**
   - Insert the longer end of a bifid spatula into the client's vagina.
   - Advance the fingerlike projection of the bifid end gently into the cervical os.
   - Allow the shorter end to rest on the outer ridge of the cervix.
   - Rotate the applicator one full 360-degree turn clockwise to scrape cells from the cervix (Figure 16.6).

▶ If the client has had a hysterectomy, obtain the scrape from the surgical stump.

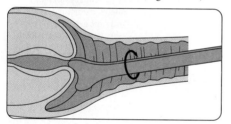

Figure 16.6 • The cervical scrape.

- Do not rotate the applicator more than once or turn it in a counterclockwise manner.
- Spread a thin smear across the slide labeled *cervical* from each side of the applicator.
- Spray fixative on the slide immediately or place in a container filled with fixative.

3. **Obtain a vaginal pool sample.**
   - Insert the paddle end of the spatula into the vaginal recess area (fornix). Alternatively, you may use a saline-moistened cotton applicator.
   - Gently rotate the spatula back and forth to obtain a sample.
   - Apply the specimen to the slide labeled *vaginal.*
   - Spray fixative on the slide immediately.

TECHNIQUES AND NORMAL FINDINGS	ABNORMAL FINDINGS SPECIAL CONSIDERATIONS

4. Obtain a gonorrhea culture.
- Obtain a gonorrhea culture if the assessment findings indicate.
- Insert a saline-moistened cotton applicator into the cervical os.
- Leave the applicator in place for 20 seconds to allow full saturation of the cotton.
- Using a Z-shaped pattern, roll a thin coat of the secretions onto the Thayer-Martin culture plate labeled *cervical*.

▶ Nurses must be sure to check with the laboratory in their institution because techniques and protocols may differ.

5. Remove the speculum.
- Gently loosen the thumbscrew on the speculum while holding the handles securely.
- Slant the speculum from side to side as you slide it from the vaginal canal.
- While you withdraw the speculum, note that the vaginal mucosa is pink, consistent in texture, rugated, and nontender. Discharge is thin or stringy, and clear or opaque.
- Close the speculum blades before complete removal.

▶ The infections that contribute to the development of discolored or foul-smelling vaginal discharge are the same as those listed in the previous section on identifying cervical discharge.

BIMANUAL PALPATION

Stand at the end of the examination table. The client remains in the lithotomy position.

1. Palpate the cervix.
- Lubricate the index and middle fingers of your gloved dominant hand.
- Inform the client that you are going to palpate her cervix.
- Place your nondominant hand against the client's thigh, then insert your lubricated index and middle fingers into her vaginal opening.
- Proceed downward at a 45-degree angle until you reach the cervix.
- Keep the other fingers of that hand rounded inward toward the palm and put the thumb against the mons pubis away from the clitoris.
- Palpate the cervix. It should feel firm and smooth, somewhat like the tip of a nose.

▶ Pressure on the clitoris may be painful for the client.

▶ Nodules, hardness, or lack of mobility suggest a tumor.

TECHNIQUES AND NORMAL FINDINGS	ABNORMAL FINDINGS SPECIAL CONSIDERATIONS

- Gently try to move it. It should move easily about 1 to 2 cm in either direction.

2. **Palpate the fornices.**
   - Slip your fingers into the vaginal recess areas, called the fornices.
   - Palpate around the grooves.
   - Confirm that the mucosa of the vagina and cervix in these areas is smooth and nontender.
   - Leave your fingers in the anterior fornix when you have checked all sides.

3. **Palpate the uterus.**
   - Place the fingers of your nondominant hand on the client's abdomen.

   - Invaginate the abdomen midway between the umbilicus and the symphysis pubis by pushing with your fingertips downward toward the cervix (Figure 16.7).

▶ If the woman is pregnant, the cervix will be soft. This is a normal finding and is called Goodell's sign.

▶ Note any tenderness, which could be indicative of inflammation.
▶ Note any tenderness, masses, nodules, or bulging. These findings may indicate inflammation, infection, cysts, tumors, or wall prolapse. Note size, shape, consistency, and mobility of nodules and masses.

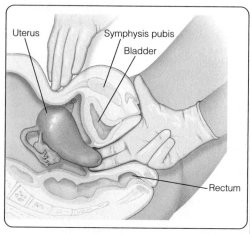

Figure 16.7 • Palpating the uterus.

- Palpate the front wall of the uterus with the hand that is inside the vagina.

TECHNIQUES AND NORMAL FINDINGS	**ABNORMAL FINDINGS** **SPECIAL CONSIDERATIONS**

- As you palpate, note the position of the uterine body to determine that the uterus is in a normal position. When in a normal position, the uterus is tilted slightly upward above the bladder, and the cervix is tilted slightly forward.

▶ In the obese female, it may be difficult to clearly differentiate the uterine structures, and an ultrasound study may be needed.

- Move the inner fingers to the posterior fornix, and gently raise the cervix up toward your outer hand.
- Palpate the front and back walls of the uterus as it is sandwiched between the two hands.

▶ Masses, tenderness, nodules, or bulging require further evaluation.

4. Palpate the ovaries.
- While positioning the outer hand on the left lower abdominal quadrant, slip the vaginal fingers into the left lateral fornix.
- Push the opposing fingers and hand toward one another, and then use small circular motions to palpate the left ovary with your intravaginal fingers (Figure 16.8).

▶ Extreme tenderness, nodularity, and masses are suggestive of inflammation, infection, cysts, malignancies, or tubal pregnancy.

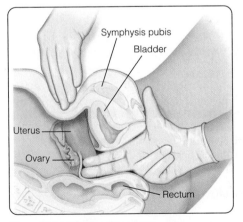

Figure 16.8 • Palpating the ovaries.

TECHNIQUES AND NORMAL FINDINGS	ABNORMAL FINDINGS SPECIAL CONSIDERATIONS

- If you are able to palpate the ovary, it will feel mobile, almond shaped, smooth, firm, and nontender to slightly tender. Often you will be unable to palpate the ovaries, especially the right ovary.
- Slide your vaginal fingers around to the right lateral fornix and your outer hand to the lower right quadrant to palpate the right ovary.
- Confirm that the uterine tubes are not palpable.

- Remove your hand from the vagina and put on new gloves.

5. Perform the rectovaginal exam.
- Tell the client that you are going to insert one finger into her vagina and one finger into her rectum in order to perform a rectovaginal exam. Tell her that this maneuver may make her feel as though she needs to have a bowel movement.
- Lubricate the gloved index and middle fingers of the dominant hand.
- Ask the client to bear down.
- Touch the client's thigh with your nondominant hand to prepare her for the insertion.
- Insert the index finger into the vagina (at a 45-degree downward slope) and the middle finger into the rectum.
- Compress the rectovaginal septum between your index and middle fingers.
- Confirm that it is thin, smooth, and nontender.
- Place your nondominant hand on the client's abdomen.
- While maintaining the position of your intravaginal hand, press your outer hand inward and downward on the abdomen over the symphysis pubis.
- Palpate the posterior side of the uterus with the pad of the rectal finger while continuing to press down on the abdomen (Figure 16.9).

▶ In obese females, it may not be possible to palpate the ovaries.

▶ In the female client who has been postmenopausal for more than 2 1/2 years, palpable ovaries are considered abnormal because the ovaries usually atrophy with the postmenopausal decrease in estrogen.

▶ If the uterine tubes are palpable, an inflammation or some other disease process such as salpingitis or ectopic pregnancy may be present.

▶ This prevents cross-contamination from the vagina to the rectum.

▶ Note any tenderness, masses, nodules, bulging, and thickened areas.

TECHNIQUES AND NORMAL FINDINGS

ABNORMAL FINDINGS
SPECIAL CONSIDERATIONS

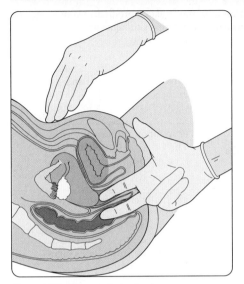

Figure 16.9 • Rectovaginal palpation.

- Confirm that the uterine wall is smooth and nontender.
- If the ovaries are palpable, note that they are normal in size and contour.
- Remove your fingers from the vagina and rectum slowly and gently.

▶ Tenderness, masses, nodules, bulging, or thickened areas require further evaluation.

6. **Examine the stool.**
   - Remove your gloves.
   - Assist the client into a comfortable position.

▶ Rectal bleeding is suspected when bright red blood is on the surface of the stool. Feces mixed with blood signals bleeding above the rectum.

   - Inspect feces remaining on the glove. Feces are normally brown and soft. Test feces for occult blood. Normally the test is negative.
   - Wash your hands.
   - Give the client tissues to wipe the perineal area. Some clients may need a perineal pad.
   - Inform the client that she may have a small amount of spotting for a few hours after the speculum examination.

▶ Black, tarry stool indicates upper gastrointestinal tract bleeding.

Abnormal Findings

Abnormal findings from assessment of the female reproductive system include but are not limited to problems with the external genitalia and internal reproductive organs.

EXTERNAL GENITALIA

Pediculosis Pubis

Nits are on and around roots of pubic hair and cause itching. The area is reddened and excoriated.

Herpes Simplex

Small vesicles appear on genitalia and may spread to the inner thigh. Ulcers are painful and erupt upon rupture of vesicles. The virus may be dormant for long periods.

Syphilitic Lesion

A syphilitic lesion is a nontender solitary papule that gradually changes to a draining ulcer.

Human Papillomavirus (HPV)

Wartlike, painless growths appear in clusters. These are seen on the vulva, inner vagina, cervix, or anal area.

Abscess of Bartholin's Gland

An abscess of Bartholin's gland includes labial edema and erythema with a palpable mass. There is purulent drainage from the duct.

CERVIX

Cyanosis

Cyanosis associated with hypoxic conditions such as congestive heart failure (CHF) can cause this. Blue coloring of the cervix is normal in pregnancy.

Carcinoma

Ulcerations with vaginal discharge, postmenopausal bleeding or spotting, or bleeding between menstrual periods are characteristics of cervical carcinoma. Diagnosis is confirmed by Pap smear.

Erosion

Inflammation and erosion are visible on the surface of the cervix. It is difficult to distinguish this from carcinoma without a biopsy.

Polyp

A soft growth extends from the os. A polyp is usually bright red and may bleed.

Diethylstilbestrol (DES) Syndrome

Abnormalities of the cervix arise in females who had prenatal exposure to DES. Epithelial abnormalities occur as granular patchiness extending from the cervix to the vaginal walls.

INTERNAL REPRODUCTIVE ORGANS

Common problems of the internal reproductive organs include myomas, fibroids, or uterine carcinoma, ovarian cysts, and cancer.

17

Musculoskeletal System

The primary function of the musculoskeletal system is to provide structure and movement for the human body. The bones and skeletal muscles allow the body to stand erect, move, and support and protect body organs.

ANATOMY AND PHYSIOLOGY REVIEW

The musculoskeletal system consists of the body's bones, skeletal muscles, and joints. The bones support and provide a framework for the soft tissues and organs of the body. They are classified according to shape and composition. Bone shapes include *long bones* (femur, humerus), *short bones* (carpals, tarsals), *flat bones* (parietal bone of the skull, sternum, ribs), and *irregular bones* (vertebrae, hip bones).

A skeletal muscle is composed of hundreds of thousands of elongated muscle cells or fibers arranged in striated bands that attach to skeletal bones. Although some skeletal muscles react by reflex, most skeletal muscles are voluntary and are under an individual's conscious control.

A **joint** (or *articulation*) is the point where two or more bones in the body meet. Joints may be classified structurally as fibrous, cartilaginous, or synovial. Bones joined by fibrous tissue, such as the sutures joining the bones of the skull, are called **fibrous joints.** Bones joined by cartilage, such as the vertebrae, are called **cartilaginous joints.** Bones separated by a fluid-filled joint cavity are called **synovial joints.** The structure of synovial joints allows tremendous freedom of movement, and all joints of the limbs are synovial joints. Most synovial joints are reinforced and strengthened by a system of *ligaments,* which are bands of flexible tissue that attach bone to bone. Some ligaments are protected from friction by small, synovial-fluid-filled sacs called **bursae. Tendons** are tough, fibrous bands that attach muscle to bone, or muscle to muscle. Tendons, subjected to continuous friction, develop fluid-filled bursae called *tendon sheaths* to protect the joint from damage. Table 17.1 describes the classification of synovial joints, and Table 17.2 describes the movements of the joints.

SPECIAL CONSIDERATIONS

There are a variety of factors or special considerations that contribute to health status. Among these are age, developmental level, race, ethnicity, work history, living conditions, socioeconomics, and emotional well-being.

INFANTS AND CHILDREN

Fetal positioning and the delivery process may cause musculoskeletal anomalies in the infant. Newborns normally have flat feet; arches develop gradually during the preschool years. Before learning to walk, infants tend to exhibit genu varum (bowlegs). The nurse should inspect the newborn's spine. Any tuft of hair, cyst, or mass may indicate spina bifida and requires further evaluation. The infant is assessed for congenital hip dislocation at every office visit until 1 year of age. Additionally, *Allis' sign* is used to detect unequal leg length. Shoulder muscle strength is present if the infant remains upright between the nurse's

Table 17.1 Classification of Synovial Joints

TYPE OF JOINT

In *plane joints*, the articular surfaces are flat, allowing only slipping or gliding movements. Examples include the intercarpal and intertarsal joints, and the joints between the articular processes of the ribs.

Carpals

A Plane joint

In *hinge joints*, a convex projection of one bone fits into a concave depression in another. Motion is similar to that of a mechanical hinge. These joints permit flexion and extension only. Examples include the elbow and knee joints.

Humerus

Ulna

B Hinge joint

In *pivot joints*, the rounded end of one bone protrudes into a ring of bone (and possibly ligaments). The only movement allowed is rotation of the bone around its own long axis or against the other bone. An example is the joint between the atlas and axis of the neck.

Ulna
Radius

C Pivot joint

(continued)

Table 17.1 Classification of Synovial Joints (continued)

TYPE OF JOINT

In *condyloid joints*, the oval surfaces of two bones fit together. Movements allowed are flexion and extension, abduction, adduction, and circumduction. An example is the radiocarpal (wrist) joints.

Metacarpal
Phalanx

D Condyloid joint

In *saddle joints*, each articulating bone has both concave and convex areas (resembling a saddle). The opposing surfaces fit together. The movements allowed are the same as for condyloid joints, but the freedom of motion is greater. The carpometacarpal joints of the thumbs are an example.

Carpal
Metacarpal 1

E Saddle joint

In *ball-and-socket joints*, the ball-shaped head of one bone fits into the concave socket of another. These joints allow movement in all axes and planes, including rotation. The shoulder and hip joints are the only examples in the body.

Head of humerus
Glenoid cavity of scapula

F Ball-and-socket joint

Table 17.2 Joint Movement

TYPE OF MOVEMENT

Gliding movements are the simplest type of joint movements. One flat bone surface glides or slips over another similar surface. The bones are merely displaced in relation to one another.

Flexion is a bending movement that decreases the angle of the joint and brings the articulating bones closer together. **Extension** increases the angle between the articulating bones. (**Hyperextension** is a bending of a joint beyond 180 degrees.)

Flexion of the ankle so that the superior aspect of the foot approaches the shin is called **dorsiflexion.** Extension of the ankle (pointing the toes) is called **plantar flexion.**

Abduction is movement of a limb away from the midline or median plane of the body, along the frontal plane. When the term is used to describe movement of the fingers or toes, it means spreading them apart. **Adduction** is the movement of a limb toward the body midline. Bringing the fingers close together is adduction.

Circumduction is the movement in which the limb describes a cone in space: while the distal end of the limb moves in a circle, the joint itself moves only slightly in the joint cavity.

Rotation is the turning movement of a bone around its own long axis. Rotation may occur toward the body midline or away from it.

The terms **supination** and **pronation** refer only to the movements of the radius around the ulna. Movement of the forearm so that the palm faces anteriorly or superiorly is called *supination.* In *pronation,* the palm moves to face posteriorly or inferiorly.

(continued)

Table 17.2	**Joint Movement** (*continued*)

TYPE OF MOVEMENT

The terms **inversion** and **eversion** refer to movements of the foot. In *inversion*, the sole of the foot is turned medially. In *eversion*, the sole faces laterally.

Protraction is a nonangular anterior movement in a transverse plane.
Retraction is a nonangular posterior movement in a transverse plane.

Elevation is a lifting or moving superiorly along a frontal plane. When the elevated part is moved downward to its original position, the movement is called **depression**. Shrugging the shoulders and chewing are examples of alternating elevation and depression.

Opposition *of the thumb* is only allowed at the saddle joint between metacarpal 1 and the carpals. It is the movement of touching the thumb to the tips of the other fingers of the same hand.

hands. Bone growth is rapid during infancy and continues at a steady rate during childhood until adolescence, at which time both girls and boys experience a growth spurt. The child's spine is assessed for scoliosis at each office visit. It is also important to inspect the child's shoes for signs of abnormal wear, and assess the child's gait.

THE PREGNANT FEMALE

Estrogen and other hormones soften the cartilage in the pelvis and increase the mobility of the joints, especially the sacroiliac, sacrococcygeal, and symphysis pubis joints. As the pregnancy progresses, lordosis (exaggeration of the lumbar spinal curve) compensates for the enlarging fetus. The female's center of gravity shifts forward, and she shifts her weight farther back on her lower extremities. This shift strains the lower spine, causing the lower back pain that is so common during late pregnancy. As the pregnancy progresses, she may develop a waddling gait because of her enlarged abdomen and the relaxed mobility in her joints. Typically, a female resumes her normal posture and gait shortly after the pregnancy.

THE OLDER ADULT

Bone changes include decreased calcium absorption and reduced osteoblast production. If the older adult has a chronic illness, such as chronic obstructive lung disease or hyperthyroidism, or takes medications containing glucocorticoids, thyroid hormone preparation, or anticonvulsants, bone strength may be greatly compromised because of decrease in the bone density. Elderly persons who are housebound and immobile or whose dietary intake of calcium and vitamin D is low may also experience reduced bone mass and strength. During aging, bone resorption occurs more rapidly than new bone growth, resulting in the loss of bone density typical of osteoporosis. The entire skeleton is affected, but the vertebrae and long bones are especially vulnerable.

The decreased height of the aging adult occurs because of a shortening of the vertebral column. Thinning of the intervertebral disks during middle age and an erosion of individual vertebrae due to osteoporosis contribute to this shortening. Kyphosis, an exaggerated convexity of the thoracic region of the spine, is common. The size and quantity of muscle fibers tend to decrease by as much as 30% by the 80th year of life. The amount of connective tissue in the muscles increases, and they become fibrous or stringy. Tendons become less elastic. The older client experiences a progressive decrease in reaction time, speed of movements, agility, and endurance.

Degeneration of the joints causes thickening and decreased viscosity of the synovial fluid, fragmentation of connective tissue, and scarring and calcification in the joint capsules. Both males and females tend to walk slower, supporting themselves as they move. Elderly males tend to walk with the head and trunk in a flexed position, using short, high steps, a wide gait, and a smaller arm swing. The bowlegged stance that is observed in older females is due to reduced muscular control, thus altering the normal angle of the hip and leading to increased susceptibility to falls and subsequent fractures.

PSYCHOSOCIAL CONSIDERATIONS

Psychosocial problems such as anxiety, depression, fear, altered body image, or a disturbance in self-esteem may promote inactivity or isolation, which in turn may lead to musculoskeletal degeneration.

CULTURAL CONSIDERATIONS

Assessment and findings are influenced by culture. See the cultural considerations box for specific examples.

Health assessment of the musculoskeletal system includes the gathering of subjective and objective data. Subjective data collection occurs during the client interview before the physical assessment.

Cultural Considerations

- Asians and Caucasians have a higher incidence of osteoporosis than African Americans.
- African Americans have greater bone density compared to Caucasians or Asians.
- Ankylosing spondylitis occurs more frequently in males than in females, and in individuals who are of Native American or European descent.
- Systemic lupus erythematosus occurs more frequently in females, and with greater frequency and severity in African Americans than in Hispanics or Caucasians.

- Sickle cell anemia, which can result in joint disruption, occurs in descendants of individuals from sub-Saharan Africa, South America, Cuba, Central America, Saudi Arabia, India, and Mediterranean countries such as Turkey, Greece, and Italy. In the United States, it occurs most frequently in African Americans.
- Osteoarthritis occurs more frequently in African American males than in Caucasian males and develops twice as frequently in African American females as in Caucasian females.
- Paget's disease occurs more frequently in Caucasians than in other cultural groups.

Gathering the Data

FOCUSED INTERVIEW QUESTIONS

1. Describe your mobility today, 2 months ago, and 2 years ago. Are you able to carry out all of your regular activities?
2. Do you or any members of your family have any musculoskeletal problem or any chronic diseases such as diabetes mellitus, hypothyroidism, sickle cell anemia, lupus erythematosus, or rheumatoid arthritis?
3. Have you had any fractures or penetrating wounds?
4. Do you have or have you had any swelling, heat, redness, or stiffness in your muscles or joints? If the response is yes, additional questions are needed.

QUESTIONS REGARDING INFANTS AND CHILDREN

1. Were you told about any trauma to the infant during labor and delivery?
2. Have you noticed any deformity of the child's spine or limbs, or any unusual shape of the child's feet and toes?
3. Please describe any dislocations or broken bones the child has had, including any treatment.
4. *For the school-age child:* Do you play any sports at school or after school?

QUESTION FOR THE PREGNANT FEMALE

1. Please describe any back pain you are experiencing.

QUESTIONS FOR THE OLDER ADULT

1. Have you noticed any muscle weakness over the past few months?
2. Have you fallen in the past 6 months?
3. Do you use any walking aids such as a cane or walker to help you get around?
4. Are you currently taking any medications such as steroids, estrogen, muscle relaxants, or any other drugs?
5. *For postmenopausal females:* Do you take calcium supplements?

Physical Assessment

Physical assessment of the musculoskeletal system requires the use of inspection and palpation. During each of the procedures the nurse is gathering data related to the client's skeleton, joints, musculature, strength, and mobility.

EQUIPMENT

examination gown
clean, nonsterile examination gloves
examination light

skin marking pen
goniometer
tape measure

HELPFUL HINTS

- Age and agility influence the client's ability to participate in the assessment.
- It is often more helpful to demonstrate the movements you expect of the client during this assessment than to use easily misunderstood verbal instructions. A "Simon Says" approach works well, especially with children.
- When assessing range of motion, do not push the joint beyond its normal range.
- Stop when the client expresses discomfort.
- Measure the joint angle with a goniometer when range of motion appears limited.
- Use an orderly approach: head to toe, proximal to distal, compare the sides of the body for symmetry.
- The musculoskeletal assessment may be exhausting for some clients. Provide rest periods or schedule two sessions.
- Use Standard Precautions.

TECHNIQUES AND NORMAL FINDINGS	ABNORMAL FINDINGS SPECIAL CONSIDERATIONS

ASSESSMENT OF THE JOINTS

1. **Inspect the temporomandibular joint on both sides.**
   - The joints should be symmetric and not swollen or painful.

   ▶ An enlarged or swollen joint shows as a rounded protuberance.

2. **Palpate the temporomandibular joints.**
   - Place the finger pads of your index and middle fingers in front of the tragus of each ear. Ask the client to open and close the mouth while you palpate the temporomandibular joints.
   - As the client's mouth opens, your fingers should glide into a shallow depression of the joints. Confirm the smooth motion of the mandible.
   - The joint may audibly and palpably click as the mouth opens. This is normal.

   ▶ Discomfort, swelling, crackling sounds, and limited movement of the jaw are unexpected findings that require further evaluation for dental or neurologic problems or TMJ syndrome.

3. **Palpate the muscles of the jaw.**
   - Instruct the client to clench the teeth as you palpate the masseter and temporalis muscles. Confirm that the muscles are symmetric, firm, and nontender.

   ▶ Swelling and tenderness suggest arthritis and myofascial pain syndrome.

4. **Test for range of motion of the temporomandibular joints.**
   - Ask the client to open the mouth as wide as possible. Confirm that the mouth opens with ease to as much as 3 to 6 cm between the upper and lower incisors.

   ▶ Temporomandibular joint dysfunction should be suspected if facial pain and limited jaw movement accompany clicking sounds as the jaw opens and closes.

TECHNIQUES AND NORMAL FINDINGS	ABNORMAL FINDINGS SPECIAL CONSIDERATIONS

- With the mouth slightly open, ask the client to push out the lower jaw, and return the lower jaw to a neutral position. The jaw should protrude and retract with ease.
- Ask the client to move the lower jaw from side to side. Confirm that the jaw moves laterally from 1 to 2 cm without deviation or dislocation.
- Ask the client to close the mouth. The mouth should close completely without pain or discomfort.

5. **Test for muscle strength and motor function of cranial nerve V.**
   - Instruct the client to repeat the movements in step 4 as you provide opposing force. The client should be able to perform the movements against your resistance. The strength of the muscles on both sides of the jaw should be equal.

THE SHOULDERS

1. **With the client facing you, inspect both shoulders.**
   - Compare the shape and size of the shoulders, clavicles, and scapula. Confirm that they are symmetric and similar in size both anteriorly and posteriorly.

   ▶ Swelling, deformity, atrophy, and misalignment, combined with limited motion, pain, and crepitus (a grating sound caused by bone fragments in joints), suggest degenerative joint disease, traumatized joints (strains, sprains), or inflammatory conditions (rheumatoid arthritis, bursitis, or tendinitis).

2. **Palpate the shoulders and surrounding structures.**
   - Begin palpating at the sternoclavicular joint; then move laterally along the clavicle to the acromioclavicular joint.
   - Palpate downward into the subacromial area and the greater tubercle of the humerus.
   - Confirm that these areas are firm and nontender, the shoulders symmetric, and the scapulae level and symmetric.

   ▶ Shoulder pain without palpation or movement may result from insufficient circulation to the myocardium. This cue, known as *referred pain,* can be a precursor to a myocardial infarction (heart attack). If the client exhibits other symptoms such as chest pain, indigestion,

TECHNIQUES AND NORMAL FINDINGS

ABNORMAL FINDINGS
SPECIAL CONSIDERATIONS

and cardiovascular changes, medical assistance must be obtained immediately.

3. **Test the range of motion of the shoulders.**
   - Instruct the client to use both arms for the following maneuvers:
     - Shrug the shoulders by flexing them forward and upward.
     - With the elbows extended, raise the arms forward and upward in an arc. (The client should demonstrate a forward flexion of 180 degrees.)
     - Return the arms to the sides. Keeping the elbows extended, move the arms backward as far as possible (Figure 17.1). (The client should demonstrate an extension of as much as 50 degrees.)

▶ If the client expresses discomfort, it is important to determine if the pain is referred. Conditions that increase intra-abdominal pressure, such as hiatal hernia and gastrointestinal disease, may cause pain in the shoulder area. When limitation or increase in range of motion (ROM) is assessed, the goniometer should be used to precisely measure the angle.

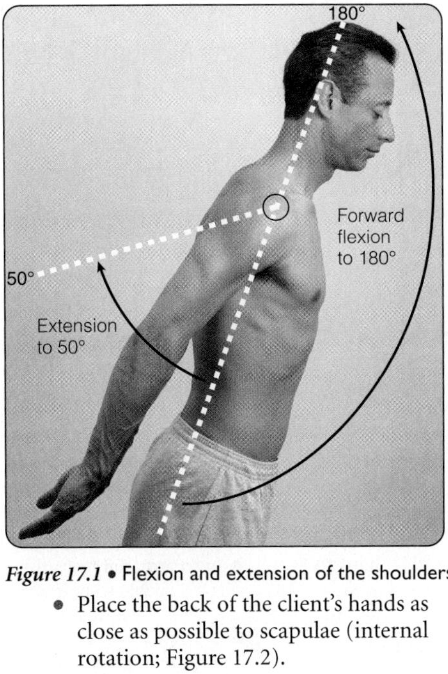

Figure 17.1 • Flexion and extension of the shoulders.

   - Place the back of the client's hands as close as possible to scapulae (internal rotation; Figure 17.2).

TECHNIQUES AND NORMAL FINDINGS

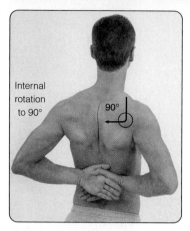

Figure 17.2 • Internal rotation of the shoulders.

- Ask the client to clasp his or her hands behind the head (external rotation; Figure 17.3).

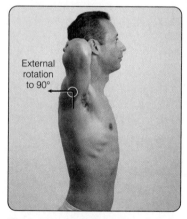

Figure 17.3 • External rotation of the shoulders.

- With elbows extended, ask the client to swing the arms out to the sides in arcs, touching the palms together above the head. The client should demonstrate abduction of 180 degrees.

▶ In rotator cuff tears, the client is unable to perform abduction without lifting or shrugging the shoulder. This sign is accompanied by pain, tenderness, and muscle atrophy.

TECHNIQUES AND NORMAL FINDINGS	**ABNORMAL FINDINGS SPECIAL CONSIDERATIONS**

- With the elbows extended, ask the client to swing each arm toward the midline of the body.
- The client should demonstrate adduction of as much as 50 degrees.

4. **Test for strength of the shoulder muscles.**
   - Instruct the client to repeat the movements in step 3 as you provide opposing force. The client should be able to perform the movements against your resistance. The strength of the shoulder muscles on both sides should be equal.
   - Muscle strength is rated on a scale of 0 to 5 with 0 representing absence of strength and 5 indicating maximum or normal strengths. Table 17.3 includes information about rating muscle strength.

▶ Full resistance during the shoulder shrug indicates adequate cranial nerve XI (spinal accessory) function.

Table 17.3	**Rating Muscle Strength**	
RATING	**DESCRIPTION OF FUNCTION**	**CLASSIFICATION**
5	Full range of motion against gravity with full resistance	Normal
4	Full range of motion against gravity with moderate resistance	Good
3	Full range of motion with gravity	Fair
2	Full range of motion without gravity (passive motion)	Poor
1	Palpable muscle contraction but no movement	Trace
0	No muscle contraction	Zero

ELBOWS

1. **Support the client's arm and inspect the lateral and medial aspects of the elbow.**
   - The elbows should be symmetric.

▶ Swelling, deformity, or malalignment requires further evaluation. If there is a subluxation (partial dislocation), the elbow looks deformed, and the forearm is misaligned.

2. **Palpate the lateral and medial aspects of the olecranon process.**
   - Use your thumb and middle fingers to palpate the grooves on either side of the olecranon process.

▶ In the presence of inflammation, the grooves feel soft and spongy, and the surrounding tissue may be red, hot, and painful.

TECHNIQUES AND NORMAL FINDINGS	ABNORMAL FINDINGS SPECIAL CONSIDERATIONS

- The joint should be free of pain, thickening, swelling, or tenderness.

▶ Inflammatory conditions of the elbow include arthritis, bursitis, and epicondylitis. *Rheumatoid arthritis* may result in nodules in the olecranon bursa or along the extensor surface of the ulna. Nodules are firm, nontender, and not attached to the overlying skin. *Lateral epicondylitis* (tennis elbow) results from constant, repetitive movements of the wrist or forearm. Pain occurs when the client attempts to extend the wrist against resistance. *Medial epicondylitis* (pitcher's or golfer's elbow) results from constant, repetitive flexion of the wrist. Pain occurs when the client attempts to flex the wrist against resistance.

3. **Test the range of motion of each elbow.**
   - Instruct the client to perform the following movements:
     - Bend the elbow by bringing the forearm forward and touching the fingers to the shoulder. The elbow should flex to 160 degrees.
     - Straighten the elbow. The lower arm should form a straight line with the

▶ To use the goniometer, begin with the joint in a neutral position and then flex the joint as far as possible. Measure the angle with the goniometer. Fully extend the joint and measure the angle with the goniometer. Compare the goniometer measurements to the expected degree of flexion and extension. See Figure 17.4 for an example.

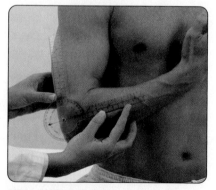

Figure 17.4 • Goniometer measure of joint range of motion.

upper arm. The elbow in a neutral
position is at 0 degree extension.
The elbow should extend to 0 degree.

- Holding the arm straight out, turn
  the palm upward facing the ceiling,
  then downward facing the floor.
  The elbow should supinate and
  pronate to 90 degrees.
- The client should be able to put each
  elbow through the normal range of
  motion without difficulty or discomfort.

4. **Test for muscle strength.**
   - Stabilize the client's elbow with
     your nondominant hand while
     holding the wrist with your
     dominant hand.
   - Instruct the client to flex the elbow
     while you apply opposing resistance
     (Figure 17.5).

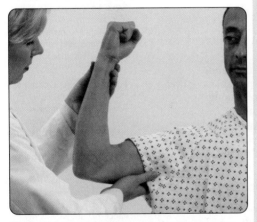

Figure 17.5 • Testing muscle strength using opposing
force.

- Instruct the client to extend the elbow
  against resistance.
- The client should be able to perform
  these movements. The strength of
  the muscles associated with flexion
  and extension of each elbow should
  be equal. Muscle strength is
  measured by testing against the
  strength of the examiner as
  resistance is applied.

TECHNIQUES AND NORMAL FINDINGS	ABNORMAL FINDINGS SPECIAL CONSIDERATIONS

WRISTS AND HANDS

1. **Inspect the wrists and dorsum of the hands for size, shape, symmetry, and color.**
   - The wrists and hands should be symmetric and free from swelling and deformity. The color should be similar to that of the rest of the body. The ends of either the ulna or radius may protrude further in some individuals.

▶ Redness, swelling, or deformity in the joints requires further evaluation. It is important to note any nodules on the hands or wrists, or atrophy of the surrounding muscles. In acute rheumatoid arthritis, the wrist, proximal interphalangeal, and metacarpophalangeal joints are likely to be swollen, tender, and stiff. As the disease progresses, the proximal interphalangeal joints deviate toward the ulnar side of the hand; the interosseous muscles atrophy, and rheumatoid nodules form, giving the rheumatic hand its characteristic appearance.

2. **Inspect the palms of the hands.**
   - There is a rounded protuberance over the thenar eminence (the area proximal to the thumb).

3. **Palpate the wrists and hands for temperature and texture.**
   - The temperature of the wrists and hands should be warm and similar to the rest of the body. The skin should be smooth and free of cuts. The skin around the interphalangeal joints may have a rougher texture.

▶ Carpal tunnel syndrome is a nerve disorder in which an inflammation of tissues in the wrist causes pressure on the median nerve (which innervates the hand). Thenar atrophy is a common finding associated with carpal tunnel syndrome; however, some atrophy of the thenar eminence occurs with aging.

4. **Palpate each joint of the wrists and hands.**
   - Move your thumbs from side to side gently but firmly over the dorsum, with your fingers resting beneath the area you are palpating. As you palpate, make sure you keep the client's wrist straight.
   - To palpate the interphalangeal joints, pinch them gently between your thumb and index finger. All joints should be firm and nontender, with no swelling.

▶ A ganglion is a typically painless, round, fluid-filled mass that arises from the tendon sheaths on the dorsum of the wrist and hand. It may require surgery. Ganglia that are more prevalent when the wrist is flexed do not interfere with range of motion or function.

| **TECHNIQUES AND NORMAL FINDINGS** | **ABNORMAL FINDINGS SPECIAL CONSIDERATIONS** |

- As you palpate, note the temperature of the client's hand.

▶ A cool temperature in the extremities may indicate compromised vascular function, which may in turn influence muscle strength.

5. **Test the range of motion of the wrist.**
   - Instruct the client to perform the following movements:
     - Straighten the hand (extension).
     - Using the wrist as a pivot point, bring the fingers backward as far as possible, and then bend the wrist downward. The wrist should hyperextend to 70 degrees and flex to 90 degrees.
     - Turn the palms down; move the hand laterally toward the fifth finger, then medially toward the thumb. Be sure the movement is from the wrist and not the elbow. Ulnar deviation should reach as much as 55 degrees, and radial deviation should reach as much as 20 degrees.
     - Bend the wrists downward and press the backs of both hands together (*Phalen's test*; Figure 17.6). This causes flexion of the wrists to 90 degrees. Normally clients experience no symptoms with this maneuver.

▶ When a Phalen's test is performed on individuals with carpal tunnel syndrome, 80% experience pain, tingling, and numbness that radiates to the arm, shoulder, neck, or chest within 60 seconds. If carpal tunnel syndrome is suspected, it is important to check for Tinel's sign by percussing lightly over the median nerve in each wrist. If carpal tunnel syndrome is present, the client feels numbness, tingling, and pain along the median nerve (Figure 17.7).

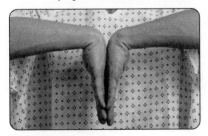

Figure 17.6 • Phalen's test.

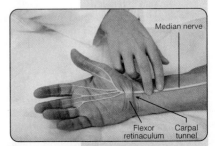

Figure 17.7 • Tinel's sign.

TECHNIQUES AND NORMAL FINDINGS	ABNORMAL FINDINGS SPECIAL CONSIDERATIONS

6. **Test the range of motion of the hands and fingers.**
   - Instruct the client to perform the following movements:
     - Make a tight fist with each hand with the fingers folded into the palm and the thumb across the knuckles (thumb flexion).
     - Open the fist and stretch the fingers (extension).
     - Point the fingers downward toward the forearm, and then back as far as possible. Fingers should flex to 90 degrees and hyperextend to as much as 30 degrees.
     - Spread the fingers far apart, then back together. Fingers should abduct to 20 degrees and should adduct fully (to touch).
     - Move the thumb toward the ulnar side of the hand and then away from the hand as far as possible.
     - Touch the thumb to the tip of each of the fingers and to the base of the little finger.

▶ In *Dupuytren's contracture,* the client is unable to extend the fourth and fifth fingers. This is a progressive, painless, inherited disorder that causes severe flexion in the affected fingers, is usually bilateral, and is more common in middle-aged and older males.

7. **Test for muscle strength of the wrist.**
   - Place the client's arm on a table with his or her palm facing up.
   - Stabilize the client's forearm with one hand while holding the client's hand with your other hand.
   - Instruct the client to flex the wrist while you apply opposing force. The client should be able to provide full resistance.

8. **Test for muscle strength of the fingers.**
   - Ask the client to spread his or her fingers, and then try to force the fingers together.
   - Ask the client to touch his or her little finger with the thumb while you place resistance on the thumb in order to prevent the movement.

▶ Clients with carpal tunnel syndrome manifest weakness when attempting opposition of the thumb.

HIPS

1. **Inspect the position of each hip and leg with the client in a supine position.**
   - The legs should be slightly apart and the toes should point toward the ceiling.

▶ External rotation of the lower leg and foot is a classic sign of a fractured femur.

TECHNIQUES AND NORMAL FINDINGS	ABNORMAL FINDINGS SPECIAL CONSIDERATIONS

2. Palpate each hip joint and the upper thighs.

- The hip joints are firm, stable, and nontender.

▶ Pain, tenderness, swelling, deformity, limited motion (especially limited internal rotation), and crepitus are diagnostic cues that signal inflammatory or degenerative joint diseases in the hip. A fractured femur should be suspected if the joint is unstable and deformed.

3. Test the range of motion of the hips.

ALERT! *Do not ask clients who have undergone hip replacement to perform these movements without the permission of the physician, because these motions can dislocate the prosthesis.*

- Instruct the client to perform the following movements:
  - Raise each leg straight off the bed or table. The other leg should remain flat on the bed. Hip flexion with straight knee should reach 90 degrees. Return the leg to its original position.

    ▶ This maneuver produces back and leg pain along the course of the sciatic nerve in the client with a herniated disk.

  - Raise the leg with the knee flexed toward the chest as far as it will go. Hip flexion with flexed knee should reach 120 degrees. Return the leg to its original position.
  - Move the foot away from the midline as the knee moves toward the midline. Internal hip rotation should reach 40 degrees.
  - Move the foot toward the midline as the knee moves away from the midline. External hip rotation should reach 45 degrees.
  - Move the leg away from the midline, then as far as possible toward the midline. Abduction should reach 45 degrees. Adduction should reach 30 degrees.
- Assist the client to turn onto his or her abdomen. An alternative position could be side lying. With the client's knee extended, ask the client to raise each leg backward and up as far as possible. Hips

TECHNIQUES AND NORMAL FINDINGS	ABNORMAL FINDINGS SPECIAL CONSIDERATIONS

should hyperextend to 15 degrees. (You may also perform this test later, during assessment of the spine, with the client standing.)

4. **Test for muscle strength of the hips.**
   - Assist the client in returning to the supine position.
   - Press your hands on the client's thighs and ask the client to raise his or her hip.
   - Place your hands outside the client's knees and ask the client to spread both legs against your resistance.
   - Place your hands between the client's knees, and ask the client to bring the legs together against your resistance.

KNEES

1. **Inspect the knees.**
   - With the client in the sitting position, inspect the knees.
   - The patella should be centrally located in each knee. The normal depressions along each side of the patella should be sharp and distinct. The skin color should be similar to that of the surrounding areas.

▶ Swelling and signs of fluid in the knee and its surrounding structures require further evaluation. Fluid accumulates in the suprapatellar bursa, the prepatellar bursa, and other areas adjacent to the patella when there is inflammation, trauma, or degenerative joint disease.

2. **Inspect the quadriceps muscle in the anterior thigh.**
   - The muscles should be symmetric.

▶ Atrophy in the quadriceps muscles occurs with disuse or chronic disorders.

3. **Palpate the knee.**
   - Using your thumb, index, and middle fingers begin palpating approximately 10 cm above the patella with your thumb, index, and middle fingers. Palpate downward, evaluating each area.
   - The quadriceps muscle and surrounding soft tissue should be firm and nontender. The suprapatellar bursa is usually not palpable.

▶ Any pain, swelling, thickening, or heat should be noted while palpating the knee. These diagnostic cues occur when the synovium is inflamed. Painless swelling frequently occurs in degenerative joint disease. A painful, localized area of swelling, heat, and redness in the knee is caused by the inflammation of the bursa (bursitis), for example, *prepatellar bursitis* (housemaid's knee).

TECHNIQUES AND NORMAL FINDINGS	ABNORMAL FINDINGS SPECIAL CONSIDERATIONS

4. **Palpate the tibiofemoral joint.**
   - With the client's knee still in the flexed position, use your thumbs to palpate deeply along each side of the tibia toward the outer aspects of the knee.
   - Then palpate along the lateral collateral ligament.
   - The joint should be firm and nontender.

▶ Signs of inflammation, including pain and tenderness, occur when the joint is inflamed or damaged and may indicate degenerative joint disease, synovitis, or a torn meniscus. Bony ridges or prominences in the outer aspects of the joint occur with osteoarthritis.

5. **Test for the bulge sign.**
   - This procedure detects the presence of small amounts of fluid (4 to 8 ml) in the suprapatellar bursa.
   - With the client in the supine position, use firm pressure to stroke the medial aspect of the knee upward several times, displacing any fluid (Figure 17.8).

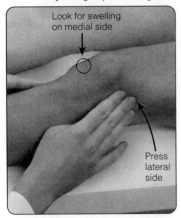

Look for swelling on medial side

Press lateral side

Figure 17.8 • Testing for the bulge sign.

   - Apply pressure to the lateral side of the knee while observing the medial side.
   - Normally no fluid is present.

▶ The medial side of the knee bulges if fluid is in the joint.

6. **Perform ballottement.**
   - **Ballottement** is a technique used to detect fluid, or to examine or detect floating body structures. The nurse displaces body fluid and then palpates the return impact of the body structure.
   - To detect large amounts of fluid in the suprapatellar bursa, with your thumb and fingers, firmly grasp the thigh just above the knee. This action causes any

▶ When there are abnormal fluid levels, fluid forced between the patella and femur causes the patella to "float" over the femur. A palpable click is felt when the patella is snapped back against the femur when fluid is present.

TECHNIQUES AND NORMAL FINDINGS	ABNORMAL FINDINGS SPECIAL CONSIDERATIONS

fluid in the suprapatellar bursa to move between the patella and the femur.

- With the fingers of your left hand, quickly push the patella downward upon the femur (Figure 17.9).

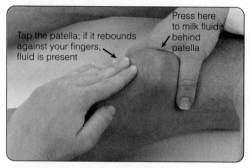

Tap the patella; if it rebounds against your fingers, fluid is present

Press here to milk fluid behind patella

Figure 17.9 • Testing for ballottement.

- Normally the patella sits firmly over the femur, allowing little or no movement when pressure is exerted over the patella.

7. Test the range of motion of each knee.
- Instruct the client to bend each knee toward the chest as far as possible and then return the knee to its extended position.

8. Test for muscle strength.
- Instruct the client to flex each knee while you apply opposing force.
- Now instruct the client to extend the knee again.
- The client should be able to perform the movement against resistance.
- The strength of the muscles in both knees is equal.

9. Inspect the knee while the client is standing.
- Ask the client to stand erect. If the client is unsteady, allow the client to hold onto the back of a chair.
- The knees should be in alignment with the thighs and ankles.
- Ask the client to walk at a comfortable pace with a relaxed gait.

▶ Look for *genu varum* (bowlegs), *genu valgum* (knock knees), or *genu recurvatum* (excessive hyperextension of the knee with weight bearing due to weakness of quadriceps muscles).

TECHNIQUES AND NORMAL FINDINGS	ABNORMAL FINDINGS SPECIAL CONSIDERATIONS

ANKLES AND FEET

1. **Inspect the ankles and feet with the client sitting, standing, and walking.**
   - The color of the ankles and feet should be similar to that of the rest of the body. They should be symmetric, and the skin should be unbroken. The feet and toes should be in alignment with the long axis of the lower leg. No swelling should be present, and the client's weight should fall on the middle of the foot.

▶ The following abnormalities require further evaluation:

Gouty arthritis: The metatarsophalangeal joint of the great toe is swollen, hot, red, and extremely painful.

Hallux valgus (bunion): The great toe deviates laterally from the midline, crowding the other toes. The metatarsophalangeal joint and bursa become enlarged and inflamed, causing a bunion.

Hammertoe: There is flexion of the proximal interphalangeal joint of a toe, while the distal metatarsophalangeal joint hyperextends. A callus or corn frequently occurs on the surface of the flexed joint from external pressure.

Pes planus (flatfoot): The arch of the foot is flattened, sometimes coming in contact with the floor. The deformity may be noticeable only when an individual is standing and bearing weight on the foot.

2. **Palpate the ankles.**
   - Grasp the heel of the foot with the fingers of both hands while palpating the anterior and lateral aspects of the ankle with your thumbs.
   - The ankle joints should be firm, stable, and nontender.

▶ Pain or discomfort on palpation and movement frequently indicates degenerative joint disease.

▶ Pain and tenderness along the tendon may indicate tendinitis or bursitis. Small nodules sometimes occur in clients with rheumatoid arthritis.

3. **Palpate the length of the calcaneal (Achilles) tendon at the posterior ankle.**
   - The calcaneal tendon should be free of pain, tenderness, and nodules.

▶ Pain and discomfort with this maneuver suggest early involvement of rheumatoid arthritis. Acute inflammation of the first metatarsophalangeal joint suggests gout.

| TECHNIQUES AND NORMAL FINDINGS | ABNORMAL FINDINGS SPECIAL CONSIDERATIONS |

4. **Palpate the metatarsophalangeal joints just below the ball of the foot.**
   - The metatarsophalangeal joints should be nontender.

   ▶ Pain, swelling, or tenderness may be associated with inflammation or degenerative joint disease.

5. **Deeply palpate each metatarsophalangeal joint.**
   - The joints should be firm and nontender.

6. **Test the range of motion of the ankles and feet.**
   - Instruct the client to perform the following movements:
     - Point the foot toward the nose. Dorsiflexion should reach 20 degrees.
     - Point the foot toward the floor. Plantar flexion should reach 45 degrees.
     - Point the sole of the foot outward, then inward. The ankle should evert to 20 degrees and invert to 30 degrees.
     - Curl the toes downward (flexion).
     - Spread the toes as far as possible (abduction), and then bring the toes together (adduction).

   ▶ Limited range of motion and painful movement of the foot and ankle without signs of inflammation suggest degenerative joint disease.

7. **Test muscle strength of the ankle.**
   - Ask the client to perform dorsiflexion and plantar flexion against your resistance.

8. **Test muscle strength of the foot.**
   - Ask the client to flex and extend the toes against your resistance.

9. **Palpate each interphalangeal joint.**
   - As you did for the hand, note the temperature of the extremity. Confirm that it is similar to the temperature of the rest of the client's body.

   ▶ Pain, swelling, or tenderness may be associated with inflammation or degenerative joint disease.

   A temperature in the lower extremities that is significantly cooler than the rest of the body may indicate vascular insufficiency, which in turn may lead to musculoskeletal abnormalities.

TECHNIQUES AND NORMAL FINDINGS	ABNORMAL FINDINGS SPECIAL CONSIDERATIONS

SPINE

1. Inspect the spine.

- With the client in a standing position, move around the client's body to check the position and alignment of the spine from all sides. Confirm that the cervical and lumbar curves are concave, and that the thoracic curve is convex (Figure 17.10).

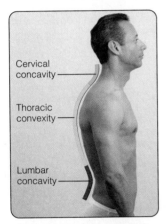

Cervical
concavity

Thoracic
convexity

Lumbar
concavity

Figure 17.10 • Lateral view of spine.

- Imagine a vertical line falling from the level of T_1 to the gluteal cleft. Confirm that the spine is straight.
- Imagine a horizontal line across the top of the scapulae. Confirm that the scapulae are level and symmetric. Similarly, check that the heights of the iliac crests and the gluteal folds are level. Ask the client to bend forward, and assess the alignment of the vertebrae.

▶ Lack of symmetry of the scapulae may indicate thoracic surgery. A scapula may appear higher if a lung has been removed on that side. In addition, the following abnormalities require further evaluation:

Kyphosis: An exaggerated thoracic dorsal curve that causes asymmetry between the sides of the posterior thorax (Figure 17.11).

Lordosis: An exaggerated lumbar curve that compensates for pregnancy, obesity, or other skeletal changes.

Flattened lumbar curve: A reduced lumbar concavity frequently occurs when spasms affect the lumbar muscles.

List: The spine leans to the left or right. A plumb line drawn from T_1 does not fall between the gluteal cleft. This condition may occur with spasms in the paravertebral muscles or a herniated disk.

Scoliosis: The spine curves to the right or left, causing an exaggerated thoracic convexity on that side (Figure 17.12). The body compensates, and a plumb line dropped from T_1 falls between the gluteal cleft. Unequal leg length may contribute to scoliosis; therefore, if scoliosis is suspected, it is necessary to measure the client's leg length. With the client supine, measure the distance from the anterior superior iliac spine to the medial malleolus, crossing the tape measure at the medial side of the knee.

| TECHNIQUES AND NORMAL FINDINGS | ABNORMAL FINDINGS SPECIAL CONSIDERATIONS |

2. **Palpate each vertebral process with your thumb.**
   - The vertebral processes should be aligned, uniform in size, firm, stable, and nontender.

▶ A *compression fracture* should be considered if the client is elderly, complains of pain and tenderness in the back, and has restricted back movement. T_8 and L_3 are the most common sites for compression fractures.

3. **Palpate the muscles on both sides of the neck and back.**
   - The neck muscles should be fully developed and symmetric, firm, smooth, and nontender.

4. **Test the range of motion of the cervical spine.**
   - Instruct the client to perform the following movements.
     - Touch the chest with the chin (flexion).
     - Look up toward the ceiling (hyperextension).
     - Attempt to touch each shoulder with the ear on that side, keeping the shoulder level (lateral bending or flexion).
     - Turn the head to face each shoulder as far as possible (rotation).

▶ *Muscle spasms* feel like hardened or knotlike formations. When they occur, the client may complain of pain and restricted movement. Muscle spasms may be associated with temporomandibular joint dysfunction or with *spasmodic torticollis*, a disorder in which the spasms cause the head to be pulled to one side.

5. **Test the range of motion of the thoracic and lumbar spine.**
   - Sit or stand behind the standing client. Stabilize the pelvis with your hands and ask the client to bend sideways to the right and to the left. Right and left lateral flexion should reach 35 degrees.
   - Ask the client to bend forward and touch the toes (flexion). Confirm that the lumbar concavity disappears with this movement and that the back assumes a single C-shaped convexity.
   - Ask the client to bend backward as far as is comfortable. Hyperextension should reach 30 degrees.
   - Ask the client to twist the shoulders to the left and to the right. Rotation should reach 30 degrees.

▶ Limited range of motion, crepitation, or pain with movement in the joint requires further evaluation. If the client complains of sharp pain that begins in the lower back and radiates down the leg, perform the straight-leg-raising test: Keeping the knee extended, raise the client's leg until pain occurs, then dorsiflex the client's foot. Record the distribution and severity of the pain and the degree of leg elevation at the time the pain occurs. Also record whether dorsiflexion increases the pain. Pain with straight-leg raising may indicate a herniated disk.

Abnormal Findings

Abnormal findings of the musculoskeletal system include rheumatic disease, abnormalities of the spine, joint disorders, and trauma-induced disorders. Table 17.4 lists and defines rheumatic diseases. Table 17.5 lists and provides definitions for trauma-induced disorders.

Table 17.4	Rheumatic Diseases
DISEASE	**DESCRIPTION**
Osteoarthritis	In osteoarthritis the joint cartilage erodes, resulting in pain and stiffness. Disability is associated with osteoarthritic changes in the spine, knees, and hips.
Rheumatoid Arthritis	Inflammation of the synovium of the joint occurs in rheumatoid arthritis. The inflammation leads to pain, swelling, damage to the joint, and loss of function. Rheumatoid arthritis affects the hands and feet symmetrically.
Juvenile Rheumatoid Arthritis	This form of arthritis can affect any body part. Inflammation causes pain, swelling, stiffness, and loss of function of joints. Symptoms may include fever and skin rash.
Systemic Lupus Erythematosus (SLE)	SLE is an autoimmune disease. The autoimmune response results in inflammation and damage to joints and other organs including the kidneys, lungs, blood vessels, and heart.
Scleroderma	In scleroderma there is an overproduction of collagen in the skin or organs, which results in damage to skin, blood vessels, and joints.
Fibromyalgia	Fibromyalgia is a chronic disease that is characterized by pain in the muscles and soft tissues that support and surround joints. Pain is experienced in tender points of the head, neck, shoulders, and hips.
Ankylosing Spondylitis	Ankylosing spondylitis is a chronic inflammatory disease of the spine. It occurs more frequently in males than in females. Fusion of the spine results in stiffness and inflexibility. This disorder may also affect the hips.
Gout	Gout is a type of arthritis caused by uric acid crystal deposits in the joints. The deposits cause inflammation, pain, and swelling in the joint.
Infectious Arthritis	Infectious arthritis refers to joint inflammatory processes that occur as a result of bacterial or viral infection. Infectious arthritis can occur as parvovirus arthritis, as gonococcal arthritis, or in Lyme disease.
Psoriatic Arthritis	Psoriatic arthritis may occur in individuals with psoriasis. Joint inflammation occurs in the fingers and toes and occasionally in the spine.

(continued)

Table 17.4	**Rheumatic Diseases (*continued*)**
DISEASE	**DESCRIPTION**
Bursitis	Bursitis refers to inflammation of the bursae (fluid-filled sacs) that surround joints. The pain of bursitis may limit range of motion of the affected area.
Tendinitis	Overuse or inflammatory processes can result in tendinitis. The inflammation of the tendon results in pain and limitation in movement.
Polymyositis	Polymyositis refers to inflammation and weakness in skeletal muscles. This disease can affect the entire body and result in disability.

Table 17.5	**Trauma-Induced Disorders**
DISORDER	**DESCRIPTION**
Dislocation	A displacement of the bone from its usual anatomic location in the joint.
Joint Sprain	A stretching or tearing of the capsule or ligament of a joint due to forced movement beyond the joint's normal range.
Fracture	A partial or complete break in the continuity of the bone from trauma.
Muscle Strain	A partial muscle tear resulting from overstretching or overuse of the muscle.

ABNORMALITIES OF THE SPINE

Kyphosis

Kyphosis is an exaggeration of the normal convex curve of the thoracic spine (Figure 17.11). It may result from congenital abnormality, rheumatic conditions, compression fractures, or other disease processes including syphilis, tuberculosis, and rickets.

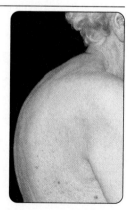

Figure 17.11 • Kyphosis (hunchback).

Scoliosis

Scoliosis is a lateral curvature of the spine (Figure 17.12). Scoliosis may occur congenitally or as a result of disease or injury. In addition, scoliosis can occur from habitual improper posture, unequal leg length, weakening of musculature, and chronic head tilting in visual disorders. Functional scoliosis is flexible. It is visible when standing.

Structural scoliosis is irreversible and visible when standing and bending.

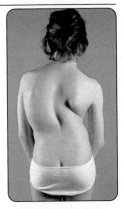

Figure 17.12 • Scoliosis.

JOINT DISORDERS

Rheumatoid Nodules

Firm, nontender subcutaneous nodules occur along the extensor surface of the ulna (Figure 17.13). They often are seen distal to the olecranon bursa in the hands and fingers.

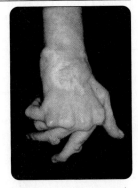

Figure 17.13 • Rheumatoid nodules.

Carpal Tunnel Syndrome

Chronic repetitive motion results in compression of the medial nerve, which lies inside the carpal tunnel. Decreased motor function leads to atrophy of the thenar eminence (Figure 17.14). Findings include pain, numbness, and positive Phalen's test.

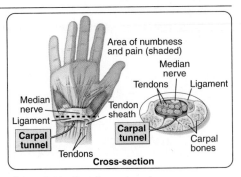

Figure 17.14 • Carpal tunnel syndrome.

Osteoarthritis

Bouchard's and Heberden's nodes occur in osteoarthritis (Figure 17.15). These nodes are hard nodules over the proximal and distal interphalangeal joints.

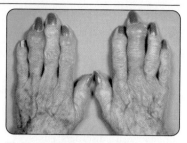

Figure 17.15 • Bouchard's. These nodes are hard nodules over the interphalangeal joints.

Bunion

Bunions are thickening and inflammation of the bursa of the joint of the great toe (Figure 17.16). There is lateral displacement of the toe with marked enlargement of the joint.

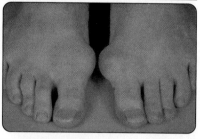

Figure 17.16 • Bunion.

Hammertoe

In hammertoe the metatarsophalangeal joint of the toe hyperextends with flexion of the interphalangeal joint of the toe (Figure 17.17).

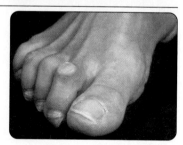

Figure 17.17 • Hammertoe.

18
Neurologic System

The complex integration, coordination, and regulation of body systems, and ultimately all body functions, are achieved through the mechanics of the nervous system. The intricate nature of the nervous system permits the individual to perform all physiological functions, perform all activities of daily living, function in society, and maintain a degree of independence.

ANATOMY AND PHYSIOLOGY REVIEW

The neurologic system, a highly integrated and complex system, is divided into two principal parts: the central nervous system (CNS) and the peripheral nervous system (PNS). The **central nervous system** consists of the brain and the spinal cord, whereas the cranial nerves and the spinal nerves make up the **peripheral nervous system.**

CENTRAL NERVOUS SYSTEM

The brain is the largest portion of the central nervous system. It is covered and protected by the meninges, the cerebrospinal fluid, and the bony structure of the skull. The **meninges** are three connective tissue membranes that cover, protect, and nourish the central nervous system. The cerebrospinal fluid also helps to nourish the central nervous system; however, its primary function is to cushion the brain and prevent injury to the brain tissue. The brain is made up of the cerebrum, diencephalon, cerebellum, and brain stem.

The **cerebrum** is the largest portion of the brain. The outermost layer of the cerebrum, the *cerebral cortex,* is composed of gray matter. Responsible for all conscious behavior, the cerebral cortex enables the individual to perceive, remember, communicate, and initiate voluntary movements. The cerebrum consists of the frontal, parietal, and temporal lobes (Figure 18.1).

The **cerebellum** is located below the cerebrum and behind the brain stem. It coordinates stimuli from the cerebral cortex to provide precise timing for skeletal muscle coordination and smooth movements. The cerebellum also assists with maintaining equilibrium and muscle tone.

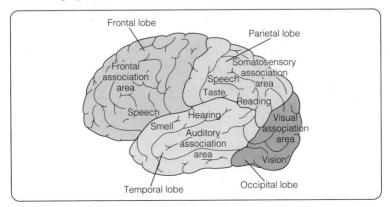

Figure 18.1 • Lobes of the cerebrum.

The **brain stem** contains the midbrain, pons, and medulla oblongata. Located between the cerebrum and spinal cord, the brain stem connects pathways between the higher and lower structures. Ten of the 12 pairs of cranial nerves originate in the brain stem.

The **spinal cord** is a continuation of the medulla oblongata. About 42 cm (17 in.) in length, it passes through the skull at the foramen magnum and continues through the vertebral column to the first lumbar vertebra.

Reflexes are stimulus-response activities of the body. They are fast, predictable, unlearned, innate, and involuntary reactions to stimuli. The individual is aware of the results of the reflex activity and not the activity itself. The reflex activity may be simple and take place at the level of the spinal cord, with interpretation at the cerebral level (Figure 18.2).

PERIPHERAL NERVOUS SYSTEM

The peripheral nervous system includes the 12 pairs of cranial nerves and the paired spinal nerves.

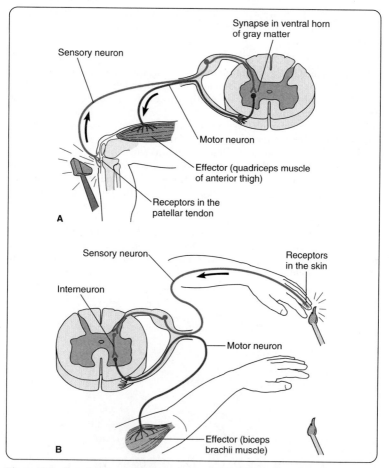

Figure 18.2 • Two simple reflex arcs. In the two-neuron reflex arc, the stimulus is transferred from the sensory neuron directly to the motor neuron at the point of synapse in the spinal cord.

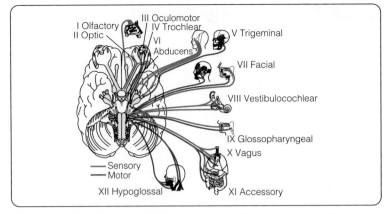

Figure 18.3 • Cranial nerves and their target regions. (Sensory nerves are shown in blue; motor nerves, in red.)

The 12 pairs of cranial nerves originate in the brain and serve various parts of the head and neck (Figure 18.3).

A summary of the name, number, function, and activity of the cranial nerves is presented in Table 18.1.

The spinal cord supplies the body with 31 pairs of spinal nerves that are named according to the vertebral level of origin. Each pair of nerves is responsible for a particular area of the body. The nerves provide some overlap of body

Table 18.1	Cranial Nerves		
NAME	**NUMBER**	**FUNCTION**	**ACTIVITY**
Olfactory	I	Sensory	Sense of smell.
Optic	II	Sensory	Vision.
Oculomotor	III	Motor	Pupillary reflex, extrinsic muscle movement of eye.
Trochlear	IV	Motor	Eye-muscle movement.
Trigeminal	V	Mixed	*Ophthalmic branch:* Sensory impulses from scalp, upper eyelid, nose, cornea, and lacrimal gland.
			Maxillary branch: Sensory impulses from lower eyelid, nasal cavity, upper teeth, upper lip, alate. *Mandibular branch:* Sensory impulses from tongue, lower teeth, skin of chin, and lower lip. Motor action includes teeth clenching, movement of mandible.
Abducens	VI	Mixed	Extrinsic muscle movement of eye.
Facial	VII	Mixed	Taste (anterior two thirds of tongue). Facial movements such as smiling, closing of eyes, frowning. Production of tears and salivary stimulation.
Vestibulocochlear	VIII	Sensory	*Vestibular branch:* Sense of balance or equilibrium. *Cochlear branch:* Sense of hearing.

(continued)

Table 18.1	Cranial Nerves *(continued)*		
NAME	**NUMBER**	**FUNCTION**	**ACTIVITY**
Glossopharyngeal	IX	Mixed	Produces the gag and swallowing reflexes. Taste (posterior third of the tongue).
Vagus	X	Mixed	Innervates muscles of throat and mouth for swallowing and talking. Other branches responsible for pressoreceptors and chemoreceptor activity.
Accessory	XI	Motor	Movement of the trapezius and sternocleidomastoid muscles. Some movement of larynx, pharynx, and soft palate.
Hypoglossal	XII	Motor	Movement of tongue for swallowing, movement of food during chewing, and speech.

segments they serve. This overlap is more complete on the trunk than on the extremities. A **dermatome** is an area of skin innervated by the cutaneous branch of one spinal nerve. All spinal nerves except the first cervical (C_1) serve a cutaneous region. The anterior and posterior views of the dermatomes of the body are shown in Figure 18.4a and Figure 18.4b.

SPECIAL CONSIDERATIONS

The nurse identifies many factors to be considered when collecting the objective and subjective data. Some of these factors include but are not limited to age, developmental level, race, ethnicity, work history, living conditions, and socioeconomics.

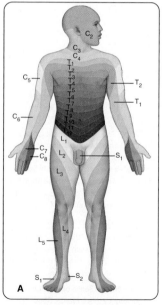

Figure 18.4A • Dermatomes of body, anterior view.

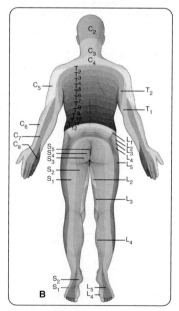

Figure 18.4B • Dermatomes of body, posterior view.

Physical and emotional wellness are also among the many factors or special considerations that impact a client's health status.

INFANTS AND CHILDREN

The maturational advances in the nervous system are responsible for the cephalocaudal and proximal-to-distal refinement of development, control, and movement. The neonate has several primitive reflexes at birth. These include but are not limited to sucking, stepping, startle (Moro), and the Babinski reflex in which stimulation of the sole of the foot from the heel toward the toes results in dorsiflexion of the great toe and fanning of other toes. The Babinski reflex and the tonic neck reflex are normal until around 2 years of age. Throughout infancy and the early childhood years, it is important to assess the fine and gross motor skills, language, and personal-social skills of the child.

THE PREGNANT FEMALE

As the uterus grows to accommodate the fetus, pressure may be placed on nerves in the pelvic cavity, thus producing neurologic changes in the legs. Changes in posture can place pressure on roots of nerves, causing sensory changes in the lower extremities. These sensory changes are reversible following relief of pressure and postural changes.

THE OLDER ADULT

In general, the aging process causes a subtle, slow, but steady decrease in neurologic function. These changes can be more pronounced and more troublesome for the individual when they are accompanied by a chronic illness such as heart disease, diabetes, or arthritis. Impulse transmission decreases, as does reaction to stimuli. Reflexes are diminished or disappear, and coordination is not as strong as it once was. Deep tendon reflexes are not as brisk. Coordination and movement may be slower and not as smooth as they were at one time.

PSYCHOSOCIAL CONSIDERATIONS

Changes in nervous system functioning may alter an individual's ability to control body movements, speech, elimination patterns, and to engage in activities of daily living. Inevitably, these changes will affect the individual's psychosocial health. Clients' self-esteem may suffer as they suddenly or progressively become unable to carry out the roles they previously assumed in their family and society. Another common psychosocial problem associated with neurologic disorders is social isolation.

CULTURAL CONSIDERATIONS

Assessment and findings are influenced by culture. See the cultural considerations box for specific examples.

Cultural Considerations

- African Americans are more likely than Caucasians to have very low birth weight babies. Very low birth weight babies are at risk for neurologic problems including intraventricular hemorrhage.
- African Americans have higher rates of Alzheimer's disease compared to Caucasians in the United States.
- There is an increased familial risk for development of Alzheimer's in African Americans.
- High blood pressure increases the risk of brain attack (stroke).
- African Americans have a higher incidence of high blood pressure.

Gathering the Data

Neurologic assessment includes gathering subjective and objective data. The subjective data collection occurs during the client interview, before the actual physical assessment.

FOCUSED INTERVIEW QUESTIONS

1. Please complete this sentence: "After I get out of bed in the morning, a typical day in my life includes _____." Have you had a change in your ability to carry out your daily activities?
2. Have you or any members of your family ever had a neurologic problem, disease, or headaches?
3. Have you ever had an injury to your head or back?
4. Do you have fainting spells? Do you have a history of seizures or convulsions?
5. Has your vision, hearing, ability to smell or taste changed in any way?
6. Do you have numbness or tingling in any part of your body?
7. Do you now use or have you ever used recreational drugs or alcohol?
8. Describe your memory.

QUESTIONS REGARDING INFANTS AND CHILDREN

1. Has the child ever had a seizure?
2. Have you noticed any clumsiness in the child's activities? For example, does the child frequently drop things, have difficulty manipulating toys, bump into things, have problems walking or climbing stairs, or fall frequently?

QUESTIONS FOR THE PREGNANT FEMALE

1. Do you have a history of seizures?

QUESTIONS FOR THE OLDER ADULT

1. When you stand up, do you have trouble starting to walk?
2. Do you notice any tremors?

Physical Assessment

Physical assessment of the neurologic system requires the use of inspection, palpation, auscultation, and special equipment and procedures to test the functions of the system.

EQUIPMENT

examination gown
percussion hammer
sterile cotton balls
ophthalmoscope
applicator
clean, nonsterile examination gloves
tuning fork
penlight
stethoscope
tongue blade
hot and cold water in test tubes
objects to touch, such as coins, paper clips, or safety pins
substances to smell, for example, vanilla, mint, and coffee
substances to taste, such as sugar, salt, lemon, and grape

HELPFUL HINTS

- Data gathering begins with the initial nurse-client interaction. As nurses meet clients, they make assessments regarding their general appearance, personal hygiene, and ability to walk and sit down. These activities are related to cerebral function.
- Physical assessment of the neurologic system proceeds in a cepahalocaudal and distal to proximal pattern, and includes comparison of corresponding body parts.
- Several assessments may occur at one time. For example, asking the client to smile tests cranial nerve VII, the ability to follow directions and initiate voluntary movements tests hearing (cranial nerve VIII) and the functions of the cerebral cortex.
- Provide specific information about what is expected of the client. Demonstrate movements.
- Explain and demonstrate the purposes and uses of the equipment.
- Use Standard Precautions.

| **TECHNIQUES AND NORMAL FINDINGS** | **ADDITIONAL ASSESSMENT TECHNIQUES** |

MENTAL STATUS

The nurse assesses the mental status of the client when meeting the client for the first time. This process begins with taking the health history and continues with each client contact.

▶ A variety of tools are available to conduct mental status assessment. These tools are described in Table 18.2.

| Table 18.2 | **Tools for Assessment of Mental Status** |

TOOL	**ASSESSMENT**
Mini-Mental State Examination (MMSE)	Cognitive status—conducted via interview
Addenbrooke's Cognitive Examination	Detects early dementia
Confusion Assessment Method (CAM)	Tests for delirium
Telephone Interview for Cognitive Status (TICS)	Similar to MMSE, cognitive function assessed via telephone interview
Cornell Scale for Depression in Dementia	Assessment of behavioral problems
Dementia Symptoms Scale	Assessment of behavioral problems
Psychogeriatric Dependency Rating Scale	Assessment of behavioral problems
Hopkins Competency Assessment Test	Assessment of ability to make decisions about health care
General Health Questionnaire	Assessment of emotional disturbance in those with normal cognitive ability
Hamilton Depression Rating Scale	Assessment of depression in clients with impaired cognition
Short Portable Mental Status Questionnaire (SPMSQ)	Assessment of organic brain deficit

1. **Observe the client.**
   - Look at the client and note hygiene, grooming, posture, body language, facial expressions, speech, and ability to follow directions.

▶ Changes could be indicative of depression, schizophrenia, organic brain syndrome, or obsessive-compulsive disorder.

TECHNIQUES AND NORMAL FINDINGS	ADDITIONAL ASSESSMENT TECHNIQUES

2. **Note the client's speech and language abilities.**
   - Throughout the assessment, note the client's rate of speech, ability to pronounce words, tone of voice, loudness or softness (volume) of voice, and ability to speak smoothly and clearly.
   - Assess the client's choice of words, ability to respond to questions, and ease with which a response is made.

▶ Changes in speech could reflect anxiety, Parkinson's disease, depression, or various forms of aphasia.

3. **Assess the client's sensorium.**
   - Determine the client's orientation to date, time, place, and reason for the assessment. Grade the level of alertness on a scale from full alertness to coma.

▶ Neurologic disease can produce a sliding or changing degree of alertness. Change in the level of consciousness may be related to cortical or brain stem disease. A stroke, seizure, or hypoglycemia could also contribute to a change in the level of consciousness.

4. **Assess the client's memory.**
   - Ask for the client's date of birth, Social Security number, names and ages of any children or grandchildren, educational history with dates and events, work history with dates, and job descriptions. Ask questions for which the response can be verified.

▶ Loss of long-term memory may indicate cerebral cortex damage, which occurs in Alzheimer's disease.

5. **Assess the client's ability to calculate problems.**
   - Start with a simple problem, such as $4 + 3, 8 \div 2$, and $15 - 4$.
   - Progress to more difficult problems, such as $(10 \times 4) - 8$, or ask the client to start with 100 and subtract 7 ($100 - 7 = 93, 93 - 7 = 86, 86 - 7 = 79$, and so on).
   - Remember to use problems that are appropriate for the developmental, educational, and intellectual level of the client.
   - Asking the client to calculate change from one dollar for the purchase of items costing 25, 39, and 89 cents is a quick test of calculation.

▶ Inability to calculate simple problems may indicate the presence of organic brain disease, or it may simply indicate lack of exposure to mathematical concepts, nervousness, or an incomplete understanding of the examiner's language. In an otherwise unremarkable assessment, a poor response to calculations should not be considered an abnormal finding.

TECHNIQUES AND NORMAL FINDINGS	ADDITIONAL ASSESSMENT TECHNIQUES

6. **Assess the client's ability to think abstractly.**
   - Ask the client to identify similarities and differences between two objects or topics, such as wood and coal, king and president, orange and apple, and pear and celery. Quote a proverb and ask the client to explain its meaning. For example:
     - "A stitch in time saves nine."
     - "The empty barrel makes the most noise."
     - "Don't put all your eggs in one basket."
   - Be aware that age and culture influence the ability to explain American proverbs and slang terms.

▶ Responses made by the client may reflect lack of education, mental retardation, or dementia. Clients with personality disorders such as schizophrenia or depression may make bizarre responses.

7. **Assess the client's mood and emotional state.**
   - Observe the client's body language, facial expressions, and communication technique. The facial expression and tone of voice should be congruent with the content and context of the communication.
   - Ask if the client generally feels this way or if he or she has experienced a change and if so over what period of time.
   - Ask the client if it is possible to identify an event or incident that fostered the change in mood or emotional state.
   - The client's mood and emotions should reflect the current situation or response to events that trigger mood change or call for an emotional response (e.g., a change in health status, a loss, or a stressful event).

▶ Lack of congruence of facial expression and tone of voice with the content and context of communication may occur with neurologic problems, emotional disturbance, or a psychogenic disorder such as schizophrenia or depression.

▶ Lack of emotional response, lack of change in facial expression, and flat voice tones can indicate problems with mood or emotional responses. Other abnormal findings in relation to mood and emotional state include anxiety, depression, fear, anger, overconfidence, ambivalence, euphoria, impatience, and irritability. Mood disorders are associated with bipolar disorder, anxiety disorders, and major depression.

TECHNIQUES AND NORMAL FINDINGS	ADDITIONAL ASSESSMENT TECHNIQUES

8. **Assess perceptions and thought processes.**
   - Listen to the client's statements. Statements should be logical and relevant. The client should complete his or her thoughts.
   - Determining the client's awareness of reality assesses perception.

▶ Disturbed thought processes can indicate neurologic dysfunction or mental disorder.

▶ Disturbances in sense of reality can include hallucination and illusion. These are associated with mental disturbances as seen in schizophrenia.

9. **Assess the client's ability to make judgments.**
   - Determine if the client is able to evaluate situations and to decide upon a realistic course of action. For example, ask the client about future plans related to employment.
   - The plans should reflect the reality of the client's health, psychologic stability, and family situation and obligations. The client's responses should reflect an ability to think abstractly.

▶ Impaired judgment can occur in emotional disturbances, schizophrenia, and neurologic dysfunction.

CRANIAL NERVES

1. **Test the olfactory nerve (cranial nerve I).**
   - If you suspect the client's nares are obstructed with mucus, ask the client to blow the nose.
   - Ask the client to close both eyes and to close one naris. Place a familiar odor under the open naris.
   - Ask the client to sniff and identify the odor. Use coffee, vanilla, perfume, cloves, and so on. Repeat with the other naris.

▶ **Anosmia**, the absence of the sense of smell, may be due to cranial nerve dysfunction, colds, rhinitis, or zinc deficiency, or it may be genetic. A unilateral change in this sense may be indicative of a brain tumor.

2. **Test the optic nerve (cranial nerve II).**
   - Test near vision by asking the client to read from a magazine, newspaper, or prepared card. Observe closeness or distance of page to face. Also note the position of the head.
   - Use the Snellen chart to test distant vision and color.

▶ Pathologic conditions of the optic nerve include retrobulbar neuritis, papilledema, and optic atrophy. **Retrobulbar neuritis** is an inflammatory process of the optic nerve behind the eyeball. Multiple sclerosis is the most common cause.

| **TECHNIQUES AND NORMAL FINDINGS** | **ADDITIONAL ASSESSMENT TECHNIQUES** |

- Use the ophthalmoscope to inspect the fundus of the eye. Locate the optic disc and describe the color and shape.

▶ **Papilledema** (or *choked disc*) is a swelling of the optic nerve as it enters the retina. A symptom of increased intracranial pressure, papilledema can be indicative of brain tumors or intracranial hemorrhage.
▶ Immediate medical attention is required if intracranial hemorrhage is suspected.
▶ **Optic atrophy** produces a change in the color of the optic disc and decreased visual acuity. It can be a symptom of multiple sclerosis or brain tumor.

3. **Test the oculomotor, trochlear, and abducens nerves (cranial nerves III, IV, and VI).**
   - Test the six cardinal points of gaze.
   - Test direct and consensual pupillary reaction to light (cranial nerve III).
   - Test convergence and accommodation of the eyes.

4. **Explain the procedure.**
   - Show the client the cotton wisp. Touch the arm with the wisp and explain that the wisp will feel like that when a body part is touched. Ask the client to close both eyes.
   - Touch the arm with the wisp. Ask the client to say "now" when the wisp is felt. Explain that further tests with the wisp will be carried out with the eyes closed, and "now" is to be stated when the wisp is felt.
   - Show the client a broken tongue blade. Explain while you touch the arm with the rounded end that the sensation is dull and with the jagged edge the sensation is sharp.
   - Tell the client that both eyes must be closed during several tests with the blade.
   - The client is expected to identify each touch or sensation as sharp or dull.
   - Discard the tongue blade at the completion of the examination.

▶ Pathologic conditions include nystagmus, strabismus, diplopia, or ptosis of the upper lid. **Nystagmus** is the constant involuntary movement of the eyeball. A lack of muscular coordination, *strabismus,* causes deviation of one or both eyes. **Diplopia** is double vision. A dropped lid, or *ptosis* of the lid, is usually related to weakness of the muscles.

TECHNIQUES AND NORMAL FINDINGS	ADDITIONAL ASSESSMENT TECHNIQUES

5. **Test the trigeminal nerve (cranial nerve V).**
   - Test the sensory function.
   - Ask the client to close both eyes.
   - Touch the face with a wisp of cotton (Figure 18.5).

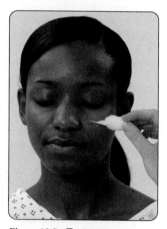

Figure 18.5 • Testing sensory function of the trigeminal nerve.

- Direct the client to say "now" every time the cotton is felt. Repeat the test using sharp and dull stimuli.
- Be random with the stimulation. Do *not* establish a pattern when testing. Be sure all three branches of the nerve are assessed.
- Test the corneal reflex.
  - Ask the client to look straight ahead.
  - Use a wisp of cotton to touch the cornea from the side.
  - Anticipate a blink.

- Test the motor function of the nerve. Ask the client to clench the teeth tightly. Bilaterally palpate the masseter and temporalis muscles, noting muscle strength.

▶ Document any loss of sensation, pain, or noted fasciculations (fine rapid muscle movements).

▶ Clients who use contact lenses need to remove them before testing. Most likely these clients will have a decreased or absent reflex because the corneal reflex has diminished in response to long-term contact lens use.

▶ Muscle pain, spasms, and deviation of the mandible with movement can indicate myofascial pain dysfunction.

TECHNIQUES AND NORMAL FINDINGS	ADDITIONAL ASSESSMENT TECHNIQUES

- Ask the client to open and close the mouth several times. Observe for symmetry of movement of the mandible without deviation from midline.

6. **Test the facial nerve (cranial nerve VII).**
   - Test the motor activity of the nerve.
   - Ask the client to perform several functions such as the following: smile, show your teeth, close both eyes, puff your cheeks, frown, and raise your eyebrows.
   - Look for symmetry of facial movements.
   - Test the muscle strength of the upper face.
   - Ask the client to close both eyes tightly and keep them closed.
   - Try to open the eyes by retracting the upper and lower lids simultaneously and bilaterally (Figure 18.6).

▶ Asymmetry or muscle weakness may indicate nerve damage. Muscle weakness includes drooping of the eyelid and changes in the nasolabial folds.

▶ Inability to perform motor tasks could be the results of a lower or upper motor neuron disease.

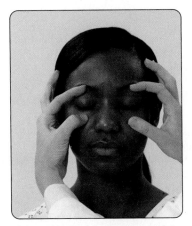

Figure 18.6 • Testing the strength of the facial muscles.

- Test the muscle strength of the lower face.
  - Ask the client to puff the cheeks.
  - Apply pressure to the cheeks, attempting to force the air out of the lips.

TECHNIQUES AND NORMAL FINDINGS	ADDITIONAL ASSESSMENT TECHNIQUES

- Test the sense of taste.
  - Moisten three applicators and dab one in each of the samples of sugar, salt, and lemon.
  - Touch the client's tongue with one applicator at a time and ask the client to identify the taste.
  - Water may be needed to rinse the mouth between tests.
- Test the corneal reflex.
  - This may have been tested with the trigeminal nerve assessment. Cranial nerve VII regulates the motor response of this reflex.

7. **Test the vestibulocochlear nerve (cranial nerve VIII).**
   - Test the auditory branch of the nerve by performing the Weber test. This test uses the tuning fork and provides lateralization of the sound.
   - Perform the Rinne test. This compares bone conduction of sound with air conduction.
   - The caloric test, or ice water test as it is sometimes called, tests the vestibular portion of the nerve.
     - This test is usually conducted only when the client is experiencing dizziness or vertigo. (Consult a neurology text for description of this technique.)
   - Romberg's test assesses coordination and equilibrium. It is discussed later in this chapter.

8. **Test the glossopharyngeal and vagus nerves (cranial nerves IX and X).**
   - Test motor activity.
     - Ask the client to open the mouth.
     - Depress the client's tongue with the tongue blade.
     - Ask the client to say "ah."
     - Observe the movement of the soft palate and uvula.
     - Normally, the soft palate rises and the uvula remains in the midline.
   - Test the gag reflex. This tests the sensory aspect of cranial nerve IX and the motor activity of cranial nerve X.

▶ Tinnitus and deafness are deficits associated with the cochlear or auditory branch of the nerve.

▶ Vertigo is associated with the vestibular portion.

▶ Unilateral palate and uvula movement indicate disease of the nerve on the opposite side.

| **TECHNIQUES AND NORMAL FINDINGS** | **ADDITIONAL ASSESSMENT TECHNIQUES** |

- Inform the client that you are going to place an applicator in the mouth and lightly touch the throat.
- Touch the posterior wall of the pharynx with the applicator.
- Observe pharyngeal movement.
- Test the motor activity of the pharynx.
  - Ask the client to drink a small amount of water and note the ease or difficulty of swallowing.

  - Note the quality of the voice or hoarseness when speaking.

▶ Clients with a diminished or absent gag reflex have an increased potential for aspiration and need medical evaluation.

▶ **Dysphagia,** difficulty with swallowing, could be related to cranial nerve disease.
▶ Vocal changes could be indicative of lesions, paralysis, or other conditions.

9. **Test the accessory nerve (cranial nerve XI).**
   - Test the trapezius muscle.
   - Ask the client to shrug the shoulders.
   - Observe the equality of the shoulders, symmetry of action, and lack of fasciculations (Figure 18.7).

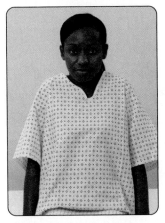

Figure 18.7 • Trapezius muscle movement.

- Test the sternocleidomastoid muscle.
  - Ask the client to turn the head to the right and then to the left.
  - Ask the client to try to touch the right ear to the right shoulder without raising the shoulder.
  - Repeat with the left shoulder.
  - Observe ease of movement and degree of range of motion.

▶ Abnormal findings include muscle weakness, muscle atrophy, fasciculations, uneven shoulders, and the inability to raise the chin following flexion.

TECHNIQUES AND NORMAL FINDINGS

- Test trapezius muscle strength.
  - Have the client shrug the shoulders while you resist with your hands.
- Test sternocleidomastoid muscle strength.
  - Ask the client to turn the head to the left to meet your hand.
  - Attempt to return the client's head to midline position (Figure 18.8).

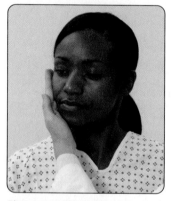

Figure 18.8 • Testing the strength of the sternocleidomastoid muscle against resistance.

- Repeat the preceding steps with the client turning to the right side.

10. **Test the hypoglossal nerve (cranial nerve XII).**
    - Test the movement of the tongue.
      - Ask the client to protrude the tongue.
      - Ask the client to retract the tongue.
      - Ask the client to protrude the tongue and move it to the right and then to the left.
      - Note ease of movement and equality of movement.
    - Test the strength of the tongue.
      - Ask the client to push against the inside of the cheek with the tip of the tongue.
      - Provide resistance by pressing one or two fingers against the client's outer cheek.
      - Repeat on the other side.

▶ Note atrophy, tremors, and paralysis. An ipsilateral paralysis will demonstrate deviation and atrophy of the involved side.

| TECHNIQUES AND NORMAL FINDINGS | ADDITIONAL ASSESSMENT TECHNIQUES |

MOTOR FUNCTION

Motor function requires the integrated efforts of the musculoskeletal and the neurologic systems. The neurologic aspect of motor function is directly related to activities of the cerebellum, which is responsible for coordination and smoothness of movement, and equilibrium. All of the following tests focus on activities of the cerebellum.

ALERT! *Be ready to support and protect the client to prevent an accident, injury, or fall.*

1. **Assess the client's gait and balance.**
   - Ask the client to walk across the room and return.
   - Ask the client to walk heel to toe (or tandem), by placing the heel of the left foot in front of the toes of the right foot, then the heel of the right foot in front of the toes of the left foot. Be sure the client is looking straight ahead and not at the floor. Continue this pattern for several yards.
   - Ask the client to walk on his or her toes.
   - Ask the client to walk on the heels. Observe the client's posture. Does the posture demonstrate stiffness or relaxation? Note the equality of steps taken, the pace of walking, the position and coordination of arms when walking, and the ability to maintain balance during all of these activities.

▶ A change in gait could be indicative of drug or alcohol intoxication, motor neuron weakness, or muscle weakness.

2. **Perform Romberg's test.**
   - **Romberg's test** assesses coordination and equilibrium (cranial nerve VIII).
   - Ask the client to stand with feet together and arms at the sides. The client's eyes are open.
   - Stand next to the client to prevent falls. Observe for swaying.
   - Ask the client to close both eyes without changing position.
   - Observe for swaying with the eyes closed. Swaying normally increases slightly when the eyes are closed (Figure 18.9).

▶ If swaying greatly increases or the client falls, suspect disease of the posterior columns of the spinal cord.

TECHNIQUES AND NORMAL FINDINGS

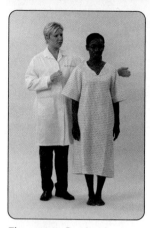

Figure 18.9 • Romberg's test for balance.

3. **Perform the finger-to-nose test.**
   - The finger-to-nose test also assesses coordination and equilibrium. It is sometimes called the pass-point test.
   - Ask the client to resume a sitting position.
   - Ask the client to extend both arms from the sides of the body.
   - Ask the client to keep both eyes open.
   - Ask the client to touch the tip of the nose with the right index finger, and then return the right arm to an extended position.
   - Ask the client to touch the tip of the nose with the left index finger, and then return the left arm to an extended position.
   - Repeat the procedure several times.
   - Ask the client to close both eyes and repeat the alternating movements.
   - Observe the movement of the arms, the smoothness of the movement, and the point of contact of finger. Does the finger touch the nose, or is another part of the face touched?
   - An alternative technique is to have the client touch the nose with the index finger and then the finger of the nurse.

▶ With the eyes closed, the client with cerebellar disease will reach beyond the tip of the nose, because the sense of position is affected.

TECHNIQUES AND NORMAL FINDINGS	ADDITIONAL ASSESSMENT TECHNIQUES

4. **Assess the client's ability to perform a rapid alternating action.**
   - Ask the client to sit with the hands placed palms down on the thighs.
   - Ask the client to turn the hands palms up.
   - Ask the client to return the hands to a palms-down position.
   - Ask the client to alternate the movements at a faster pace. If you suspect any deficit, test one side at a time.
   - Observe the rhythm, rate, and smoothness of the movements.
   - The finger-to-finger test is an alternative method to assess coordination.
   - Ask the client to touch the thumb to each finger in sequence with increasing pace.

▶ Inability to perform this task could indicate upper motor neuron weakness.

5. **Ask the client to perform the heel-to-shin test.**
   - Assist the client to a supine position.
   - Ask the client to place the heel of the left foot below the right knee.
   - Ask the client to slide the left heel along the shin bone to the ankle (Figure 18.10).

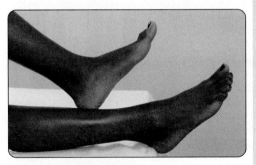

Figure 18.10 • Heel-to-shin test.

   - Ask the client to repeat the procedure, reversing the legs.
   - Observe the smoothness of the action. The client should be able to move the heel in a straight line so that it does not fall off the lower leg.

▶ Inability to perform this test could indicate disease of the posterior spinal tract.

TECHNIQUES AND NORMAL FINDINGS	ADDITIONAL ASSESSMENT TECHNIQUES

SENSORY FUNCTION

This part of the physical assessment evaluates the client's response to a variety of stimuli. This assessment tests the peripheral nerves, the sensory tracts, and the cortical level of discrimination. A variety of stimuli are used, including light touch, hot/cold, sharp/dull, and vibration. Stereognosis, graphesthesia, and two-point discrimination are also assessed. Each of these assessments is described in the following sections.

> **ALERT!** *The client may tire during these procedures. If this happens, stop the assessment and continue at a later time. Be sure to test corresponding body parts. Take a distal-to-proximal approach along the extremities. When the client describes sensations accurately at a distal point, it is usually not necessary to proceed to a more proximal point. If a deficit is detected at a distal point, then it becomes imperative to proceed to proximal points while attempting to map that specific area of the deficit. Repeat testing to determine accuracy in areas of deficits.*

Remember, always ask the client to describe the stimulus and the location. Do not suggest the type of stimulus or location. Tell the client to keep both eyes closed during testing. To promote full client understanding, you may have to demonstrate what you will do.

1. **Assess the client's ability to identify light touch.**
   - Using a wisp of cotton, touch various parts of the body, including feet, hands, arms, legs, abdomen, and face.
   - Touch at random locations and use random time intervals.
   - Ask the client to say "yes" or "now" when the stimulus is perceived. Be sure to test corresponding dermatomes.

2. **Assess the client's ability to distinguish the difference between sharp and dull.**
   - Ask the client to say "sharp" or "dull" when something sharp or dull is felt on the skin.

▶ **Anesthesia** is the inability to perceive the sense of touch. **Hyperesthesia** is an increased sensation, whereas *hypoesthesia* is a decreased but not absent sensation.

TECHNIQUES AND NORMAL FINDINGS	ADDITIONAL ASSESSMENT TECHNIQUES

- Touch the client with the jagged edge of a broken tongue blade.
- Now touch the client with the blunt end of the tongue blade.
- Alternate between sharp and dull stimulation.
- Touch the client using random locations, random time intervals, and alternating patterns.
- Be sure to test corresponding body parts.
- Discard the tongue blade.

3. **Assess the client's ability to distinguish temperature.**
   - Perform this test only if the client demonstrates an absence or decrease in pain sensation.
   - Randomly touch the client with test tubes containing warm and cold water.
   - Ask the client to describe the temperature.
   - Be sure to test corresponding body parts.

4. **Assess the client's ability to feel vibrations.**
   - Set a tuning fork in motion and place it on bony parts of the body, such as the toes, ankle, knee, iliac crest, spinal process, fingers, sternum, wrists, or elbows (Figure 18.11).

▶ The absence of pain sensation is called **analgesia.** Decreased pain sensation is called **hypalgesia.** These conditions may result from neurologic disease or circulatory problems such as peripheral vascular disease.

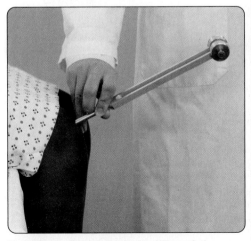

Figure 18.11 • Testing the client's ability to feel vibrations, the knee.

TECHNIQUES AND NORMAL FINDINGS	ADDITIONAL ASSESSMENT TECHNIQUES

- Ask the client to say "now" when the vibration is perceived and "stop" when it is no longer felt.
- If the client's perception is accurate when you test the most distal aspects (toes, ankles, fingers, and wrist), end the test at this time.
- Proceed to proximal points if distal perception is diminished.

5. **Test stereognosis, the ability to identify an object without seeing it.**
   - Direct the client to close both eyes. Place a safety pin in the client's right hand and ask the client to identify it.
   - Place a different object in the left hand and ask the client to identify it.
   - Place a coin in the right hand and ask the client to identify it (Figure 18.12).

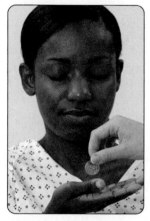

Figure 18.12 • Testing stereognosis using a coin.

- Place a different coin in the left hand and ask the client to identify it.
- The objects you use must be familiar and safe to hold (no sharp objects).
- Test each object independently.

6. **Test graphesthesia, the ability to perceive writing on the skin.**
   - Direct the client to keep both eyes closed.

▶ The inability to perceive vibration may indicate neuropathy. This may be associated with aging, diabetes, intoxication, or posterior column disease.

| TECHNIQUES AND NORMAL FINDINGS | ADDITIONAL ASSESSMENT TECHNIQUES |

- Using the noncotton end of an applicator or the base of a pen, scribe a number such as 3 into the palm of the client's right hand (Figure 18.13).

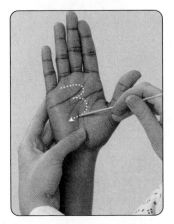

Figure 18.13 • Testing graphesthesia.

- Be sure the number faces the client.
- Ask the client to identify the number.
- Repeat in the left hand using a different number such as 5 or 2.
- Ask the client to identify the number.

▶ Inability to perceive a number on the skin may indicate cortical disease.

7. **Assess the client's ability to discriminate between two points.**
   - Simultaneously touch the client with two stimuli over a given area.
   - Use the unpadded end of two applicators.
   - Vary the distance between the two points according to the body region being stimulated. The more distal the location, the more sensitive the discrimination.
   - Normally, the client is able to perceive two discrete points at the following distances and locations:

     | Fingertips | 0.3 to 0.6 cm |
     | Hands and feet | 1.5 to 2 cm |
     | Lower leg | 4 cm |

   - Ask the client to say "now" when the two discrete points of stimulus are first perceived.

▶ An inability to perceive two separate points within normal distances may indicate cortical disease.

TECHNIQUES AND NORMAL FINDINGS	ADDITIONAL ASSESSMENT TECHNIQUES

- Note the smallest distance between the points at which the client can perceive two distinct stimuli.
- Discard the applicators.

8. **Assess topognosis, the ability of the client to identify an area of the body that has been touched.**
   - This need not be a separate test. Include it in any of the previous steps by asking the client to identify what part of the body was involved. Also ask the client to point to the area you touched.

▶ Inability of the client to identify a touched area demonstrates sensory or cortical disease.

9. **Assess position sense of joint movement.**
   - Ask the client to close both eyes. Grasp the great toe. Move the joint into dorsiflexion, plantar flexion, and abduction.
   - Ask the client to identify the movement (Figure 18.14).

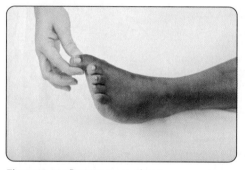

Figure 18.14 • Position sense of joint movement.

REFLEXES

Reflex testing is usually the last part of the neurologic assessment. The client is usually in a sitting position; however, you can use a supine position if the client's physical condition so requires. Position the client's limbs properly to stretch the muscle partially.

Proper use of the reflex hammer requires practice. Hold the handle of the reflex hammer in your dominant hand between your thumb and index finger. Use your wrist, not your hand or arm, to generate the striking motion. Proper wrist action will provide a brisk, direct, smooth arc for stimulation with the flat or pointed end of the hammer. Stimulate the

TECHNIQUES AND NORMAL FINDINGS	ADDITIONAL ASSESSMENT TECHNIQUES

reflex arc with a brisk tap to the tendon, not the muscle. Through continued practice and experience, you will learn the amount of force to use. Strong force will cause pain, and too little force will not stimulate the arc. After striking the tendon, remove the reflex hammer immediately.

Evaluate the response on a scale from 0 to 4+:

0	no response
1+	diminished
2+	normal
3+	brisk, above normal
4+	hyperactive

Before concluding that a reflex is absent or diminished, repeat the test. Encourage the client to relax. It may be necessary to distract the client to achieve relaxation of the muscle before striking the tendon. Distraction techniques include but are not limited to clenching the teeth, counting ceiling blocks, or humming.

1. **Assess the biceps reflex (C_5, C_6).**
   - Support the client's lower arm with your nondominant hand and arm. The arm needs to be slightly flexed at the elbow with palm up.
   - Place the thumb of your nondominant hand over the biceps tendon.
   - Using the pointed side of a reflex hammer, briskly tap your thumb (Figure 18.15).

▶ Neuromuscular disease, spinal cord injury, or lower motor neuron disease may cause absent or diminished (hypoactive) reflexes. Hyperactive reflexes may indicate upper motor neuron disease. Clonus, rhythmically alternating flexion and extension, confirms upper motor neuron disease.

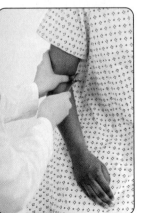

Figure 18.15 • Testing the biceps reflex.

TECHNIQUES AND NORMAL FINDINGS	ADDITIONAL ASSESSMENT TECHNIQUES

- Look for contraction of the biceps muscle and slight flexion of the forearm.

2. **Assess the triceps reflex (C_6, C_7).**
   - Support the client's elbow with your nondominant hand.
   - Sharply percuss the tendon just above the olecranon process with the flat end of the reflex hammer.
   - Observe contraction of the triceps muscle with extension of the lower arm.

3. **Assess the brachioradialis reflex (C_5, C_6).**
   - Position the client's arm so the elbow is flexed and the hand is resting on the client's lap with the palm down (pronation).
   - Using the flat end of the reflex hammer, briskly strike the tendon toward the radius (about 2 or 3 inches above the wrist).
   - Observe flexion of the lower arm and supination of the hand.

4. **Assess the patellar (knee) reflex (L_2, L_3, L_4).**
   - Palpate the patella to locate the patellar tendon inferior to the patella.
   - Briskly strike the tendon with the flat end of the reflex hammer.
   - Note extension of lower leg and contraction of the quadriceps muscle.

5. **Assess the Achilles tendon (ankle) reflex (S_1).**
   - Flex the leg at the knee.
   - Dorsiflex the foot of the leg being examined.
   - Hold the foot lightly in the nondominant hand.
   - Strike the Achilles tendon with the flat end of the reflex hammer (Figure 18.16).

▶ Flex the leg at the knee. Occasionally, the response is not obtained. Distraction may be required.

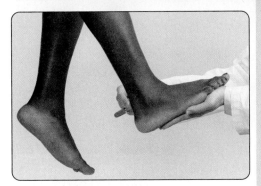

Figure 18.16 • Testing the Achilles tendon reflex with client in a sitting position.

- Observe plantar flexion of the foot; the heel will "jump" from your hand.

6. **Assess the plantar reflex (L_5, S_1).**
   - Position the leg with a slight degree of external rotation at the hip.
   - Stimulate the sole of the foot from the heel to the ball of the foot on the lateral aspect. Continue the stimulation across the ball of the foot to the big toe.
   - Observe for plantar flexion, in which the toes curl toward the sole of the foot (Figure 18.17). It may be necessary to hold the client's ankle to prevent movement.

▶ A **Babinski response** is the fanning of the toes with the great toe pointing toward the dorsum of the foot (Figure 18.18). This is called dorsiflexion of the toe and is considered an abnormal response in the adult. It may indicate upper motor neuron disease.

▶ A positive Babinski response is considered a normal response in the child until about 2 years of age.

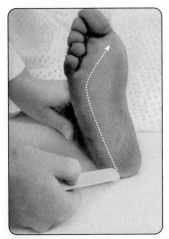

Figure 18.17 • Testing the plantar reflex.

| TECHNIQUES AND NORMAL FINDINGS | ADDITIONAL ASSESSMENT TECHNIQUES |

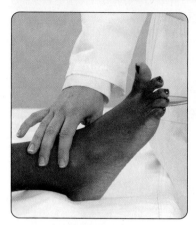

Figure 18.18 • Babinski response.

7. **Assess the abdominal reflexes (T_8, T_9, T_{10} for upper and T_{10}, T_{11}, T_{12} for lower).**
   - Using an applicator or tongue blade, briskly stroke the abdomen from the lateral aspect toward the umbilicus.
   - Observe muscular contraction and movement of the umbilicus toward the stimulus.
   - Repeat this procedure in the other three quadrants of the abdomen.

▶ Obesity and upper and lower motor neuron pathology can decrease or diminish the response.

| ADDITIONAL ASSESSMENT TECHNIQUES | ABNORMAL FINDINGS SPECIAL CONSIDERATIONS |

CAROTID AUSCULTATION

Auscultation of the carotid arteries may be performed with the assessment of the head and neck or as part of the peripheral vascular assessment. You may need to review your assessment notes for findings of carotid artery auscultation.

▶ A bruit may be indicative of an obstructive disease process such as atherosclerosis. The amount of blood flow to the brain may be diminished. This decrease in oxygen could be responsible for subtle changes in client responses.

MENINGEAL ASSESSMENT

Ask the client to flex the neck by bringing the chin down to touch the chest. Observe the degree of range of motion and the absence or presence of pain. The client should be able to flex the neck about 45 degrees without pain.

▶ When the meningeal membranes are irritated or inflamed, as in meningitis, the client will experience **nuchal rigidity** or stiffness of the neck.

ADDITIONAL ASSESSMENT TECHNIQUES	ABNORMAL FINDINGS SPECIAL CONSIDERATIONS

When the client complains of pain and has a decrease in the flexion motion, you will observe for *Brudzinski's sign.* With the client in a supine position, assist the client with neck flexion. Observe the legs. Brudzinski's sign is positive when neck flexion causes flexion of the legs and thighs.

USE OF THE GLASGOW COMA SCALE

The *Glasgow Coma Scale* assesses the level of consciousness of the individual on a continuum from alertness to coma (Figure 18.19). The scale tests three body functions: verbal response, motor response, and eye response. A maximum total score of 15 indicates the person is alert, responsive, and oriented. A total score of 3, the lowest achievable score, indicates a nonresponsive comatose individual.

▶ **Syncope** is a brief loss of consciousness and is usually sudden. **Coma** is a more prolonged state with pronounced and persistent changes.

▶ A client experiencing any loss of consciousness needs immediate medical interventions.

▶ The Glasgow Coma Scale has limitations. For example, a client with an endotracheal tube or tracheostomy cannot communicate. As a result, the score is carried out according to each individual component of the scale. The verbal response score would then indicate intubation or tracheostomy. In addition, the motor response scale is invalid in a client with a spinal cord injury, and eye opening may be impossible to assess in those individuals with severe orbital injury.

GLASGOW COMA SCALE
BEST EYE-OPENING RESPONSE
4 = Spontaneously
3 = To speech
2 = To pain
1 = No response
(Record "C" if eyes closed by swelling)
BEST MOTOR RESPONSE to painful stimuli
6 = Obeys verbal command
5 = Localizes pain
4 = Flexion—withdrawal
3 = Flexion—abnormal
2 = Extension—abnormal
1 = No response
(Record best upper limb response)
BEST VERBAL RESPONSE
5 = Oriented × 3
4 = Conversation—confused
3 = Speech—inappropriate
2 = Sounds—incomprehensible
1 = No response
(Record "E" if endotracheal tube in place, "T" if tracheostomy tube in place)

Figure 18.19 • Glasgow Coma Scale.

Abnormal Findings

Problems commonly associated with the neurologic system include changes in motor function, including gait and movement, seizures, spinal cord injury, infections, degenerative disorders, and cranial nerve dysfunction. These conditions are described in Tables 18.3 and 18.4.

Table 18.3	Problems with Motor Function
GAIT	**MOVEMENT**
Ataxic Gait	**Fasciculation**
A walk characterized by a wide base, uneven steps, feet slapping, and a tendency to sway. This type of walk is associated with posterior column disease or decreased proprioception regarding extremities. Seen in multiple sclerosis and drug or alcohol intoxication.	Commonly called a twitch, this is an involuntary, local, visible muscular contraction. It is not significant when it occurs in tired muscles. It can be associated with motor neuron disease.
Scissors Gait	**Tic**
A walk characterized by spastic lower limbs and movement in a stiff, jerky manner. The knees come together; the legs cross in front of one another; and the legs are abducted as the individual takes short, progressive, slow steps. This is seen in individuals with multiple sclerosis.	Commonly called a *habit,* a tic is usually psychogenic in nature. The involuntary spasmodic movement of the muscle is seen in a muscle under voluntary control, usually in the face, neck, or shoulders.
Steppage Gait	**Tremor**
Sometimes called the "foot drop" walk. The individual flexes and raises the knee to a higher-than-usual level yielding a flopping of the foot when walking. This usually is indicative of lower motor neuron disease. Seen in individuals with alcoholic neuritis and progressive muscular atrophy.	A rhythmic or alternating involuntary movement from the contraction of opposing muscle groups. Tremors vary in degree and are seen in Parkinson's disease, multiple sclerosis, uremia (a form of kidney failure), and alcohol intoxication.
	Athetoid Movement
Festination Gait	A continuous, involuntary, repetitive, slow, "wormlike," arrhythmic muscular movement. The muscles are in a state of hypotoxicity, producing a distortion to the limb. This movement is seen in cerebral palsy.
Referred to as the "Parkinson's walk." The individual has stooped posture, takes short steps, and turns stiffly. There is a slow start to the walk and frequent, accelerated steps. This gait is associated with basal ganglia disease.	**Dystonia**
	Similar to athetoid movements, dystonia involves larger muscle groups. The twisting movements yield a grotesque change to the individual's posture. Torticollis, or wryneck, is an example of dystonia.
	Myoclonus
	A continual, rapid, short spasm involving a muscle, part of a muscle, or even a group of muscles. Frequently occurs in an extremity as the individual is falling asleep. Myoclonus is also seen in seizure disorders.

Table 18.4	Problems Associated with Dysfunction of Cranial Nerves

CRANIAL NERVE		DYSFUNCTION
I	Olfactory	Unilateral or bilateral anosmia.
II	Optic	Optic atrophy, papilledema, amblyopia, field defects.
III	Oculomotor	Diplopia, ptosis of lid, dilated pupil, inability to focus on close objects.
IV	Trochlear	Convergent strabismus, diplopia.
V	Trigeminal	Tic douloureux, loss of facial sensation, decreased ability to chew, loss of corneal reflex, decreased blinking.
VI	Abducens	Diplopia, strabismus.
VII	Facial	Bell's palsy, decreased ability to distinguish tastes.
VIII	Vestibulocochlear	Tinnitus, vertigo, deafness.
IX	Glossopharyngeal	Loss of "gag" reflex, loss of taste, difficulty swallowing.
X	Vagus	Loss of voice, impaired voice, difficulty swallowing.
XI	Accessory	Difficulty with shrugging of shoulders, inability to turn head to left and right.
XII	Hypoglossal	Difficulty with speech and swallowing, inability to protrude tongue.

SEIZURES

Seizures are sudden, rapid, and excessive discharges of electrical energy in the brain. They are usually centered in the cerebral cortex. Some seizure disorders stem from neurologic problems that occur before or during birth, or they can develop secondary to childhood fevers. In children and adults, seizures can result from a variety of factors including trauma, infections, cerebrovascular disease, environmental toxins, drug overdose, and withdrawal from alcohol, sedatives, or antidepressants. *Epilepsy* is a chronic seizure disorder.

INFECTIONS OF THE NEUROLOGIC SYSTEM

Infections of the neurologic system include meningitis, myelitis, brain abscess, and Lyme disease. Each of these is described in the following sections.

Meningitis

Meningitis is caused by a virus or bacteria that infect the coverings, or meninges, of the brain or spinal cord. Meningitis may result from a penetrating wound, fractured skull, or upper respiratory infection, or it may occur secondary to facial or cranial surgery.

In some cases, meningitis may spread to the underlying brain tissues, causing encephalitis. *Encephalitis* is defined as an inflammation of the tissue of the brain. It usually results from a virus, which may be transmitted by ticks or mosquitoes, or it may result from a childhood illness such as chickenpox or the measles.

Myelitis

Myelitis is an inflammation of the spinal cord. Poliomyelitis and herpes zoster infection are two common causes. It may develop after an infection such as measles or gonorrhea, or it may follow vaccination for rabies.

Brain Abscess

A *brain abscess* is usually the result of a systemic infection. It is marked by an accumulation of pus in the brain cells. Most brain abscesses develop secondary to a primary infection. Others result from skull fractures or penetrating injuries, such as a gunshot wound.

Lyme Disease

Lyme disease is an infection caused by a spirochete transmitted by a bite from an infected tick that lives on deer. Its major symptoms are arthritis, a flulike syndrome, and a rash. If untreated, Lyme disease may cause severe neurologic disorders.

DEGENERATIVE NEUROLOGIC DISORDERS

Degenerative neurologic disorders include Alzheimer's disease, amyotrophic lateral sclerosis, Huntington's disease, multiple sclerosis, myasthenia gravis, and Parkinson's disease. These are discussed in the following paragraphs.

Alzheimer's Disease

Alzheimer's disease is a progressive degenerative disease of the brain that leads to dementia. Although it is more common in people over age 65, its onset may occur as early as middle adulthood. Symptoms include a loss of memory, particularly of recent events, shortened attention span, confusion, and disorientation. Eventually, the client with Alzheimer's disease may experience paranoid fantasies and hallucinations.

Amyotrophic Lateral Sclerosis

Amyotrophic lateral sclerosis, commonly known as Lou Gehrig's disease, is a chronic degenerative disease involving the cerebral cortex and the motor neurons in the spinal cord. The result is a progressive wasting of skeletal muscles that eventually leads to death. Although the cause is unknown, research has implicated viral infection.

Huntington's Disease

Huntington's disease is an inherited disorder characterized by uncontrollable jerking movements, called *chorea,* which literally means dance. It typically progresses to mental deterioration and ultimately death. Symptoms usually first appear in early middle age; thus, those with Huntington's disease often have had children before they know they have the disorder.

Multiple Sclerosis

Multiple sclerosis is the deterioration of the protective sheaths, composed of myelin, of the nerve tracts in the brain and spinal cord. The first attack usually occurs between the ages of 20 and 40. Early symptoms include temporary tingling, numbness, or weakness that may affect only one limb or one side of the body. Other symptoms include unsteadiness, blurred vision, slurred speech, and difficulty in urinating. Some individuals experience repeated attacks that progress in severity. In these individuals, permanent disability with progressive neuromuscular deficits develops.

Myasthenia Gravis

Myasthenia gravis is a chronic neuromuscular disorder involving increasing weakness of voluntary muscles with activity, and some abatement of symptoms with rest. Onset is gradual and usually occurs in adolescence or young adulthood. The precise etiology is unknown, but it is believed that myasthenia gravis is an *autoimmune* disorder, that is, the individual's immune system attacks the individual's own normal cells rather than foreign pathogens. Some of the most common symptoms include ptosis (drooping eyelids), diplopia (double vision), a flat affect, and a weak, monotone voice.

Parkinson's Disease

Parkinson's disease is a degeneration of the basal nuclei of the brain, which are collections of nerve cell bodies deep within the white matter of the cerebrum. These nuclei are responsible for initiating and stopping voluntary movement. Parkinson's disease is characterized by slow movements, continuous "pill-rolling" tremor of the forefinger and thumb, rhythmic shaking of the hands, bobbing of the head, and difficulty in initiating movement. The individual may have a masklike facial expression, difficulty in speaking clearly, and difficulty maintaining balance while walking. Although the precise etiology is unknown, research indicates that environmental toxins, such as carbon monoxide or certain metals, may cause some cases of Parkinson's disease. It may also result from previous encephalitis.

19
Putting It All Together

This chapter is designed to help the nurse utilize the concepts of health assessment. The skills and techniques discussed in the previous chapters are applied to a client situation. The collection of subjective and objective data is reflected in the health history and physical assessment (see Boxes 19.1 and 19.2). Presented in documentation format, the collected data reflect a state of wellness.

Box 19.1	Narrative Recording of the Health History

Biographic Data   Mrs. Amparo Bellisimo, age 31, comes to the health center for a health assessment. She is employed as an account representative for a large retail clothing establishment. Mrs. Bellisimo has insurance through Corporate Insurance Company, through her employer. It covers medical, dental, and eye care. She lives in a single-family residence at 22 Highland Avenue, Midland Park, New Jersey. Mrs. Bellisimo lives with her husband, who she names as her emergency contact. Mrs. Bellisimo was born on July 20, 1973, in Santa Clara, Cuba. She emigrated to the United States 9 years ago. She speaks English with an accent. Mrs. Bellisimo can read and write in English and Spanish. Mrs. Bellisimo has no immediate family in the United States. She completed 12 years of school in Cuba and took several accounting courses at a community college in New Jersey. She has no formal religious affiliations, because religious practice was not permitted in Cuba when she lived there. Some of her family were "hidden" Catholics. She states, "I am happy with my life. I have made adjustments to being in the United States. I have many Cuban friends and have a close relationship with my husband's family. I like my job, except when it gets crazy."

Present Health Status: Reason for Seeking Health Care   Mrs. Bellisimo has no complaints except "weight gain and occasional headaches relieved with aspirin." The weight gain has occurred "over 3 years since I started dating my husband and more since we got married last year." The headaches occur "when I'm tired, stressed, or reading too much."

Health Beliefs and Practices   Mrs. Bellisimo has no current health problem, except as stated above. She believes "health is important, and you need to take care of yourself, but sometimes it's out of your control." When she was a child her mother used to tell her things like "no bathing when you have your period, no water at all," and she "prepared certain foods for certain illnesses and sometimes got medicines from a botanica for ailments." Since she has been covered by health insurance and encouraged by her husband, she has had regular physical, gynecologic, dental, and eye examinations, all of which have been completed annually for 3 years.

Mrs. Bellisimo states she "sleeps well most nights, about 8 hours, unless I stay up and read." She "feels rested most mornings." She tries to exercise but finds it hard "after work and when it's cold out."

| Box 19.1 | **Narrative Recording of the Health History** (*continued*) |

Mrs. Bellisimo would like to lose weight. She would "feel healthier, my clothes would fit and I'd feel good about myself." People in Cuba would not have a problem with this weight, but "I don't like it." Eating patterns include "fast foods at lunch, bread at every meal, and dessert or snacks at night."

Medications   Mrs. Bellisimo uses oral contraceptives "for 4 years," without problems, and takes a multivitamin every day. She is not undergoing any therapy and "really have never needed any specific care."

Past History, Surgeries, and Illnesses   Mrs. Bellisimo had measles as a child. She received smallpox, polio, mumps, tetanus, and other "vaccines" as a child. She has had no major illnesses. She has never been hospitalized, received a blood transfusion, been pregnant, or had allergies. Mrs. Bellisimo cut her lower left leg on glass as a child and had sutures, and a scar remains. She had four wisdom teeth extracted 2 years ago with no complications, "no other surgery."

Emotional History   Mrs. Bellisimo states, "I miss my family and get sad when I can't see them. I get frustrated when I don't understand some American ways. I'm pretty emotional. I cry over books and movies, but I haven't had a mental problem." She doesn't smoke, but her whole family smoked when she was in Cuba. "I drink some beer, wine, and tequila on weekends or at dinner with my in-laws. I have never used drugs or anything like that."

Family History   Mrs. Bellisimo's father died at age 56 from "some cancer." "He didn't live with us, so I don't know for sure and my mother doesn't say." Her mother is 49 and well. She has a brother, 33, and a sister, 27. Both are "well." Her grandparents were not really known to her but were "old when they died."

Psychosocial History—Occupation   Mrs. Bellisimo held jobs in hotels as a teenager in Cuba. "Since coming to America, I have worked in a factory making clothes, been a receptionist in a hair salon, and in some form of accounting for the past 5 years." She states, "I have not been poor but just okay almost all my life until the last 4 or 5 years. Things are really bad in Cuba, no proper food or medicine. They were better when I was there, but not like here."

Roles and Relationships   She states, "I love my family, but I can't see them. I have friends here that are like my family. My friends were a big part of my wedding. One walked me down the aisle. I call home to Cuba, but it's hard to be far away. My husband is American and we dated for 2 years before we got engaged. He helped me a lot and we love each other a lot. His family are like my new family. We see them a lot, they help us, and they treat me like a daughter, so it's very good."

Ethnicity and Culture   Mrs. Bellisimo says she will always consider herself Cuban, but "I am an American citizen now, and am so much more of a gringo than my friends. I have come to like American food, especially pasta, but still make my beans and rice and other Cuban foods. My husband likes it too but not every day. I laugh sometimes when I call my mother in Cuba and speak English sometimes."

Spirituality   Mrs. Bellisimo states, "I have no real religion; family and honesty are important to me. I believe in God and sometimes pray, but really believe your family helps you when you are in need."

(*continued*)

Box 19.1	**Narrative Recording of the Health History** (continued)

Self-Concept Mrs. Bellisimo says of herself, "I am a good person. I worry about others. I want to have a family, with children who understand about being Cuban but who believe America is a good place. I was brainwashed and thought gringos were mean and selfish people. I have come to know better. I take care of myself and other than some extra pounds think I look pretty good."

Review of Systems

Skin, Hair, and Nails
No reported problems. "I use sunscreen, shower daily, use conditioner on my hair and lotion to prevent dry skin. I would like to have a professional manicure more often, but keep my nails looking nice."

Head and Neck
No reported problems except "occasional headache relieved by aspirin."

Eyes
Annual eye exam for 3 years. Glasses for "driving."

Ear, Nose, Mouth, and Throat
No problems with hearing, has "never had an official exam." Regular dental exams. Wisdom teeth extracted with no problems. No trouble eating or swallowing.

Respiratory
No reported problems. "A cold once a year." No exposure to pollutants. No history of tobacco use. Exposure to secondhand smoke from birth to 22 years of age at home. Denies cough, difficulty breathing.

Breasts and Axillae
"I have large breasts and have since I was 12. I don't like to examine my breasts; I get scared I might find something. I do get them checked every year by the doctor." No changes, discharge, discomfort.

Cardiac
No reported problems. No history of heart disease. Never has palpitations.

Peripheral Vascular
No reported problems. "The doctor says my blood pressure is fine. I have two veiny spots on my legs, but they don't hurt. They are flat and stringy."

Gastrointestinal
No reported problems. "My bowels move every day with no problem. I get diarrhea when I'm nervous sometimes."

Urinary
No reported problems. "I pass urine five or six times a day and more if I drink more."

Reproductive
Onset of menses age 11. "Regular every 28 days for 3 or 4 days. I take birth control pills." Denies pregnancy, abortion. "Relations are good with my husband."

Musculoskeletal
No reported problems. "I don't get enough exercise."

Neurologic
No history of head injury, seizure, tremor, loss of consciousness. "Other than headache, I'm okay."

Box 19.2	**Physical Assessment**

General Survey

Dress clean and appropriate for situation and weather. Hair neat, nails manicured, breath fresh, no body odor. Gait coordinated and smooth, posture erect, body build symmetric and proportional. Mood and affect appropriate for situation. Sitting quietly, rates anxiety as 3 on a scale of 0 to 10. Oriented to person, place, time, speech clear, accent, moderate volume.

Height and Weight

61 inches, 132 pounds

Vital Signs

Temperature 98.4 F, pulse 80, regular, Blood Pressure Left 128/76, Right 126/74, Respirations 18, regular.

Skin, Hair, and Nails

Skin color light tan, pink undertone, even pigment, no odor. Warm, moist, smooth, no areas of thickness or thinness. Turgor elastic and mobile. No superficial vasculature.
Linear scar, 4 cm. near lateral femoral condyle, left leg. No sensitive areas.
Hair clean, no nits. Dark brown, uniform, curly, soft with even distribution. No alopecia or scalp lesions.
Nails Fingernails and toenails clean, trimmed. Nail beds pink, white crescents at bases, capillary refill immediate. Surface slightly convex, base angle 160. Nail texture smooth, strong, regular, firm attachment at base. Cuticles smooth and flat.

Head, Neck, and Related Lymphatics

Head Normocephalic, all facial structures symmetric. Movements symmetric and smooth. Temporal Artery smooth, no bruit. TMJ full ROM, no pain.
Neck Color consistent with face, symmetric. Full ROM. Pulsation of carotids visible, jugulars not visualized. Trachea midline, distance to sternocleidomastoids equal, C-Rings palpable, mobile. Thyroid visible on swallow, nonpalpable, no bruits. Lymph nodes nonpalpable.

Eye

Distant Vision 20/50 without correction, 20/30 with correction bilaterally. Near vision 14/14 Jaeger bilaterally. Visual Fields full by confrontation. EOM intact, no nystagmus. Corneal Light Reflex symmetric. PERRLA.
Eyebrows, lashes brown, no flaking, symmetric, upper lids cover small arc of iris, palpebral fissures equidistant from midline, corneas clear. Eyeball firm, no swelling or tenderness, conjunctiva pink, sclera no lesions. Fundus disc oval, creamy pink, distinct margins, physiologic cup ½ disc diameter; Arterioles: Veins = 2:1, no hemorrhage, no lesions.

Ears, Nose, Mouth, and Throat

Ears symmetric, helices at level of eye canthus, no lesions. Tragus nontender, mastoid smooth and nontender. Canal patent, no drainage, small amount cerumen in canal, tympanic membrane intact, no scars, cone of light at 5 o'clock right, 7 o'clock left. Rinne AC>BC 2:1 bilaterally. Weber no lateralization.

(continued)

Box 19.2	Physical Assessment (*continued*)

Nose and Sinuses Nose straight, septum midline, nares equal, patent, no drainage, mucosa pink. Sinuses nontender.

Mouth and Throat Lips smooth, symmetric, no lesions. Teeth 28 intact, clean, smooth edges. Oral mucosa pink, intact. Tongue mobile, white coating. Gums intact, no swelling. Salivary ducts visible, productive, no swelling or pain. Palates smooth, continuous, uvula midline, rises with "aah." Tonsils intact behind pillars, pharyngeal mucosa pink, smooth, no lesions.

Respiratory

Respirations 18, regular and deep, with no use of accessory musculature. Skin color consistent. Chest 2:1 Transverse to AP diameter. Clavicles and scapulae symmetric, vertebrae midline, ribs intact. Symmetric thoracic expansion. Tactile fremitus symmetric, strong over trachea, diminishing to bases. Resonance to percussion throughout. Diaphragmatic excursion 5 cm bilaterally. Clear vesicular sounds on auscultation. No adventitious breath sounds throughout.

Breasts and Axillae

Large, pendulous, color consistent, freely mobile. Nipples equal in size, shape, color, consistent with areolae. Mild venous patterns. No palpable lesions, dimpling, or discharge. Axillae shaved, clean, no palpable nodes.

Cardiovascular

Chest color consistent, no edema, no visible pulsations, heaves, thrills. Carotid pulsations visible, jugular veins not visible. Heart Sounds: aortic S2>S1, pulmonic S2>S1, Erb's point S1=S2, tricuspid S1>S2, mitral S1>S2. No extra sounds auscultated. Carotid pulse = Apical pulse.

Peripheral Vascular

Extremities color consistent, warm. No edema, superficial vessels, or varicosities. Sensation intact for pain and temperature. Pulses: All strong and regular. Epitrochlear and inguinal nodes nonpalpable. Allen Test ulnar and radial patency. Manual Compression Test no valve incompetence. Trendelenburg Test no valve incompetence. Homans' Sign negative, bilateral venous stars.

Abdomen

Shape and contour round, symmetric, smooth, no lesions, bulges, pulsations, or visible peristalsis. Umbilicus midline, inverted. Skin color consistent. Bowel sounds present all quadrants. No bruits, venous hums, or friction rubs. Tympany throughout to percussion. Abdomen soft, smooth, nontender to palpation. Liver, spleen, urinary bladder nonpalpable. No rebound tenderness. Aorta width = 3 cm. Psoas Sign no pain with hip flexion. Murphy's Sign negative.

Urinary

No CVA tenderness to palpation or percussion. Lower pole of kidneys, bladder nonpalpable. No bruits auscultated.

Box 19.2 **Physical Assessment (*continued*)**

Reproductive

Full distribution of clean pubic hair. Labia majora symmetric, round, smooth, no swelling, lesions. Labia minora smooth, pink, no redness, swelling, bruising, lesions. Clitoris midline no tears. Urethral orifice midline, pink, slitlike, patent, no urine leakage, discharge. Vaginal opening pink, smooth and round. Vaginal walls rugated, soft, no bulges. Vaginal fornices smooth, nontender. Urethra, Skene's glands, Bartholin glands no masses, pain, or discharge. Cervix pink, round, mobile, central opening, scant clear odorless secretions. Pap smear obtained. Uterus anteverted, smooth, nontender, no masses. Uterine tubes nonpalpable. Ovaries mobile, smooth, nontender. Perineum smooth. Rectum smooth, sphincter intact, no occult blood.

Musculoskeletal

All joints and bones symmetrical, full ROM. No edema, visible deformities, crepitus, crackling, clicking, pain or discomfort. Muscles symmetric, firm, nontender and strong. Phalen's Test no pain, tingling, or numbness. Tinel's Sign no pain, tingling, or numbness. Bulge sign negative. Ballottement No patellar movement. Spinal alignment normal curvatures, vertebral processes aligned. Scapulae, iliac crests and gluteal folds level and symmetric, leg length equal.

Neurologic

Recent and remote memory intact. Calculates backwards from 100 by 7s. Abstract reasoning can state differences and similarities in several categories. Facial expression congruent with topic. Maintains eye contact throughout interaction. Follows directions. Cranial Nerves intact. Romberg test slight sway. Walks heel to toe, tandem, tiptoe, and on heels without difficulty. Finger to nose with smooth movements with eyes open and closed. Able to perform alternating movements rapidly and smoothly. Able to perform heel to shin test smoothly. Able to identify light touch and variations in temperature. Able to discriminate between sharp and dull sensations. Able to identify onset and cessation of vibrations. Stereognosis and Graphesthesia intact.

Two-Point Discrimination: Fingertips = 0.4 cm, Hands = 1.5 cm, Feet = 2 cm, Legs = 3.5 cm.

Reflexes all 2+. Brudzinski sign negative. Glascow Coma Scale Score 15.

20
The Complete Health Assessment

INTRODUCTION

This chapter is designed to help the student perform a complete health assessment. Conducting a complete health assessment requires effective communication, organization, use of knowledge from the natural and behavioral sciences and nursing, efficient and accurate performance of physical assessment techniques, recognition of verbal and nonverbal client cues, and the abilities to interpret and document findings. For the student, a complete health assessment may seem difficult. However, learning to conduct a complete health assessment is essential in developing plans to meet the health care needs of clients.

Planning and organization are steps to a successful assessment. Plan the sequence of steps, gather necessary equipment, review documentation forms, and have pen and paper prepared for recording data or to write reminders or notes for oneself to clarify points, to prompt follow-up in specific areas, and to help in orderly and concise documentation.

The complete health assessment includes the interview, general survey, assessment of vital signs, and physical assessment of all body systems. Recall that findings are influenced by a number of factors, which include age, gender, developmental level, genetic makeup, culture, religion, psychologic and emotional status, and the client's internal and external environments.

The following pages describe one sequence for the complete health assessment. This sequence minimizes the number of position changes for the client. There are a variety of sequences that may be employed. The complete health assessment should be approached with confidence and a professional demeanor. This important part of professional nursing will become easier with practice.

The complete health assessment begins with the first client encounter. Observations made during your introduction and settling down for the interview provide data as part of the general survey and may provide cues about the client. Always begin by introducing yourself, state the purpose of the complete health assessment, and include assurances regarding the confidentiality of the information. Follow guidelines for client safety and Standard Precautions throughout the assessment. In the initial encounter and during the interview the client is clothed and sits facing the nurse.

SEQUENCE

1. **The Health History**
   The client will be sitting.

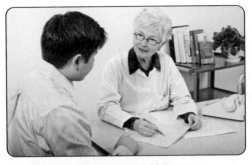

The client participating in the health history.

   Complete the interview.
   Include all areas and address cultural and spiritual assessments.
   The data is subjective; document in the client's own words.

2. **Appearance and Mental Status**

   Compare stated age with appearance.
   Assess level of consciousness.
   Observe body build, height, and weight in relation to age, lifestyle, and health.
   Observe facial expression, posture, position, and mobility.
   Observe overall hygiene and grooming.
   Note body odor and breath odor.
   Note signs of health or illness (skin color, signs of pain).
   Assess attitude, attentiveness, affect, mood, and appropriateness of responses.
   Listen for quantity, quality, relevance, and organization of speech.

   At the completion of the interview have the client change into an examination gown. Have the client empty the bladder; if required, provide a container and instructions for collecting a urine specimen.

3. **Measurements**

   Measure height.
   Measure weight.

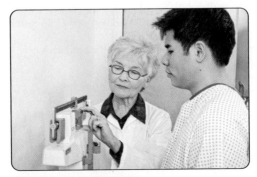

Measuring the client's weight.

Measure skinfold thickness.
Calculate the BMI.
Assess vision with Snellen Chart and Jaeger Card. (Cranial Nerve II)

4. Vital Signs

Assess the radial pulses.
Count respirations.
Take the temperature.
Measure the blood pressure bilaterally.
Assess for pain.

5. Skin, Hair, and Nails

Inspect the skin on the face, neck, upper and lower extremities. (Other skin areas will be assessed as part of the systems assessment.)
Inspect for color and uniformity of color.

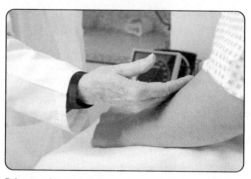

Palpating skin moisture.

Inspect and palpate skin moisture.
Palpate for skin temperature, moisture, turgor, and edema.
Inspect, palpate, measure, and describe lesions.
Inspect the hair on the scalp and body.
Palpate scalp hair for texture, moisture.
Inspect the fingernails for curvature, angle, and color.
Palpate the nails for texture and capillary refill.

6. Head, Neck, and Related Lymphatics

Inspect the skull for size, shape, and symmetry.
Observe facial expressions and symmetry of facial features and movements. (Cranial Nerve V and VII)
Palpate the skull and lymph nodes of the head and neck.

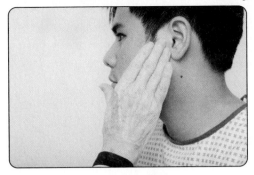

Palpating the preauricular lymph nodes.

Inspect the neck for symmetry, pulsations, swelling, or masses.

Assess range of motion and strength of muscles against resistance. Observe as client moves the head forward and back and side to side and shrugs the shoulders. (Cranial Nerve XI)

Palpate the trachea.

Palpate the thyroid for symmetry and masses.

Palpate and auscultate the carotid arteries one at a time.

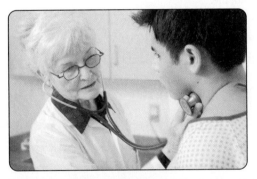

Auscultation of the carotid artery.

Palpate the muscles of the face. (Cranial Nerve V)

Assess facial response to sensory stimulation. (Cranial Nerve V)

7. The Eye

Inspect the external eye.

Inspect the pupils for color, size, shape, equality.

Test the visual fields. (Cranial Nerve II)

Test extraocular movements. (Cranial Nerves III, IV, VI)

Test pupillary reaction to light and accommodation. (Cranial Nerve III)

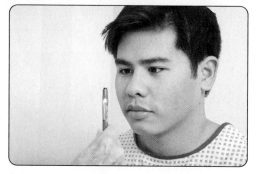

Testing for accommodation.

Darken the room and use the ophthalmoscope to assess the red reflex, optic disc, retinal vessels, retinal background, macula, and fovea centralis.

8. Ears, Nose, Mouth, and Throat

Inspect the external ears.
Palpate the auricle and tragus of each ear.
Use an otoscope to inspect each external ear canal and the tympanic membrane.

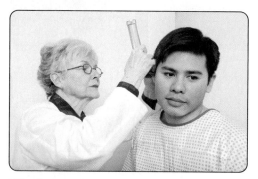

Using the otoscope.

Test hearing using the whisper, Weber, and Rinne tests. (Cranial Nerve VIII)
Assess patency of nares.
Test sense of smell. (Cranial Nerve I)
Use a speculum to inspect the internal nose.
Palpate the nose and sinuses.
Palpate the temporal artery.
Palpate the TMJ as client opens and closes the mouth.
Inspect the lips.
Use a penlight to inspect the tongue, palates, buccal mucosa, gums, teeth, the opening to the salivary glands, tonsils, oropharynx.
Test the sense of taste. (Cranial Nerve VII)

Wearing gloves, palpate the tongue, gums, and floor of the mouth.

Observe the uvula for position and mobility as the client says "ah" and test the gag reflex. (Cranial Nerves IX, X)

Observe as the client protrudes the tongue. (Cranial Nerve XII)

9. **The Respiratory System, Breasts, and Axillae**

Inspect the skin of the posterior chest.

Inspect the posterior chest for symmetry, musculoskeletal development, and thoracic configuration.

Inspect and palpate the scapula and spine.

Palpate and percuss the costovertebral angle for tenderness.

Observe respiratory excursion.

Palpate for thoracic expansion and tactile fremitus.

Percuss over all lung fields.

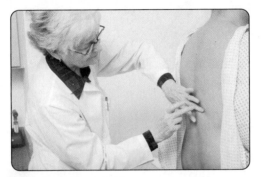

Percussing the posterior thorax.

Percuss for diaphragmatic excursion.

Auscultate breath sounds.

Inspect the skin of the anterior chest.

Inspect the anterior chest for symmetry and musculoskeletal development.

Assess range of motion and movement against resistance of the upper extremities.

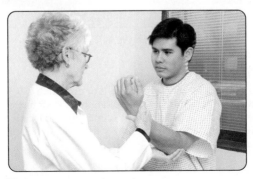

Testing movement against resistance.

Inspect the breasts for symmetry, mobility, masses, dimpling, and nipple retraction. Ask the female to lift arms over her head, press her hands on her hips, and lean forward as you inspect.

Palpate the axillary, supraclavicular, and infraclavicular lymph nodes.

The patient will now be assisted to supine position for breast assessment.

Palpate the breasts and nipples.

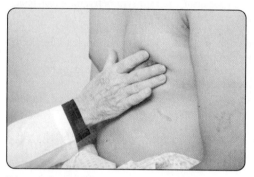

Palpating the nipple.

Palpate the anterior chest.

Percuss over all lung fields.

Auscultate for breath sounds.

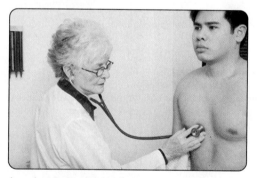

Auscultating the anterior thorax.

10. The Cardiovascular System

Inspect the neck for jugular pulsations or distention.

Inspect and palpate the chest for pulsations, lifts, or heaves.

Palpate the apical pulse and note the intensity and location.

Use the bell and diaphragm of the stethoscope to auscultate for heart sounds.

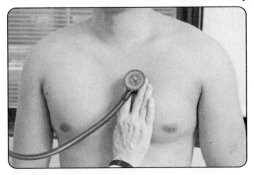

Using the bell to auscultate the pulmonic area.

At each area of auscultation distinguish rate, rhythm, and location of S1 and S2 sounds.

11. The Abdomen

Inspect the skin of the abdomen.

Inspect the abdomen for symmetry, contour, and movement or pulsation.

Auscultate the abdomen for bowel sounds.

Auscultate the abdomen for vascular sounds.

Percuss the abdomen in all quadrants.

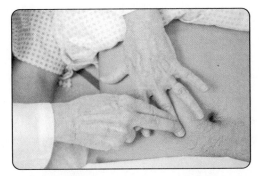

Percussing the abdomen.

Percuss the abdomen to determine liver and spleen size.

Palpate the liver, spleen, and kidneys.

Palpate to determine if tenderness, masses, or distention are present.

Palpate the inguinal region for pulses, lymph nodes, and presence of hernias.

12. The Musculoskeletal System

Test range of motion and strength in hips, knees, ankles, and feet.

Assist the client to a standing position.

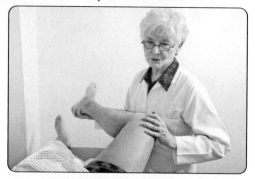

Testing range of motion of the lower extremity.

Inspect the skin of the posterior legs.

Perform the Romberg test.

Observe as the client walks in a natural gait.

Observe the client walking heel to toe.

Observe the client stand on the right foot, then the left foot with eyes closed.

Observe as the client performs a shallow knee bend.

Stand behind the client, observe the spine as the client touches the toes.

Test range of motion of the spine.

13. **The Neurologic System**

Assess sensory function. Include light touch, tactile location, pain, temperature, vibratory sense, kinesthetic sensation, and tactile discrimination.

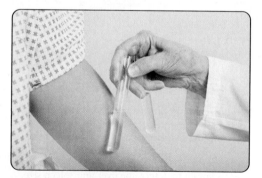

Testing temperature sensation.

Test position sense.

Test cerebellar function with finger to nose test.

Test cerebellar function with heel-shin test.

Test stereognosis and graphesthesia.

Test tendon reflexes bilaterally and compare.

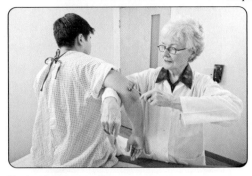

Testing the triceps reflex.

14A. The Female Reproductive System

Inspect the amount, distribution, and characteristics of pubic hair.
Inspect the clitoris, urethral orifice, and vaginal orifice.
Palpate Bartholin's glands.
Assess the integrity of the pelvic musculature.
Insert a speculum and examine the internal genitalia.
Inspect the cervix for shape of the os, color, size, and position.
Obtain a specimen for a Papanicolaou smear.
Inspect the vaginal walls.
Perform a bimanual examination.
Palpate the rectum and rectovaginal walls.
Observe and test stool for occult blood.
Inspect the sacrococcygeal and perianal areas.
Palpate the rectal walls and prostate gland.
Observe any stool and test for occult blood.

14B. The Male Reproductive System

Observe the amount, distribution, and characteristics of pubic hair.
Inspect penile shaft, glans, and urethral meatus.
Observe the color and position of the urethral meatus.

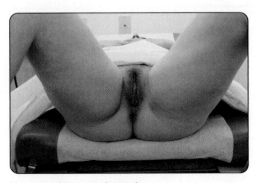

Inspecting the external genitalia.

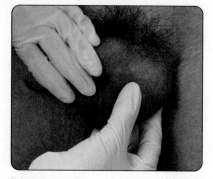

Palpating the testes.

Inspect the scrotum for appearance, size, and symmetry.
Palpate the scrotum, testicles, epididymis, and spermatic cord. If a mass is present, then transilluminate.

SUMMARY

This chapter presents information related to the complete health assessment. This assessment requires application of knowledge and skills acquired in the study and practice of the individual elements of the interview, general survey, assessment of vital signs, and physical assessment of all body systems. You are reminded to consider the characteristics of the individual client, including, but not limited to, age, gender, and developmental level in planning and organizing your approach to the assessment. One sequence, minimizing the number of position changes for the client, is presented. The sequence begins with the first client encounter and then follows an organized approach to collection of subjective and objective data. Conducting a complete health assessment becomes easier with practice, and learning to conduct a complete health assessment is essential to meeting the specific healthcare needs of clients of all ages and in varied settings.

21
The Hospitalized Client

Nursing process has been recognized as the systematic and cyclic process used by the nurse to plan and provide care for clients. Assessment, the first step of the nursing process, is a dynamic and fluid activity. Analysis of the data gathered in the assessment phase of the nursing process requires critical thinking and application of knowledge about health, illness, and the factors that influence a person's response to changes in their health status. Only with detailed assessment and accurate analysis of data can nursing care plans to meet the specific needs of the client be developed.

The depth and breadth of assessment of the hospitalized client varies with both the purpose of the assessment and the health status of the client. In nonemergent situations, nurses conduct complete (comprehensive) health assessments of clients on admission.

When the client is in distress, or in special circumstances, such as following surgery, a more focused and limited assessment is carried out. Routine, or ongoing, assessments occur throughout the client's hospital stay. These ongoing assessments include shift by shift assessments and those to ascertain response to a treatment or intervention. In practice, each client encounter includes assessment in relation to current and expected status, change, and progress.

Hospitalized clients undergo frequent assessments; therefore, it is important that the nurse communicate effectively regarding the type of assessment and the purpose of the assessment. In addition, the nurse must be sure to have all of the required equipment and be able to use physical assessment techniques with efficiency and competence. Hospitals often have policies to guide the types and frequencies of assessments required in accordance with medical diagnoses or parameters for laboratory findings, monitor readings, client condition, or administration of medication.

Application of the nursing process is specific for each client. Integration of assessment data with other knowledge about a client is essential to planning care. The knowledge base about the client will include the health problems; that is, current and coexisting medical diagnoses, age, gender, nutritional status, results of laboratory and diagnostic testing, documentation and communication with other members of the healthcare team, medication regimes, and functional capabilities. Additionally, the knowledge base includes psychosocial factors and concerns, for example, presence of a support system, knowledge about the health problems, coping abilities, culture, and spirituality. This knowledge base assists the nurse to make judgments about assessment findings in relation to expected norms in each client encounter.

The following pages present two types of assessment of the hospitalized client. The first is a rapid assessment, requiring one minute or less to complete. This type of assessment is often used as an initial assessment of a group of clients in a nursing assignment. The nurse uses the collected data to prioritize her actions and interventions. As a beginning student, the rapid assessment of a single client assessment is helpful in reducing anxiety because priorities can be established alone or in collaborative discussion with the faculty, preceptor, or staff. In addition, documentation of data from the rapid assessment establishes a baseline for ongoing client interaction and care.

The second type of assessment is referred to here as a routine or initial assessment. This assessment is used to gather more in-depth data about a client for whom care will be provided. Data gathered in the initial assessment guide the direction of care and informs the nurse about the need for as well as the type and frequency of continuing assessment.

Remember to apply all concepts of client safety, Standard Precautions, and professional standards in each client encounter, in professional communication, and in documentation of assessment data.

The Rapid Assessment

SEQUENCE

Wash your hands.

Note isolation precautions, latex allergies, or fall precautions.

Enter the room.

Identify yourself and explain that you will be providing care for a given time period.

Ask the client's name and identify the client using the identification band and number.

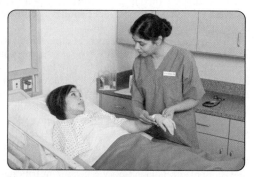

The nurse confirms the client's identification.

Note the location of the client (bed, chair, bathroom).

If in bed, is the bed in the lowest position, is the call bell in reach?

Observe for level of consciousness.

Observe for signs of distress.

Observe skin color and respiratory effort.

Observe posture, facial expression, and symmetry.

Observe client's response to your introduction.

Observe speech for clarity.

Place a hand on the client, assess skin temperature.

Note any equipment that is immediately visible.

Explain that you will return shortly.

Discuss with faculty, preceptor, or staff, as needed.

Document findings.

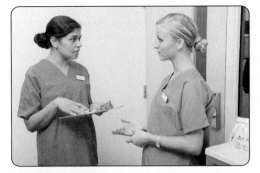

Discussion of client assessment.

The Routine or Initial Assessment

1. Introduction

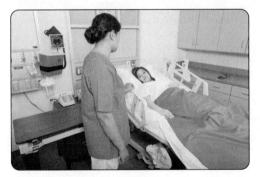

The nurse observing the client in bed.

Wash your hands.

Enter the room.

Identify yourself and that you will be providing care for a given length of time.

Ask the client's name and identify the client with the wristband and identification number.

Note the client's location (bed, chair, bathroom).

Note that call bell is in reach.

2. General Appearance

Observe the following:

Level of consciousness

Respiratory status

Skin color

Nutritional status

Facial expression—symmetry and appropriateness

Body posture and position, relaxation, comfort, or pain
Clarity, fluency, quality, and appropriateness of speech
Hygiene and grooming
Response to your introduction in relation to hearing and congruence
with situation.

3. Measurement

Temperature
Pulses—radial, dorsalis pedis bilaterally

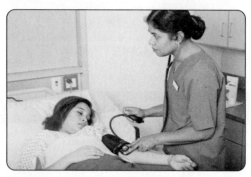

The nurse checking vital signs.

Respiration
Blood pressure (bilaterally if not contraindicated)
Pain—Use of rating scale—Correlate with administration of pain medication if so indicated.
Pulse oximetry

4. Respiratory System

Respiratory effort
Oxygen therapy—mask, nasal cannula, check placement and flow meter.
Auscultate breath sounds posterior and anterior. Seek assistance for positioning if required.
Assess for coughing; if productive, assess sputum.

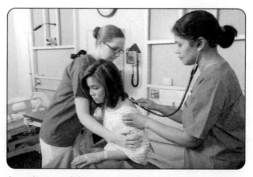

Auscultation of the posterior thorax.

5. Cardiovascular System

Auscultate apical pulse for rate, rhythm.

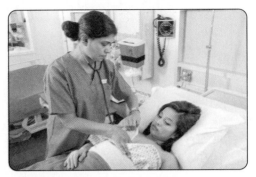

Auscultation of the apical pulse.

Assess heart sounds in five auscultatory areas.
Assess for capillary refill.

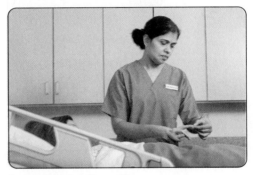

Assessment of capillary refill.

Assess for peripheral edema.
Assess intravenous site and if IV fluid is running verify that it is the correct solution and rate.

6. Abdomen

Inspect for contour, skin color, pulsations.
Auscultate bowel sounds.
Palpate and percuss.
Assess time of most recent bowel elimination and /or flatus.
Assess drains, tubes, dressings, when indicated.

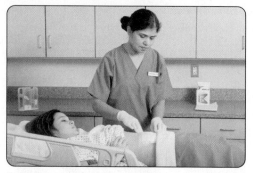

Assessment of an abdominal dressing.

7. Genitourinary

Assess urine output—voiding—frequency and amount, or catheter drainage amount.

Assess color and clarity of urine.

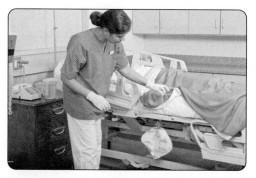

Assessment of urinary catheter drainage.

8. Skin

Palpate skin temperature, moisture.
Assess skin turgor.

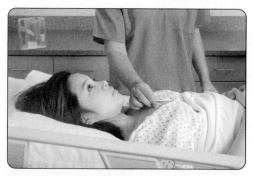

Assessment of skin turgor.

Assess for lesions.

Assess wounds and incision lines if present.

Utilize standardized tools to determine risk for skin problems (scales/questionnaires).

Assess functioning of any devices applied on skin or used to prevent pressure.

9. **Activity**

Assess symmetry and coordination of movements throughout assessment.

Assess ability to move self to sitting and standing positions.

Assess presence of and use of assistive devices.

Use standardized measures to evaluate risk for falls.

Assess the environment for hazards for mobility.

10. **Documentation**

Document findings according to agency policy.

SUMMARY

This chapter presents an overview of several types of assessments required when applying the nursing process in the care of the hospitalized client. Hospitalized clients undergo frequent assessments; therefore, it is important that the nurse communicates effectively and uses physical assessment techniques with efficiency and competence. Two types of assessments of the hospitalized client are presented in the chapter. The first is a rapid assessment, requiring 1 minute or less to complete. This type of assessment is often used as an initial assessment to prioritize actions and interventions. The second type of assessment is a routine or initial assessment and is used to gather more in-depth data about a client for whom care will be provided.

The chapter reminds you that analysis of the data requires critical thinking and application of knowledge about health, illness, and the factors that influence a person's response to changes in his or her health status. Only with detailed assessment and accurate analysis of data can nursing care plans to meet the specific needs of the client be developed.

Photo Credits

Chapter 5: Skin, Hair, and Nails
5-7: Logical Images/Logical Images, Inc.; 5-17: Charles Stewart & Associates; 5-18: Charles Stewart & Associates; 5-19: Logical Images, Inc.; 5-20 P. Barber/Custom Medical Stock Photo, Inc.; 5-21: Logical Images, Inc.; 5-22: Logical Images/Logical Images, Inc.; 5-23: Custom Medical Stock Photo, Inc.; 5-24: Custom Medical Stock Photo, Inc.; 5-25: SIU Bio Med/Custom Medical Stock Photo, Inc.; 5-26: Logical Images/Logical Images, Inc.; 5-27: NMSB/Custom Medical Stock Photo, Inc.; 5-28: NMSB/Custom Medical Stock Photo, Inc.; 5-30: National Archives and Records Administration; 5-31: Edward H. Gill/Custom Medical Stock Photo, Inc.; 5-32: Courtesy of Jason L. Smith, MD; 5-33: Dr. P. Marazzi/Photo Researchers, Inc.; 5-34: Dr. Steve Kraus/Centers for Disease Control and Prevention (CDC); 5-35: SPL/Photo Researchers, Inc.; 5-36: Courtesy of Dr. Hikka Helovuo, K. Kakkarainen, and K. Pannio. Oral Microbiol. Immuno. 75–79, (1993); 5-37: Logical Images/Logical Images, Inc.; 5-38: Logical Images/Logical Images, Inc.

Chapter 6: Head, Neck, and Related Lymphatics
6-8: Dr. P. Marazzi/Photo Researchers, Inc.; 6-9: Scott Cunningham/Merrill Education; 6-12: NMSB/Custom Medical Stock Photo, Inc.

Chapter 7: Eye
7-5: Don Wong/Photo Researchers, Inc.; 7-10: NMSB/Custom Medical Stock Photo, Inc.; 7-11: Biophoto Associates/Science Source/Photo Researchers, Inc.; 7-12: ©Dorling Kindersley/Dorling Kindersley Media Library; 7-14: Science Source/Science Photo Library/Photo Researchers, Inc.; 7-15: Paul Parker/Photo Researchers, Inc.

Chapter 8: Ears, Nose, Mouth, and Throat
8-8: Janet Hayes/Medical Images Inc.; 8-9: Professor Tony Wright/Photo Researchers, Inc.; 8-12: Dr. P. Marazzi/Science Photo Library/Custom Medical Stock Photo, Inc.; 8-13: Dr. R. Gottsegen/Peter Arnold, Inc.; 8-14: E. H. Gill/Custom Medical Stock Photo, Inc.; 8-15: Dr. P.Marazzi/Science Photo Library/Custom Medical Stock Photo, Inc.; 8-16: Logical Images/Logical Images Inc.; 8-17: O. J. Staats/Custom Medical Stock Photo, Inc.; 8-18: Courtesy PD Dr. P. Itin, Kantonsspital Basel.

Chapter 15: Male Reproductive System
T 15-01: From Van Wieringen et al.: Growth Diagrams 1965. Courtesy of Wolters-Noordhoff, the Netherlands.

Chapter 16: Female Reproductive System
T 16-01: From Van Wieringen et al.: Growth Diagrams 1965. Courtesy of Wolters-Noordhoff, the Netherlands.

Chapter 17: Musculoskeletal System
17-11: Dr. P. Marazzi/Photo Researchers, Inc.; 17-12: Princess Margaret Rose Orthopaedic Hospital, Edinburgh, Scotland/Science Photo Library/Photo Researchers, Inc.; 17-13: Princess Margaret Rose Orthopaedic Hospital/Photo Researchers, Inc.; 17-15: ©1972–2004 American College of Rheumatology Clinical Slide Collection. Used with permission; 17-16: Biophoto Associates/Science Source/Photo Researchers, Inc; 17-17: M. English/Stockphoto.com/Medichrome/The Stock Shop, Inc.

Index

Page numbers followed by *f* indicate figures and those followed by *t* indicate tables.

A

ABCDE criteria, melanoma assessment, 49
Abdomen:
    abnormal findings, 172–83, 180*t*, 181*t*
    anatomy and physiology, 168, 168*f*
    assessment in hospitalized client, 315, 316*f*
    auscultation, 173–74
    cultural considerations, 170
    focused interview, 170–71
    hints for physical assessment, 171
    in infants and children, 169, 171
    inspection, 172–73
    landmarks, 168
    in older adults, 169
    palpation, 176–77, 177*f*
    percussion, 174, 178, 307*f*
    in pregnant female, 169, 171
    psychosocial considerations, 170
    quadrants, 168, 169*f*
    sequence for physical assessment, 171, 307
Abdominal pain, 181*t*
Abdominal reflexes, 288
Abducens nerve (cranial nerve VI), 263*t*, 271, 291*t*
Abduction, 235*t*
Accessory nerve (cranial nerve XI):
    dysfunction, 243, 291*t*
    function and activity, 264*t*
    testing, 275–76, 275*f*, 276*f*
Accommodation testing, 87, 304*f*
Achilles tendon, 253
Achilles tendon reflex, 286–87, 287*f*
Addison's disease, 41*t*
Adduction, 235*t*
Adie's (tonic) pupil, 92, 92*f*
Adolescents. *See also* Children
    breasts, 133
    female reproductive system, 212, 213*t*, 215

male reproductive system, 197, 198*t*, 200
    skin, hair, and nails, 37–38
Adventitious breath sounds, 124*t*
African Americans:
    breast cancer, 133
    cardiovascular disease, 145
    diabetes, 145
    ears, nose, mouth, and throat, 98
    eye disorders, 80
    female reproductive system, 214
    fetal alcohol syndrome, 67
    gastrointestinal disorders, 170
    hypertension, 145, 155, 185, 265
    low birth weight rates, 265
    male reproductive system, 199
    musculoskeletal system, 237
    neurologic system, 265
    obesity, 155, 170
    respiratory system, 116
    skin, hair, and nails, 42
    smoking, 155
Alaska Natives, 67
Albinism, 39*t*
Allen's test, 160
Allergic rhinitis, 110, 110*f*
Allis' sign, 23
Alopecia areata, 50
Alzheimer's disease, 265, 268, 292
Amplitude (intensity), 14
Amyotrophic lateral sclerosis, 292
Analgesia, 281
Anesthesia, 280
Ankles, 253–54
Ankyloglossia, 111, 111*f*
Ankylosing spondylitis, 237, 257*t*
Annular lesions, 56, 56*f*
Anosmia, 270
Anus, 197, 208
Aorta, 177
Aortic aneurysm, 173
Apical pulse, 21, 21*f*, 151, 315*f*
Apocrine glands, 36
Appendicitis, 178, 181*t*

Aqueous humor, 79
Arcus senilis, 80
Areola, 130
Arms:
    arteries, 153*f*
    lymph nodes, 154*f*
    vascular assessment, 159–61, 160*t*
    veins, 154*f*
Ascites, 178
Asians:
    ears, nose, mouth, and throat, 98
    musculoskeletal system, 237
    preventive care, 133
    respiratory system, 116
    skin, hair, and nails, 42
Assessment. *See also specific body systems*
    health. *See* Health assessment
    in nursing process, 3
Asthma, 116, 128, 128*f*
Astigmatism, 92
Asystole, 150
Ataxic gait, 290*t*
Atelectasis, 128, 128*f*
Athetoid movement, 290*t*
Atlas, 64
Atrial fibrillation, 152, 152*f*
Atrial flutter, 152, 152*f*
Atrial gallop, 142
Atrioventricular (AV) node, 143
Atrioventricular (AV) valves, 141
Attending, 27*t*
Auricle, 95
Auscultation, 14
    abdomen, 173–74
    anterior thorax, 126–28, 127*f*, 306*f*
    cardiovascular system, 150–51, 307*f*
    carotid artery, 151, 158, 288, 303, 303*f*
    posterior thorax, 122–24, 122*t*, 124*t*
    renal artery, 188
    sounds, 14
Autoimmune disorder, 293
Axillae, 138, 139, 154*f*, 161
Axillary tail, 130, 136
Axis, 64

B

Babinski reflex, 265
Babinski response, 287, 288*f*
Bacterial vaginitis, 223
Balance, 277
Ball-and-socket joint, 234*t*
Ballottement, 251–52, 251*f*, 252*f*
Bartholin's gland, 217, 220, 220*f*, 230
Behavior assessment, 19–20
Bell's palsy, 75, 75*f*
Biceps reflex, 285–86, 285*f*
Biferiens pulse, 166*t*
Bladder, 193, 194
Bladder cancer, 199
Blindness, 80
Blood pressure, 22, 145, 157, 157*t*
Blumberg's sign, 178
Blunt percussion, 12, 12*f*
Body odor, 44
Body piercing, 42
Bones, 232
Bouchard's nodules, 260, 260*f*
Bounding pulse, 166*t*
Bowel sounds, 180*t*
Brachial pulse, 160
Brachioradialis reflex, 286
Brain abscess, 292
Brain attack (stroke), 76, 76*f*
Brain stem, 262
Breast cancer, 132, 133, 135–36, 138
Breasts:
    abnormal findings, 135–36, 138–39, 140
    anatomy and physiology, 130, 130*f*, 131*f*
    cultural considerations, 133
    equipment for physical assessment, 134
    focused interview, 133
    hints for physical assessment, 134
    in infants and children, 131, 133
    inspection, 134–36, 134*f*
    male, 139, 140
    in older adults, 131, 133
    palpation, 136–38, 137*f*, 306*f*
    in pregnant female, 131, 133
    psychosocial considerations, 132
    self-examination, 132*t*
Breath sounds, 122–24, 122*t*, 124*t*
Bronchi, 113

Brudzinski's sign, 289
Bruit:
    abdominal, 174, 180*t*
    carotid artery, 151, 159
    definition, 69, 151, 159
Bulbourethral glands, 197, 208–9
Bulge sign, 251, 251*f*
Bulla, 55, 55*f*
Bundle branches, 143
Bundle of His, 143
Bunion (hallux valgus), 253, 260, 260*f*
Bursae, 232
Bursitis, 250, 258*t*

C

Calcaneal (Achilles) tendon, 253
Caloric test, 274
Cancer/carcinoma:
    bladder, 199
    breast, 132, 133, 135–36, 185
    cervical, 214, 230
    gastrointestinal, 170
    oral, 112, 112*f*
    penile, 199
    prostate, 199, 209
    testicular, 199
    thyroid, 77
Candidiasis, 223
Capillary refill, 51, 159, 315*f*
Cardiac conduction system, 142–43
Cardiac cycle, 143
Cardinal fields of gaze, 84–85, 85*f*
Cardiovascular system:
    abnormal findings, 147–52
    anatomy and physiology, 141, 141*f*
    assessment in hospitalized client, 315, 315*f*
    auscultation, 150–51, 307*f*
    cardiac conduction system, 142–43
    cultural considerations, 145
    equipment for physical assessment, 147
    focused interview, 146
    heart sounds, 141–42, 142*t*
    hints for physical assessment, 147
    in infants and children, 144
    inspection, 147–49, 148*f*, 149*f*
    landmarks, 143, 143*f*, 149*f*
    in older adults, 145
    palpation, 149–50
    in pregnant female, 145

    psychosocial considerations, 145
    sequence for physical assessment, 306–7
Carotenemia, 41*t*
Carotid artery:
    auscultation, 151, 158, 288, 303, 303*f*
    bruit, 151, 159
    inspection, 70, 149
    palpation, 158
Carotid pulse, 150, 151, 158
Carpal tunnel syndrome, 246, 247, 248, 259, 259*f*
Cartilaginous joints, 232
Cataract, 93, 93*f*
Caucasians:
    breast cancer, 133
    cardiovascular disease, 145
    ears, nose, mouth, and throat, 98
    eye disorders, 80
    male reproductive system, 199
    musculoskeletal system, 237
    respiratory system, 116
    skin, hair, and nails, 42
Central nervous system, 261–62, 261*f*. *See also* Neurologic system
Central venous pressure, 148, 148*f*
Cerebellum, 261
Cerebrum, 261, 261*f*
Cerumen, 98
Cervical cancer, 214
Cervical spine, 256
Cervix:
    abnormal findings, 230–31
    palpation, 225–26
    Pap smear procedure, 223–24
    visualization with speculum, 222–23
Chadwick's sign, 223
Charting by exception, 8
Chickenpox (varicella), 60, 60*f*
Children:
    abdomen/gastrointestinal tract, 169
    breasts, 133
    cardiovascular system, 146
    ear, nose, mouth, and throat, 100
    eyes and vision, 80, 81
    female reproductive system, 212, 213*t*, 215
    male reproductive system, 197, 198*t*, 200
    musculoskeletal system, 232, 236, 238
    neurologic system, 265, 266

peripheral vascular system, 155, 156

respiratory system, 115, 117

skin, hair, and nails, 37–38, 43

Cholecystitis, 181*t*

Choroid, 78

Chronic obstructive pulmonary disease (COPD), 118

Circumcision, 199

Circumduction, 235*t*

Cleft lip and palate, 98

Client record, 7

Clitoris, 217–18, 218*f*

Clonus, 285

Clubbing, fingernails, 52, 52*f*, 63, 63*f*

Cluster headache, 74

Cochlea, 96

Cold sores, 107, 112*f*

Colostrum, 131

Coma, 289

Communication, 26

Compression fracture, 256

Condyloid joint, 234*t*

Confluent lesions, 57, 57*f*

Congenital hypothyroidism, 77

Congestive heart failure, 129, 129*f*, 148

Conjunctiva, 88–89

Conjunctivitis, 93, 93*f*

Contact dermatitis, 217

Convergence, 87

Coping strategies, for pain, 24

Cornea, 78

Corneal light reflex, 85

Corneal reflex, 272

Corrigan's pulse, 167*t*

Costovertebral angle (CVA), 184, 189, 189*f*

Cover test, 85–86

Cranial nerves. *See also specific nerves*
   dysfunction, 291*t*
   functions and activities, 263–64*t*
   target regions, 263–64, 263*f*
   testing, 270–76, 272*f*, 273*f*, 275*f*, 276*f*

Cremasteric reflex, 205

Crepitation, 69

Crepitus, 240

Critical thinking, 5–7, 5*f*

Crohn's disease, 183*t*

Cross-examination, 29

Cues, 16–17

Cullen's sign, 48

Cultural considerations:
   breasts, 133
   cardiovascular system, 145

ear, nose, mouth, and throat, 98

eye and vision, 80

female reproductive system, 214

gastrointestinal tract, 170

head and neck, 67

male reproductive system, 199

musculoskeletal system, 237

neurologic system, 265

in nurse-client interactions, 29

peripheral vascular system, 155

respiratory system, 116

skin, hair, and nails, 38, 39–41*t*, 42

urinary system, 185

Cutaneous glands, 36

Cuticle, 37

Cyanosis, 39*t*, 45, 230

Cystocele, 219

D

Dandruff, 50

Data, 2, 3

Database, 9

Deep palpation, 11, 11*f*

Deep percussion, 181*t*

Depression (joint movement), 236*t*

Depression (mental), 269

Dermatomes, 264, 264*f*

Dermis, 36

Deviated septum, 105, 110, 110*f*

Diabetes, 185

Diabetic acidosis, 109

Diabetic retinopathy, 94, 94*f*

Diagnosis, in nursing process, 4

Diaphoresis, 46

Diastolic pressure, 22

Diethylstilbestrol (DES) syndrome, 231

Diplopia, 271

Direct leading, 27*t*

Direct percussion, 12, 12*f*

Discrete lesions, 57, 57*f*

Dislocation, 258*t*

Diversity, 29

Diverticulitis, 181*t*

Documentation, 7–8, 35, 294–96*t*

Doppler ultrasonic stethoscope, 15

Dorsalis pedis pulse, 164

Dorsiflexion, 235*t*

Down syndrome, 75, 75*f*

Dry skin, 46

Ductus arteriosus, 144

Dullness, 14

Duodenal ulcer, 181*t*

Dupuytren's contracture, 248

Duration, of sound, 14

Dysphagia, 275

Dyspnea, 113

Dysreflexia, 195

Dystonia, 290*t*

E

Ear:
   abnormal findings, 100–102, 109–10
   anatomy and physiology, 95–96, 95*f*
   cultural considerations, 98
   equipment for physical assessment, 100
   focused interview, 99
   hearing assessment, 102–4, 104*f*
   hints for physical assessment, 100
   in infants and children, 98
   inspection, 100–102, 101*f*
   in older adults, 98
   in pregnant female, 98
   sequence for physical assessment, 304–5

Ecchymosis, 48

Eccrine glands, 36

Ectopic pregnancy, 181*t*

Edema, 47, 48*f*, 165, 165*f*

Elbows, 243–45, 244*f*, 245*f*

Electrocardiogram (ECG), 143, 144*f*

Elevation, 236*t*

Emmetropia, 91

Emphysema, 121, 129, 129*f*

Encephalitis, 291

Endocardium, 141

Environment, for physical assessment, 17

Epicardium, 141

Epididymis, 199, 205

Epididymitis, 203

Epilepsy, 291

Epispadias, 202

Equilibrium, assessment of, 104

Erythema, 40*t*

Esophagitis, 182

Eupnea, 113

Eustachian tube, 96

Evaluation, in nursing process, 5

Eversion, 236*t*

Extension, 235*t*

Eye. *See also* Vision
   abnormal findings, 84–88, 90–94
   accessory structures, 79
   anatomy and physiology, 78, 78*f*, 79*f*

Eye. *See also* Vision (*Continued*)
cardinal fields of gaze
testing, 84–85
conjunctiva and sclera
examination, 88–89
corneal light reflex
testing, 85
cover test, 85–86
cultural considerations, 80
equipment for physical
assessment, 81
focused interview, 81
fundus examination with
ophthalmoscope,
89–91, 90f
hints for physical
assessment, 82
in infants and children,
79–80, 81
inspection, 87–88
in older adults, 80, 81
palpation, 88
in pregnant female, 80, 81
psychosocial
considerations, 80
pupils assessment, 86–87
refraction, 79
sequence for physical
assessment, 303–4

F

Facial nerve (cranial nerve
VII), 263t, 273–74,
273f, 291t
False reassurance, 26
Fasciculation, 290t
Feet, 253–54
Female genital mutilation, 214
Female reproductive system:
abnormal findings, 216–31
anatomy and physiology,
211, 211f, 212f
cultural considerations,
214
equipment for physical
assessment, 215
focused interview, 214–15
hints for physical
assessment, 216
in infants and children,
212, 213t
inspection, 216–19, 218f
in older adults, 214
palpation, 219–20, 225–29
in pregnant female, 214
psychosocial
considerations, 214
sequence for physical
assessment, 309
speculum examination,
220–23, 222f
Femoral hernia, 207, 210t
Femoral pulse, 163
Festination gait, 290t

Fetal alcohol syndrome, 67
Fever blisters, 107, 112, 112f
Fibromyalgia, 257t
Fibrous joints, 232
Findings, interpretation of, 3
Finger-to-nose test, 278
Fingers. *See* Hand and fingers
Flanks, 188
Flatness, 14
Flexion, 235t
Flow sheets, 8
Focus documentation, 8
Focused interview, 2–3, 31
Focusing, 27t
Folliculitis, 63, 63f
Fontanels, 66
Foramen ovale, 144
Fovea centralis, 78
Fracture, 258t
Fremitus, 10, 121
Frequency (pitch), 14
Friction rub, 124t, 180t
Functional assessment, in
general survey, 25
Functional incontinence, 195

G

Gag reflex, 274–75
Gait, 277, 290t
Galactorrhea, 138
Ganglion, 246
Gardasil, 212
Gastric bubble, 176
Gastritis, 181t
Gastroenteritis, 173
Gastroesophageal reflux
disorder (GERD), 181t
Gastrointestinal tract. *See*
Abdomen
General survey:
age-related
considerations, 20
components, 19–20
functional assessment, 25
height and weight
measurement, 20–21
pain assessment, 22–25,
23f, 24f
vital signs, 21–22, 21f, 22f
Genital warts, 217
Genogram, 33, 34f
Genu recurvatum, 252
Genu valgum (knock
knees), 252
Genu varum (bowlegs),
232, 252
German measles (rubella),
60, 60f
Gingival hyperplasia,
111, 111f
Gingivitis, 111, 111f
Glasgow Coma Scale,
289, 289t
Glaucoma, 93, 93f

Gliding movement, 235t
Glomerulonephritis, 194
Glossopharyngeal nerve
(cranial nerve IX), 264t,
274–75, 291t
Goiter, 76
Golfer's elbow (medial
epicondylitis), 244
Goniometer, 244, 244f
Gonorrhea, 204, 220, 225
Goodell's sign, 226
Gout, 257t
Gouty arthritis, 253
Graphesthesia, 282–83, 282f
Graves' disease, 71, 76
Grey Turner's sign, 48, 188
Grouped lesions, 57, 57f
Gynecomastia, 131, 139
Gyrate lesions, 58, 58f

H

Hair:
abnormal findings, 50–51,
62–63, 62f, 63f
anatomy and physiology,
36f, 37
cultural considerations, 42t
focused interview, 43
loss, 50
physical assessment,
50–51, 302
special considerations, 37
Hallux valgus (bunion), 253,
256, 256f
Hammertoe, 253, 260, 260f
Hand and fingers, 9, 10f,
246–48
Hashimoto's thyroiditis, 77
Head:
abnormal findings, 69,
74–76, 75–76f
anatomy and physiology,
64, 64f, 65f
cultural considerations, 67
equipment for physical
assessment, 68
focused interview, 67
hints for physical
assessment, 68
psychosocial
considerations, 67
sequence for physical
assessment, 302–3
special considerations, 66
Headaches, 74
Health, 1
Health assessment:
components, 2–3
definition, 2
planning, 300
sequence, 301–10
Health history:
components, 31–35, 32t
definition, 26

documentation, 7–8, 35, 294–96*t*
purpose, 2
Health history interview:
barriers to effective interaction in, 26, 29
for clients who do not speak English, 30*t*
communication skills for, 26, 27–28*t*
cultural influences on interactions in, 29
phases, 31
primary source, 29–30
secondary sources, 30–31
Health pattern, 33
Hearing assessment, 102–4, 104*f*
Heart, 141, 141*f*
Heart block, 152, 152*f*
Heart murmurs, 142, 142*t*
Heart sounds, 141–42, 142*t*
Heel-to-shin test, 279, 279*f*
Height, 20
Helicobacter pylori, 170
Helix, 95
Hematuria, 190
Hepatitis, 182
Hepatitis A virus, 182
Hepatitis B virus, 182
Hepatitis C virus, 170, 182
Hepatitis D virus, 182
Hepatitis E virus, 182–83
Hernia, 180, 182, 197, 210*t*
Herpes simplex:
genital, 217, 230
oral/facial, 61, 61*f,* 112, 112*f*
Herpes zoster (shingles), 61, 61*f*
Hiatal hernia, 182
Hinge joint, 233*t*
Hips, 248–50
Hispanics:
breast cancer, 133
diabetes, 145
eye disorders, 80
female reproductive system, 214
gastrointestinal disorders, 170
hypertension, 145
obesity, 155, 170
preventive care, 133
respiratory system, 116
smoking, 155
Homans' sign, 163
Hospitalized client:
nursing process in assessment, 311
rapid assessment, 312–13, 312*f*
routine or initial assessment, 313–17, 313*f,* 314*f,* 315*f,* 316*f*

Human papillomavirus, 212, 230
Huntington's disease, 292
Hypalgesia, 281
Hyperemia, 40*t*
Hyperesthesia, 280
Hyperextension, 235*t*
Hyperopia (farsightedness), 92
Hyperresonance, 14
Hypertension, 145, 157, 157*t,* 185
Hypertensive retinopathy, 94
Hyperthyroidism, 71, 76, 77
Hypodermis (subcutaneous tissue), 36
Hypoesthesia, 280
Hypoglossal nerve (cranial nerve XII), 264*t,* 276, 291*t*
Hypospadias, 202
Hypothyroidism, 67, 71, 77

I

Impetigo, 61, 61*f*
Implementation, in nursing process, 4–5
Incisional hernia, 182
Incontinence:
fecal, 208
urinary, 195, 218
Indians, 42
Indirect percussion, 12–13, 13*f*
Infants:
abdomen/gastrointestinal system, 169, 171
cardiovascular system, 144, 146
ear, nose, mouth, and throat, 98
eyes, 79–80, 81
female reproductive system, 212, 215
head and neck, 66, 67
height and weight measurements, 21
male reproductive system, 197, 200
musculoskeletal system, 238
neurologic system, 265
peripheral vascular system, 155, 156
respiratory system, 115
skin, hair, and nails, 37–38, 43
urinary system, 184–85, 186
Infectious arthritis, 257*t*
Inguinal areas, 197, 203–4, 206, 206*f*
Inguinal hernia, 197, 206, 207, 210*t*
Inguinal lymph nodes, 163, 207

Initial assessment, of hospitalized client, 313–17, 313*f,* 314*f,* 315*f,* 316*f*
Initial interview, 31
Inspection, 9
Intensity:
of pain, 24, 24*f*
of sound, 14
Interactional skills, 26, 27–28*t*
Interphalangeal joint, 246, 254
Interpretation of findings, 3
Interview, 2. *See also* Health history interview
Intestinal obstruction, 181*t*
Intra-atrial conduction pathway, 143
Inversion, 236*t*
Iris, 78
Irritable bowel syndrome, 181*t*

J

Japanese, 170
Jaundice, 40*t*
Jaw, 239–40
Jewish Americans, 170
Joints (articulations), 232
assessment, 239–40
movements, 235–36*t*
synovial, 233–34*t*
trauma-induced disorders, 258*t*
Jugular veins, 70, 147–48, 148*f*
Juvenile rheumatoid arthritis, 257*t*

K

Kaposi's sarcoma, 62, 62*f*
Keloid, 56, 56*f*
Kidneys:
abnormal findings, 190–92, 194
palpation, 190–92
percussion, 188–90, 189*f*
Knees, 250–52, 251*f,* 252*f*
Kyphosis, 255, 258, 258*f*

L

Labia majora, 217
Labia minora, 217
Lactose intolerance, 170
Lanugo, 37
Lateral epicondylitis, 244
Legs:
arteries, 153*f*
lymph nodes, 154*f*
vascular assessment, 160*t,* 161–65
veins, 154*f*
Leiomyosarcoma, 214
Lens, 79

Leukoplakia, 112, 112*f*
Lichenification, 55, 55*f*
Ligaments, 232
Light palpation, 10, 10*f*
Linear lesions, 58, 58*f*
List, spinal, 255
Liver, 174–75
Lobar pneumonia, 129, 129*f*
Lobule, 95
Lordosis, 255
Lou Gehrig's disease, 292
Lumbar curve, flattened, 255
Lumbar spine, 256
Lungs, 113
Lunula, 37
Lyme disease, 292
Lymph nodes, 154*f*, 161, 163
Lymphadenopathy, 73
Lymphatics, 66, 73, 73*f*

M
Macula, 78
Macular degeneration,
    94, 94*f*
Macule, 54, 54*f*
Male reproductive system:
    abnormal findings, 201–10
    anatomy and physiology,
        196–97, 196*f*
    cultural considerations,
        199
    equipment for physical
        assessment, 200
    focused interview, 200
    hints for physical
        assessment, 201
    in infants and children,
        197, 198*t*, 200
    inspection, 201–4, 202*f*
    maturation stages, 198*t*
    in older adults, 197–98,
        200
    palpation, 204–9,
        204*f*, 206*f*
    psychosocial
        considerations, 198–99
    sequence for physical
        assessment, 309–10
    testicular self-examination,
        199*t*
Mammography, 132
Manual compression test, 162
Mapping, abdomen, 169
Mastoiditis, 101
McBurney's point, 178
Measles (rubeola), 60, 60*f*
Medial epicondylitis, 244
Median nerve, 247, 247*f*
Mediastinal space, 141
Mediastinum, 113
Melanoma, 49
Melasma, 42*t*, 66
Meninges, 261, 288–99
Meningitis, 291

Mental status assessment,
    19, 267–70, 267*t*
Metatarsophalangeal
    joint, 254
Migraine, 74
Milia, 37
Miosis, 92, 92*f*
Mobility, assessment, 19
Moderate palpation, 11, 11*f*
Molding, 66
Mongolian spots, 37
Montgomery's glands, 130
Mood disorders, 269
Motor function, 277–79,
    278*f*, 290*t*
Mouth and throat:
    abnormal findings, 107–9,
        111–12
    anatomy and physiology,
        96–97
    focused interview, 99
    physical assessment,
        107–9, 304–5
    psychosocial
        considerations, 98
Multiple sclerosis, 270, 293
Murphy's sign, 179
Muscle spasms, 256
Muscle strain, 258*t*
Muscle strength, 243, 243*t*
    ankles and feet, 254
    elbow, 245, 245*f*
    fingers, 248
    hips, 250
    knees, 252
    shoulder, 243
    sternocleidomastoid
        muscle, 276, 276*f*
    trapezius muscle, 276
    wrist, 248
Musculoskeletal system:
    anatomy and physiology,
        232
    ankles and feet, 253–54
    cultural considerations, 237
    elbows, 243–45,
        244*f*, 245*f*
    equipment for physical
        assessment, 238
    focused interview, 238
    hints for physical
        assessment, 239
    hips, 248–50
    in infants and children,
        232, 236
    joints, 232, 233–34*t*,
        235–36*t*, 239–40
    knees, 250–52,
        251*f*, 252*f*
    muscle strength rating,
        243, 243*t*
    in older adults, 236–37
    in pregnant female, 236
    psychosocial
        considerations, 237

rheumatic diseases,
    257–58*t*
sequence for physical
    assessment, 307–8
shoulders, 240–43,
    241*f*, 242*f*
spine, 255–56, 255*f*
trauma-induced
    disorders, 258*t*
wrists and hands,
    246–48, 247*f*
Muslims, 42, 67
Myasthenia gravis, 293
Mydriasis, 92, 92*f*
Myelitis, 292
Myocardial infarction (heart
    attack), 240
Myocardium, 141
Myoclonus, 290*t*
Myopia (nearsightedness),
    80, 90, 92
Myxedema, 77

N
Nabothian cysts, 223
Nails:
    abnormal findings, 51–53,
        52*f*, 63, 63*f*
    anatomy and physiology,
        37, 37*f*
    focused interview, 43
    in older adults, 38
    physical assessment,
        51–53, 52*f*, 165
Narrative notes, 8
Nasal polyps, 105
Native Americans:
    cardiovascular
        disease, 145
    diabetes, 145
    ears, nose, mouth, and
        throat, 98
    eye disorders, 80
    female reproductive
        system, 214
    fetal alcohol syndrome, 67
    gastrointestinal
        disorders, 170
    respiratory system, 116
    skin, hair, and nails, 42
Neck. *See also* Thyroid gland
    abnormal findings, 69–71
    anatomy and physiology,
        64–65, 64*f*, 65*f*, 66*f*
    cultural considerations, 67
    focused interview, 67
    inspection, 69–70
    palpation, 70–73
    psychosocial
        considerations, 67
    range of motion, 70
    sequence for physical
        assessment, 302–3
    special considerations, 66

Neuroblastoma, 188
Neurologic system:
    anatomy and physiology,
        261–64, 261*f,* 262*f*
    cranial nerves. *See*
        Cranial nerves
    cultural considerations,
        265
    degenerative disorders,
        292–93
    equipment for physical
        assessment, 266
    focused interview, 266
    hints for physical
        assessment, 267
    in infants and children,
        265, 266
    infections, 291–92
    mental status assessment,
        19, 267–70, 267*t*
    motor function
        assessment, 277–79,
        278*f,* 290*t*
    in older adults, 265, 266
    in pregnant female,
        265, 266
    psychosocial
        considerations, 265
    reflexes, 262, 262*f,* 284–88,
        285*f,* 287*f,* 288*f*
    seizures, 291
    sensory function
        assessment, 280–84,
        281*f,* 282*f,* 283*f,* 284*f*
    sequence for physical
        assessment, 308
Nipples, 135, 138, 139
Nocturia, 185
Nodule, 54, 54*f*
Nose and sinuses:
    abnormal findings,
        105–7, 110
    anatomy and physiology,
        96, 96*f*
    focused interview, 99
    physical assessment,
        105–7, 304
Nuchal rigidity, 288
Nurse-client interactions:
    barriers to, 26, 29
    cultural influences on, 29
    skills for effective, 26,
        27–28*t*
Nursing process, 3–5, 4*f*
Nystagmus, 271

O

Obese client:
    abdominal assessment, 173
    cardiovascular assessment,
        150
    fecal incontinence, 208
    female reproductive
        system, 216, 228

male reproductive
    system, 201
neck assessment, 70
peripheral vascular
    assessment, 155,
    157, 158
respiratory system
    assessment, 122, 124
techniques and equipment
    for assessment, 17–18
urinary incontinence, 218
Obesity, 155, 170
Objective data, 3
Obstructive sleep apnea, 116
Oculomotor nerve (cranial
    nerve III):
    dysfunction, 88, 92,
        92*f,* 291*t*
    function and activity, 263*t*
    testing, 271
Oil (sebaceous) glands, 36
OLDCART & ICE acronym,
    for pain history, 23*f*
Older adults:
    abdomen, 169
    breasts, 133
    cardiovascular system,
        145, 146
    ear, nose, mouth, and
        throat, 98, 100
    eyes and vision, 80, 81
    female reproductive
        system, 214, 215,
        217, 228
    head and neck, 66
    male reproductive system,
        197–98
    middle-aged adults, 200
    musculoskeletal system,
        236–37, 238
    neurologic system, 265,
        266
    peripheral vascular system,
        155
    respiratory system, 117
    skin, hair, and nails,
        38, 43
    urinary system, 185
Olecranon process, 243–44
Olfactory nerve (cranial
    nerve I), 263*t,* 270, 291*t*
Oliguria, 190
Onycholysis, 53
Ophthalmoscope, 15–16,
    89–91, 90*f,* 94*f*
Opposition, of thumb, 236*t*
Optic atrophy, 271
Optic disc, 78, 90*f*
Optic nerve (cranial nerve II),
    263*t,* 270–71, 291*t*
Oral cavity. *See* Mouth and
    throat
Orchitis, 203
Orthodox Jews, 42
Ossicles, 95

Osteoarthritis, 237, 251, 257*t,*
    260, 260*f*
Otitis media, 98, 109, 109*f*
Otoscope, 16, 101–2, 101*f,*
    304*f*
Ovaries, 227–28, 227*f*
Oxygen saturation, 22

P

Pacific Islanders, 80, 116
Paget's disease, 237
Pain assessment, 22–25,
    23*f,* 24*f*
Pain history, 23–25, 23*f*
Pain rating scales, 24, 24*f*
Palate, 97
Pallor, 39*t*
Palpation, 9–12
    abdomen, 176–77, 177*f*
    ankles and feet, 253–54
    anterior thorax, 124–26
    bladder, 193
    breasts, 136–38, 137*f,* 306*f*
    cardiovascular system,
        149–50
    carotid artery, 158
    deep, 11, 11*f*
    elbow, 243–44
    eye, 88
    female reproductive
        system, 219–20, 225–29
    hip, 249
    jaw, 239
    kidneys, 190–92
    knee, 251–52
    light, 10, 10*f*
    lymph nodes, 73, 73*f*
    male reproductive system,
        204–9, 204*f,* 206*f*
    moderate, 11, 11*f*
    neck, 70–73
    posterior thorax,
        119–21, 305*f*
    shoulder, 240
    skin, 45–49, 46*f,* 47*f*
    spine, 256
    temporomandibular
        joint, 239
    wrists and hands,
        246–47
Pancreatitis, 181*t*
Pap smear, 223–24, 224*f*
Papilledema, 271
Papule, 54, 54*f*
Paranasal sinuses, 96
Paraphimosis, 202
Paraphrasing, 27*t*
Parkinson's disease, 75,
    75*f,* 293
Paronychia, 53, 63, 63*f*
Patch, 54, 54*f*
Patellar reflex, 286
Peau d'orange, 135
Pediculosis capitis, 51

Pediculosis pubis (pubic lice), 201, 216, 230
Penile cancer, 199
Penis, 197, 201–2, 204–5, 204f
Percussion:
  abdomen, 174, 178, 307f
  anterior thorax, 126
  bladder, 193
  blunt, 12, 12f
  direct, 12, 12f
  gastric bubble, 176
  indirect, 12–13, 13f
  kidneys, 188–90, 189f
  liver, 174–75
  posterior thorax, 126
  sinuses, 106
  sounds, 13–14
  spleen, 175
Perianal area, 197, 207
Perineum, 197, 218
Peripheral nervous system, 262–64, 263f, 264–65t. *See also* Neurologic system
Peripheral pulses, 21, 22f
Peripheral vascular system:
  abnormal findings, 157–65, 166–67t
  anatomy and physiology, 153, 153f, 154f
  arms, 159–61, 160t
  blood pressure measurement, 157, 157t
  cultural considerations, 155
  equipment for physical assessment, 156
  focused interview, 156
  hints for physical assessment, 157
  in infants and children, 155
  legs, 161–65
  in older adults, 155
  in pregnant female, 155
  psychosocial considerations, 155
Peritonitis, 182
Pes planus (flatfoot), 253
Phalen's test, 247, 247f
Pharyngitis, 109
Phimosis, 202
Physical abuse, 49
Physical appearance, assessment, 19
Physical assessment. *See also specific body systems*
  definition, 3
  documentation, 297–99t
  equipment, 15–18, 15t
  professional responsibilities, 16–18
  rapid, for hospitalized client, 312–13, 312f
  routine or initial, for hospitalized client, 313–17, 313f, 314f, 315f, 316f

sequence, 302–10
  techniques, 9–14
Pilonidal cyst, 207
Pinna, 95
Pitch (frequency), 14
Pitcher's elbow (medial epicondylitis), 244
Pivot joint, 233t
Plane joint, 233t
Planning, in nursing process, 4
Plantar flexion, 235t
Plantar reflex, 287–88, 287f
Plaque, 54, 54f
Pleural membranes, 113
Pleximeter, 12
Plexor, 12
Pneumonia, 129, 129f
Pneumothorax, 120
Polycyclic lesions, 59, 59f
Polycystic kidney disease, 192
Polycythemia vera, 40t, 51
Polymyositis, 258t
Polyps, cervical, 230
Popliteal pulse, 163
Posterior tibial pulse, 164
Postpartum thyroiditis, 77
Preauricular lymph nodes, 303f
Pregnant female:
  abdomen/gastrointestinal tract, 169, 171
  breasts, 133
  cardiovascular system, 145, 146
  ear, nose, mouth, and throat, 98, 99
  eyes and vision, 80, 81
  female reproductive system, 214
  head and neck, 66, 67
  musculoskeletal system, 236, 238
  neurologic system, 265, 266
  peripheral vascular system, 155, 156
  respiratory system, 115, 117
  skin, hair, and nails, 38, 43
  urinary system, 186
Preinteraction phase, interview, 31
Prepatellar bursitis (housemaid's knee), 250
Presbyopia, 80, 92
Primary source, 29–30
Problem-oriented charting, 8
Prolapsed uterus, 219
Pronation, 235t
Prostate cancer, 199, 209
Prostate gland, 197, 208–9
Prostate specific antigen (PSA), 199
Protraction, 236t

Pseudofolliculitis, 42t
Psoas sign, 178–79, 179f
Psoriatic arthritis, 257t
Ptosis, 88, 271
Puberty:
  female, 212, 213t, 216
  male, 197, 198t
Pubic hair, 201, 216
Pubic lice (pediculosis pubis), 201, 216, 230
Pulse, 21, 166–67t
Pulse points, 21, 21f, 22f, 159–60
Pulse rate, 21, 158
Pulsus alternans, 167t
Pulsus bigeminus, 167t
Pulsus paradoxus, 167t
Pupils, 86–87
Purkinje fibers, 143

Q

Quadriceps muscle, 250
Quality, of sound, 14
Questioning, 28t

R

Radial pulse, 159
Rales/crackles, 124t
Range of motion:
  ankles and feet, 254
  cervical spine, 256
  elbow, 244–45, 244f
  hands and fingers, 248
  hips, 249–50
  knees, 252
  neck, 70
  shoulders, 241–43, 241f, 242f
  thoracic and lumbar spine, 256
  wrist, 247, 247f
Rapid assessment, of hospitalized client, 312–13, 312f
Rebound tenderness, 178
Rectal bleeding, 209, 229
Rectocele, 219
Rectovaginal examination, 228–29, 229f
Red reflex, 79, 90
Referred pain, 179, 240
Reflecting, 28t
Reflex incontinence, 195
Reflexes, 262, 262f, 284–88, 285f, 287f, 288f
Refraction, 79
Renal arteries, 188
Renal calculi, 189, 194
Renal failure, 194
Renal tumor, 194
Resonance, 13
Respiratory cycle, 113

Respiratory disorders, 128–29
Respiratory rate, 22
Respiratory system:
    abnormal findings,
        118–26, 128–29
    anatomy and
        physiology, 113
    assessment in hospitalized
        client, 314, 314*f*
    auscultation of anterior
        thorax, 126–28,
        127*f*, 306*f*
    auscultation of posterior
        thorax, 122–24,
        122*t*, 124*t*
    cultural considerations, 116
    equipment for physical
        assessment, 117
    focused interview,
        116–117
    hints for physical
        assessment, 117
    in infants and
        children, 115
    inspection of posterior
        thorax, 118–19
    landmarks, 113–14, 114*f*
    in older adults, 116
    palpation of anterior
        thorax, 124–26
    palpation of posterior
        thorax, 119–21, 305*f*
    percussion of anterior
        thorax, 126
    percussion of posterior
        thorax, 121
    in pregnant female, 115
    psychosocial
        considerations, 116
    sequence for physical
        assessment, 305–6
Retina, 78
Retraction, 236*t*
Retrobulbar neuritis, 270
Review of body systems, 35, 35*t*
Rheumatic diseases, 257–58*t*
Rheumatoid arthritis, 244, 246
Rheumatoid nodules, 259, 259*f*
Rhinitis, 110, 110*f*
Rhonchi, 124*t*
Rinne test, 103, 274
Romberg's test, 104, 274,
    277, 278*f*
Rotation, 235*t*
Rotator cuff tear, 242
Rubella (German measles),
    60, 60*f*
Rubeola (measles), 60, 60*f*

S

S₁, 141, 142*t*
S₂, 141, 142*t*
Saddle joint, 234*t*
Salivary glands, 108

Sarcoidosis, 116
Scales, 55, 55*f*
Schamroth technique, nail
    inspection, 52, 52*f*
Schizophrenia, 269, 270
Scissor gait, 290*t*
Sclera, 78, 88–89
Scleroderma, 257*t*
Scoliosis, 255, 259, 259*f*
Scrotum, 196, 203, 205
Sebaceous (oil) glands, 36
Secondary sources, 30–31
Seizures, 291
Semilunar valves, 141
Seminal vesicles, 197
Sensitive issues, 29
Sensory function testing,
    280–84, 281*f*, 282*f*,
    283*f*, 284*f*
Sexual abuse, 217, 218
Shifting dullness, 178
Shingles (herpes zoster),
    61, 61*f*
Shoulders, 240–43,
    241*f*, 242*f*
Sickle cell anemia, 237
Sikhs, 42, 67
Sinoatrial (SA) node, 142
Sinuses. *See* Nose
    and sinuses
Skene's glands, 219
Skin:
    abnormal findings, 44–49.
        See also Skin lesions
    anatomy and physiology,
        36–37, 36*f*
    assessment in hospitalized
        client, 316–17, 316*f*
    color variations in light
        and dark skin, 39–41*t*
    cultural considerations,
        38, 42*t*
    equipment for physical
        assessment, 44
    focused interview, 42–43
    hints for physical
        assessment, 44
    inspection, 44–45
    palpation, 45–49,
        46*f*, 47*f*
    psychosocial
        considerations, 38
    sequence for physical
        assessment, 302
    special considerations,
        37–38
Skin lesions:
    common, 59–61, 59–61*f*
    configurations and shapes,
        56–59, 56–59*f*
    malignant, 62, 62*f*
    primary, 48, 54–55,
        54–55*f*
    secondary, 48, 55–56,
        55–56*f*

Smegma, 202
Smoking, 145, 155
Sounds:
    in auscultation, 14.
        See also Auscultation
    breath, 122–24, 122*t*, 124*t*
    heart, 141–42, 142*t*
    in percussion, 13–14.
        See also Percussion
Spastic colon, 181*t*
Speculum, 220–23, 222*f*
Spermatic cord, 196, 205
Spermatocele, 203
Spina bifida, 232
Spinal cord, 262
Spine:
    abnormal findings,
        255–56, 258–59,
        258*f*, 259*f*
    inspection, 255, 255*f*
    palpation, 256
    range of motion, 256
Spleen, 175
Spoon nails, 53
Squamous cell carcinoma,
    62, 62*f*
Standard precautions, 18
Steppage gait, 290*t*
Stereognosis, 282, 282*f*
Sternocleidomastoid muscle,
    275, 276, 276*f*
Stethoscope, 15
Stool examination, 209, 229
Strabismus, 271
Straight-leg-raising test, 256
Stress incontinence, 195
Striae, 172
Stridor, 124*t*
Stroke (brain attack), 76, 76*f*
Subcutaneous tissue
    (hypodermis), 36
Subjective data, 2
Subluxation, 243
Summarizing, 28*t*
Supination, 235*t*
Sutures, 64
Syncope, 289
Synovial joints, 232, 233–34*t*
Syphilitic lesion, 230
Systemic lupus erythematosus
    (SLE), 237, 257*t*
Systolic pressure, 22

T

Tachycardia, 151, 151*f*
Tactile fremitus, 121
Target lesions, 58, 58*f*
Tattoos, 42
Teeth, 107
Temperature, 21
Temporal artery, 69
Temporomandibular joint
    (TMJ), 69, 239–40
Tendinitis, 258*t*

Tendon sheaths, 232
Tendons, 232
Tennis elbow (lateral epicondylitis), 244
Tension headache, 74
Testes, 196, 199, 203, 204, 310*f*
Testicular cancer, 199
Thenar atrophy, 246
Thoracic spine, 256
Thrills, 149
Throat. *See* Mouth and throat
Thyroid gland:
    abnormalities, 71, 76–77
    anatomy, 65, 66*f*
    physical assessment, 71–73, 72*f*
Thyroiditis, 77
Tibiofemoral joint, 251
Tic, 290*t*
Tinea, 59
Tinea capitis, 62, 62*f*
Tinea corporis, 59, 59*f*
Tinea versicolor, 39*t*
Tinel's sign, 247, 247*f*
Toenails, 165
Tongue, 108
Tonic (Adie's) pupil, 92, 92*f*
Tonsillitis, 111, 111*f*
Topognosis, 284
Torticollis, 76, 76*f*
Trachea, 70, 113
Tragus, 95
Trapezius muscle, 275, 276
Tremor, 290*t*
Trendelenburg's test, 162
Triceps reflex, 286, 309*f*
Trichomoniasis, 223
Trigeminal nerve (cranial nerve V):
    dysfunction, 291*t*
    function and activity, 263*t*
    testing, 240, 272–73, 272*f*
Trochlear nerve (cranial nerve IV), 263*t*, 271, 291*t*
Tumor, 54, 54*f*
Turgor, skin, 47
Tympanic membrane, 95, 102, 110, 110*f*
Tympany, 13

U

Ulcer:
    duodenal, 181*t*
    skin, 56, 56*f*
Ulcerative colitis, 182
Umbilical hernia, 182
Umbilicus, 172
Uremia, 41*t*
Urethra, 197, 218, 219
Urethral stricture, 202, 204
Urethritis, 204
Urge incontinence, 195
Urinary retention, 195
Urinary system:
    abnormal findings, 187–95
    anatomy and physiology, 184, 184*f*
    assessment in hospitalized client, 316, 316*f*
    bladder palpation and percussion, 193
    cultural considerations, 185
    equipment for physical assessment, 186
    focused interview, 186
    hints for physical assessment, 187
    in infants and children, 184–85, 186
    inspection, 187–88
    kidney palpation, 190–92
    kidney percussion, 188–90, 189*f*
    in older adults, 185, 186
    in pregnant female, 185, 186
    psychosocial considerations, 185
    renal artery auscultation, 188
Urinary tract infection, 194
Uterus, 219, 226–27, 226*f*
Uvula, 97

V

Vagina, 218, 219
Vagus nerve (cranial nerve X), 264*t*, 274–75, 291*t*
Varicella (chickenpox), 60, 60*f*
Varicocele, 205

Varicosities, 162
Venous hum, 180*t*
Ventral hernia, 182
Ventricle tachycardia, 151, 151*f*
Ventricular fibrillation, 152, 152*f*
Ventricular gallop, 142
Vernix caseosa, 37
Vertigo, 274
Vesicle, 55, 55*f*
Vestibulocochlear nerve (cranial nerve VIII), 263*t*, 274, 291*t*
Vietnamese, 42
Vision:
    abnormal findings, 83, 91–92
    acuity testing, 82–83, 82*f*
    visual fields testing, 83–84
Vital signs:
    blood pressure, 22
    pulse, 21, 21*f*, 22*f*
    respiratory rate, 22
    temperature, 21
Vitiligo, 39*t*, 45
Vitreous humor, 79

W

Water-hammer pulse, 167*t*
Weber test, 103–4, 104*f*, 274
Weight, 20–21
Wheeze, 124*t*
Whisper test, 102
Wilms' tumor, 188
World Health Organization (WHO), definition of health, 1
Wrists, 246–48, 247*f*

Z

Zosteriform lesions, 59, 59*f*